CANCER ETIOLOGY, DIAGNOSIS AND TREATMENTS

NEW APPROACHES IN THE TREATMENT OF CANCER

MA. DEL CARMEN MEJIA VAZQUEZ
AND
SAMUEL NAVARRO
EDITORS

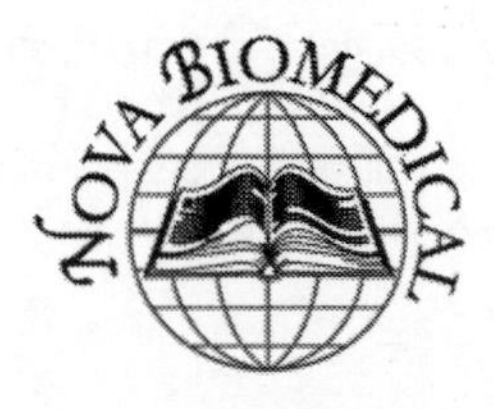

Nova Science Publishers, Inc.
New York

For permission to use material from this book please contact us:
Telephone 631-231-7269; Fax 631-231-8175
Web Site: http://www.novapublishers.com

LIBRARY OF CONGRESS CATALOGING-IN-PUBLICATION DATA

New approaches in the treatment of cancer / editors, Ma. del Carmen Mejma
Vazquez, Samuel Navarro.
p. ; cm.
Includes bibliographical references and index.
ISBN 978-1-62100-067-9 (softcover)
1. Cancer--Treatment. I. Mejma Vazquez, Ma. del Carmen. II. Navarro,
Samuel.
[DNLM: 1. Neoplasms--therapy. 2. Antineoplastic Agents--therapeutic use.
3. Biological Therapy--methods. QZ 266 N5308 2010]
RC270.8.N46 2010
616.99'406--dc22
2010013743

Published by Nova Science Publishers, Inc. † New York

CONTENTS

In: New Approaches in the Treatment of Cancer
Editors: Carmen Mejia Vazquez et al. pp.1-31
ISBN 978-1-62100-067-9

Chapter I

A LOOK AT CANCER

J. Christian Moreno-Vargas[1], Perla Reyes-Fernandez[1], Melissa Pamela Monroy-Romo P[1], Samuel Navarro[2] and Carmen Mejia[1,*,#]

[1]Instituto de Investigaciones Biomédicas, UNAM, México
[2]University of Valencia, Spain

ABSTRACT

In the present update, the authors review the current state of the art in cancer. Epidemiology of the neoplastic disease is reviewed considering the incidence and prevalence of the different and most frequent types of cancer as well as their mortality rates. Moreover, comments of costs and prevention have been reviewed. A second part of this chapter is the review of the causes of cancer. The aetiology of the neoplastic processes is developed, taking into account the environmental factors such as industrial environment, ultra-light and irradiation, cigarette smoking and the effects of diet. The authors also review the action of drugs, hereditary factors, oncogenes and viruses. Finally, an exhaustive review of the different therapeutic strategies including chemotherapy, radiotherapy, and other new treatments such as gene therapy, hormone therapy, targeted therapy or immunotherapy are discussed.

---

* Correspondence concerning this article should be addressed to: Carmen Mejia, Instituto de Investigaciones Biomédicas, Departamento de Medicina Genómica y Toxicología Ambiental, Lab. A-119, Universidad Nacional Autónoma de México, Avenida Universidad 3000, C. P. 04510, D.F., México. Tel. (+52-55) 5622-3144; E-mail: maria.c.mejia@uv.es,

Grant sponsors: CONACYT Investigación Básica 55464, CONACYT-REDES 60085, and RD06/0020/0102 from RTICC, Instituto Carlos III, Spanish Ministry of Science and Innovation.

Introduction

Cancer is a diverse set of diseases characterized by uncontrolled cell division and cell growth. If its spreading is not controlled, it can result in death. Current evidence supports the concept of carcinogenesis as a multistage process genetically regulated [1]. In the first step or *initiation* a normal cell is exposed to carcinogenic substances, and it can produce genetic damage that, if not repaired, results in irreversible cellular mutations. In the second phase or *promotion*, carcinogens alter the environment to favour the growth of the mutated cell population over normal cells giving it the potential to develop into a clonic population of neoplastic cells. The difference between initiation and promotion is that the first is a reversible process. Finally, in the last step or *progression* the malignant cells can travel to distant places resulting in metastasis [2].

There is increasing evidence that aetiological factors may interact with each other resulting in a more than additive cancer risk. This has been demonstrated for example with hepatitis B virus and aflatoxins in hepatocellular carcinoma [3] and alcohol and tobacco in cancer of the oesophagus [4]. This has long been known from animal experiments but human cancer susceptibility is a complex genetic trait involving genes responsible for carcinogen metabolism, DNA repair, and as yet unidentified cell specific susceptibility genes. With the progress in our understanding of the molecular mechanisms and underlying etiology of cancer there is much hope in the development of specific targeted treatment that will substantially reduce the cancer mortality rate.

Epidemiology of Cancer: Incidence, Mortality, Costs and Prevention

Global epidemiologic studies have identified environmental and occupational chemicals as potential carcinogens. The fact that genetic changes in individual cancer cells are essentially irreversible, and that malignant changes are transmitted from one generation of cells to another strongly points to DNA as the critical cellular target modified by tobacco smoke and environmental chemicals. DNA damage by chemicals occurs randomly; the phenotypes of associated carcinogenic changes are determined by selection [5]. Demographic shift, urbanization, industrialization, changes in lifestyles, population growth and aging all have contributed for epidemiological transition in the country. The number of new cancer cases is increasing rapidly, due to the growth in the size of population, and increase in the proportion of the elderly as a result of improved life expectancy following control of communicable diseases [6]. One in eight deaths worldwide is due to cancer, which causes more deaths than AIDS, tuberculosis, and malaria combined. Cancer is the second leading cause of death in economically developed countries, following heart diseases, and the third leading cause of death in developing countries, following heart diseases and enteric syndromes causing diarrhea [7]. According with the National Cancer Institute (NCI) 1,437,180 patients (745,180 men and 692,000 women) will be diagnosed with cancer and 565,650 of them will die of it in 2009 [8].

CANCER ETIOLOGY, DIAGNOSIS AND TREATMENTS

NEW APPROACHES IN THE TREATMENT OF CANCER

CANCER ETIOLOGY, DIAGNOSIS AND TREATMENTS

Additional books in this series can be found on Nova's website under the Series tab.

Additional E-books in this series can be found on Nova's website under the E-book tab.

The burden of cancer is increasing in developing countries as childhood mortality and deaths from infectious diseases decline and more people live to older ages. Furthermore, as people in developing countries adopt western lifestyle behaviors, such as cigarette smoking, higher consumption of saturated fat and calorie-dense foods, and reduced physical activity, rates of cancers common in western countries will raise if preventive measures are not widely applied [7]. Cancer accounted for 7.9 million deaths (or around 13% of all deaths worldwide) in 2007. The main types of cancer leading to overall cancer mortality each year are: lung (1.4 million deaths/year), stomach (866,000 deaths), liver (653,000 deaths), colon (677,000 deaths), and breast (548,000 deaths). About 72% of all cancer deaths in 2007 occurred in low- and middle-developed countries. Deaths from cancer worldwide are projected to continue rising, with an estimated 12 million deaths in 2030 [9], of which 5.4 million will occur in economically developed countries and 6.7 million in economically developing countries [7]. From 2001-2005, the median age at diagnosis for cancer of all sites was 67 years of age [8].

Approximately 1.1% was diagnosed under age 20; 2.7% between 20 and 34; 5.9% between 35 and 44; 13.8% between 45 and 54; 21.3% between 55 and 64; 25.3% between 65 and 74; 22.4% between 75 and 84; and 7.5% 85+ years of age. The age-adjusted incidence rate was 467.4 per 100,000 men and women per year. These rates are based on cases diagnosed in 2001-2005 from 17 SEER (Surveillance, Epidemiology, and End Results, Program of the National Cancer Institute) geographic areas. From 2002-2006, the median age at diagnosis for cancer of all sites was 66 years of age.

The age-adjusted incidence rate was 462.9 per 100,000 men and women per year. These rates are based on cases diagnosed in 2002-2006 from 17 SEER geographic areas. From 2002-2006, the median age at death for cancer of all sites was 73 years of age.

Approximately 0.4% died under age 20; 0.8% between 20 and 34; 2.7% between 35 and 44; 9.0% between 45 and 54; 17.5% between 55 and 64; 25.2% between 65 and 74; 29.9% between 75 and 84; and 14.6% 85+ years of age. By 2050, the global burden is expected to grow to 27 million new cancer cases and 17.5 million cancer deaths simply due to the growth and aging of the population. In economically developed countries, the three most commonly diagnosed cancers are prostate, lung and bronchus and colorectal among men, and breast, colorectal and lung and bronchus among women. In economically developing countries, the three most commonly diagnosed cancers are lung and bronchus, stomach, and liver in men, and breast, cervix uteri, and stomach in women. In both economically developed and developing countries, the three most common cancer sites are also the three leading causes of cancer deaths [7].

Factors that contribute to regional differences in the cancer types include regional variations in the prevalence of major risk factors, availability and use of medical practices such as cancer screening, availability and quality of treatment, completeness of reporting, and age structure. Approximately 15% of all worldwide cancer incidents are attributable to infections [10]. This percentage is about three times higher in developing countries (26%) than in developed countries (8%). Tobacco is the most important identified cause of cancer followed by dietary practices, inadequate physical activity, alcohol consumption, infections due to viruses and sexual behavior [6]. Studies show that 19% of breast cancer deaths and 26% of colorectal cancer mortality are attributable to increased weight and physical inactivity [11]. Armstrong and Doll [12] conducted an epidemiologic study to relate dietary factors to cancer incidence and mortality in various places. In general, fat was the dietary component that most highly correlated with risk of cancers of the colon, rectum, breast, ovary, and prostate. Several years later, Doll and Peto [13] listed a dozen possible factors as avoidable cancer risks. Diet was estimated to have caused the most cancer deaths. The best estimate was that dietary factors contributed to 35% of cancer deaths but the confidence limits were 10–70% [14]. An epidemiologic study examined the association between dietary fiber intake and the incidence of colon cancer in 591,978 European subjects and concluded that increasing the fiber intake of subjects presently consuming a low fiber diet could result in a 40% reduction of their risk of colorectal cancer [15]. Increased alcohol consumption is causally associated with cancers in various places, mainly oral [16] and pharynx, larynx, esophagus, liver, or colorectal [17] and breast [18]. Harmful alcohol causes 351,000 cancer deaths and chronic hepatitis B virus infection causes about half the world's liver cancer deaths, killing 340,000 people annually [11]. The frequency of commonly diagnosed cancer cases or deaths also varies by geographic areas. Currently, two of the three leading cancers in men (stomach and liver) and women (cervix and stomach) in developing countries are related to infection. Stomach cancer continues to be the most common infection-related cancer worldwide, followed closely by liver and cervix. The most commonly diagnosed cancer is cervix uteri in Eastern and Southern Africa, breast cancer in Northern and Western Africa [19], and Kaposi's sarcoma in Middle Africa [20].

Anyone can develop cancer; however, the risk of being diagnosed with cancer increases with age. In economically developed countries, 78% of all newly diagnosed cancer cases occur at age 55 or older compared with 58% in developing countries. The difference is largely due to variations in age structure of the populations. The populations of developing countries are younger and have a smaller proportion of older individuals in whom cancer most frequently occurs. The risk of developing any form of cancer is nearly twice as high in economically developed countries as in economically developing countries in both men (14.8% vs. 8.5%) and women (13.1% vs. 8.1%). In contrast, the risk of dying before age 65 from cancer is similar between developed and developing countries (7.2% vs. 6.1% in men and 4.8% vs. 4.9% in women). These differences relate to variations in the type of major cancers and to the availability of early detection and treatment services between economically developed and developing countries.

Incidence and mortality rates are the two most frequently used parameters of cancer occurrence. These statistics factors quantify the number of newly diagnosed cancer cases or deaths, respectively, in a specified population over a defined time period. Incidence and death rates are usually expressed per 100,000 people per year. It is estimated that 5%-10% of all cancers are strongly hereditary, meaning that individuals who inherit a specific genetic alteration have a very high risk of developing a particular cancer. It is thought that many cancers result from a combination of hereditary and environmental factors [7]. The total number of cancer survivors in the world is unknown because many areas lack cancer registries and information on survival. However, the International Agency for Research on Cancer (IARC) estimates that in 2002 there were approximately 24.6 million cancer survivors worldwide who had been diagnosed within the past five years. Some of these individuals were cancer free, while others still had evidence of cancer and may have been undergoing treatment. The number of people with a history of cancer is expected to increase during the coming years because of improvements in survival and the anticipated growth and aging of the population [21].

The corresponding estimates for the total number of cancer deaths in 2007 is 7.6 million (about 20,000 cancer deaths a day), 2.9 million in economically developed countries and 4.7

million in economically developing countries [7]. In addition to the human toll of cancer, the financial cost of cancer is substantial. The direct costs include payments and resources used for treatment, as well as the costs of care and rehabilitation related to the illness. Indirect costs include the loss of economic output due to days missed from work (morbidity costs) and premature death (mortality costs). There are also hidden costs of cancer, such as health insurance premiums and nonmedical expenses (transportation, child or elder care, housekeeping assistance, wigs, etc.) [22]. Data limitations do not allow estimating the worldwide economic costs of cancer. However, the costs of cancer are staggering. With the growth and aging of the population, prevention efforts are important in order to reduce new cancer cases, human suffering, and economic costs [7].

Advances in cancer biology offer enormous potential to improve clinical practice and public health. More selective targeting of molecular phenomena implicated in tumorigenesis and metastasis may enable more effective and less toxic interventions. Enhanced assessment modalities promise earlier and more definitive identification and quantification of risk, as well as enhanced means of assessing and monitoring the effectiveness of interventions across the spectrum of neoplastic development and progression. Ultimately, new knowledge of molecular, cellular, and systems biology may lead to more effective preventive interventions targeted at individuals with defined cancer risk [23].

Epidemiological studies have shown that many cancers may be avoidable. It is widely held that 80–90% of human cancers may be attributable to environmental and lifestyle factors. About 30% of cancer could be prevented and up to 40% of all cancer deaths can be avoided by modifying or avoiding key risk factors, according to a 2005 study by international cancer collaborators [6,9]. Cancer prevention includes primary and secondary prevention measures such as public education on 'tobacco and its health hazards' and alcohol consumption, recommended dietary guidelines, safe sexual practices, and lifestyle modifications form the main features of primary prevention of cancer. Incorporating screening for cancer of cervix, breast and oral cancers into peripheral health infrastructure can have a significant effect on reducing mortality from these diseases.

Factors on Cancer Etiology

Cancer aetiology is related to causal agents, processes, and cells involved in early events in carcinogenesis. The areas include gene regulation [24], DNA damage and repair mechanisms related to carcinogenesis [25]; chemical and environmental induced carcinogenesis; identification of causal agents such as xenobiotics [26], DNA adducts [27]; responses to stress such as free radicals, oxidative stress and reactive oxygen species as they contribute to the carcinogenic process [28]; metabolism of endogenous and exogenous compounds that lead to carcinogenesis and contribution of viruses, other than HIV, to carcinogenesis [29].

There exist several groups whose goal is to initiate, foster, and conduct basic and applied research in the etiology, surveillance, prevention, and control of cancer and its risk factors that, independently or in combination with biomedical approaches, reduce cancer risk, incidence and mortality. Environmental factors may be important in a significant percentage of human cancers. Such factors as exposure to radiation [30], nickel [31], uranium dust [32], strontium [33], and cigarette smoking [34] are all suspected causes of cancer. Dietary factors [35], immunosuppressive and cytotoxic drugs, and hormones [36] also play a role.

It is believed that heredity plays a role in developing cancer. Statistical evidence supports a genetic etiology of some cancers in humans. Some scientists think that cancer is not caused by a single agent or factor, but by the interplay of several factors that combine to cause the "normal" cell to change into a "malignant" cell. It's generally believed that transformation of the normal cell into a malignant cell occurs when one or more oncogenes are activated. The role of genetics in cancer etiology can be loosely grouped into the following two categories: the single (rare) genes and the more common susceptibility genes. When present, they confer a high relative and absolute risk of a particular cancer. Over a dozen genes have been identified and studied in the family setting [37]. These include Rb (retinoblastoma), WT1 (Wilms tumor) and p53 (Li-Fraumeni syndrome). The second type is composed of the more common, low penetrance genes thought to play a role in many or even most human diseases. These genes are characterized by a high gene frequency (1– 90% or more), low relative and absolute risk, but potentially high population attributable risk. The role of exposure is critical for the susceptibility genes but may be only modest for the single gene [38]. In the majority of cases in which diet is involved in the carcinogenic process, the susceptibility genes are thought to be most relevant [39].

Historically, early studies established that carcinogens require metabolic activation, and it was proposed that genetic control of activation [40] or elimination [41], might account for genetically mediated variation in tobacco and diet-related cancer susceptibility. A broader appreciation of human carcinogenesis suggests categories of genes that go beyond metabolic activation/detoxification. These include genes that influence DNA repair, chromosome stability, the activity of oncogenes or tumor suppressor genes, cell cycle control or signal transduction, hormonal or vitamin metabolism pathways, immune function and receptors or neurotransmitter action. There are also other polymorphic enzymes that may interact with various dietary components and play a role in human carcinogenesis [42].

Some occupations have been implicated in the etiology of cancer [43]. For example, workers in the aniline dye industry have an increased risk of developing bladder cancer. Lung cancer is more prevalent among those who mine or work with asbestos and those working with chromate or uranium ores, especially if they also smoke cigarettes [44]. Workers in nickel-refining plants are more likely to develop cancer of the nasal sinuses [45] than are average individuals. Exposure to certain solvents such as benzene has been associated with an incidence of leukemia [46], and asbestos workers may develop mesotheliomas of the pleural or peritoneal cavities [47]. Excessive exposure to sunlight is responsible for a high incidence of skin cancer among farmers and other outdoor workers. Fair-skinned individuals who sunburn easily also are at high risk for developing skin cancer. Cancer of the thyroid is more common in individuals who received irradiation to the neck as children [48]. The survivors of the A-bomb explosions at Hiroshima and Nagasaki are subject to an increased incidence of cancers, particularly acute myelocytic leukemia [49]. Although not a common cause of cancer, radiation exposure does increase the risk of lung cancer in the uranium, strontium, nickel, and beryllium industries. An increased incidence of leukemia has been reported after exposure to radiation [50].

Increasing incidence of lung cancers in women is directly linked to the increase in smoking of this population. Smoking-related illnesses cause more than 419,000 premature deaths every year. Smoking is also implicated in the risk of developing bladder cancer, the exact mechanism is unknown, but statistics show that there is a correlation between smoking and an increased incidence of bladder cancer [51]. Alcohol is thought to be a carcinogen or cocarcinogen (along with cigarette smoke) for cancers of the head, neck, and esophagus, and it may also play a role in the etiology of liver cancer [52].

Aside from prostate cancer in men and breast cancer in women, the yearly number of new cases of colorectal cancer in the US is second after lung cancer. It is suspected that this high incidence is due, in part, to diet. As refrigeration and processed food have led to a reduction in roughage and bulk (non-digestible complex carbohydrates) in the typical Western diet, the incidence of colon cancer has increased and stomach cancer decreased. Populations who traditionally have a non-Western diet high in fiber have a very low incidence of colorectal cancer but a high incidence of stomach cancer. Research in Africa, England, and India by Dr. Denis Burkitt and others has shown a direct relationship between the fiber content of food and intestinal bulk [53]. Bulk fiber represents non-absorbable sugars which increase intestinal mass and may actually change the intestinal milieu, particularly the transit time of carcinogens and the type of bacteria present. Unlike low-fiber foods, those with a high fiber content produce greater waste bulk, which moves through the intestine faster and produces large and soft stools that are easy to excrete. Low-fiber foods may produce a reverse effect, resulting in greater formation of potential carcinogens in the large bowel by the action of certain bacteria on bile salts. Burkitt postulates that bile salts in the colon may be increased by the greater consumption of fat in Western countries. It is not known whether bacteria may be affected by changes in fat, fiber, or both food constituents. In any event, a low-residue (low bulk fiber) diet produces a small stool that tends to take longer to pass through the intestine, allowing the bacteria more time to degrade bile salts. Thus, any carcinogen formed has longer contact with the bowel mucosa and a greater opportunity to cause cancer [53].

Diet also seems to be related to the high incidence of liver cancer among certain groups of black Africans living in Africa, compared to American blacks. The high incidence among black Africans in Africa correlates with the eating of foods (especially peanuts) contaminated with fungus *Aspergillus flavus*. This fungus produces aflatoxin, a highly carcinogenic substance. On the other hand, chronic hepatitis is known to predispose to the development of liver cancer, and chronic hepatitis is very common in Africa and Asia [54]. An association between high-fat diets and breast cancer has been suggested from several different sources of data. Epidemiologic data cannot, however, establish a firm cause-effect relationship, and the resolution of this issue must await clinical studies of the influence of a reduced-fat diet on breast cancer incidence [55, 56]. Lung cancer has been associated with low intake of vitamin A. Attempts to reduce the incidence of lung cancer by administration of vitamin A–like compounds have not been successful [57].

The parasite *Schistosoma haematobium*, common in Egypt, can cause bladder cancer. The parasite enters the body through the skin as workers stand in infested waters. It then migrates to the bladder where it deposits the eggs in the mucosa and sub-mucosa of the bladder and lower ureters developing squamous cell carcinoma (SCC) of the bladder as a long-term sequel of the chronic infection. Parasite antigens might induce alterations in epithelial cells towards cancer. An *in vitro* study with CHO cells treated with *S. haematobium* total antigen (Sh), showed increase in proliferation and S-phase, decrease of apoptosis with up-regulation of Bcl-2, down-regulation of tumor suppressor p27, as well as increased migration and invasion [58].

A number of drugs in clinical use have also been rarely associated with cancer. The majority of the highly implicated agents are immunosuppressive agents, principally the antimetabolites and glucocorticosteroids. It should be kept in mind that the risk of developing drug-induced cancer is dependent on several nondrug factors: 1) age at first exposure (younger age increases risk); 2) the long latency period between exposure and cancer development (an average of 40–50 years in industrial exposures, 5–10 years for drugs); and 3) the presence of cocarcinogens (such as cigarette smoking or ionizing radiation). The most highly implicated carcinogenic drugs are anticancer agents, and the major cancers produced are leukemia and lymphomas. Acute myelocytic leukemia is an unfortunate and rare complication of alkylating agents [59] such as melphalan and cyclophosphamide. The drugs most commonly associated with second neoplasm are the alkylating agents. These drugs bind to DNA and induce mutations. As well, radiotherapy could potentiate the leukemogenic action of alkylating agents [60].

Some hormones are thought to possess carcinogenic potential and this is important in several cancers. *Breast Cancer:* Large doses of estrogens, when administered continuously can cause breast cancer in susceptible strains of mice. Animal studies also show that estrogens are cocarcinogens; e.g., they are carcinogenic when administered experimentally along with another cancer-causing agent such as X-rays or the chemical methylcholanthrene [61]. The animal data has raised concern that women who take birth control pills, or who receive estrogen supplements at menopause, might incur in an increased risk of cancer. Most of the large scale studies suggest that exogenous estrogen probably is not a significant factor in human breast cancer, although some experts still feel that the safety of estrogen has not been proven [62]. *Endometrial Cancer:* Many scientists now suspect that estrogen increases the hazard of developing cancer of the endometrium. This is based upon case-control studies reporting an increased risk of malignancy in women receiving estrogen supplements—though other studies report no such increases, and still other studies find an actual decrease in the risk [63]. *Vaginal Adenocarcinoma:* In 1938 it was thought that synthetic estrogens such as DES (diethylstilbestrol) were well tolerated in pregnancy, safe for the fetus, and effective for preventing abortion. As a result, DES and related synthetic estrogens were widely prescribed until a published study in 1971 showed that the daughters of DES-treated mothers had an increased incidence of cell adenocarcinoma of the vagina and cervix [64]. Because the use of DES in pregnancy has been stopped, this complication will cease to be a problem in a few years. *Prostate Cancer:* The most important risk factor in prostate cancer is age, but testosterone after being metabolized to dihydrotestosterone (DHT) is a potent stimulator of cell division in prostate cells. Dihydrotestosterone may be involved in malignant transformation, and studies are under way to determine whether inhibition of DHT production will reduce the incidence of prostate cancer [65].

Breeding experiments with mice led to the development of mouse families with very high incidences of specific cancers, such as lung and breast cancer. Other selected mating of mice produced families that were essentially cancer-free. Statistical evidence supports the genetic etiology of cancer in humans. The best example of a hereditary cancer in man is retinoblastoma, a relatively uncommon neoplasm of children. However, genetic factors probably play an important role in the familial tendencies toward some common cancers such as cancer of the colon (familial polyposis), hereditary non-polyposis colorectal cancer (HNPCC), breast cancer, and stomach cancer. A genetic history is an essential part of every cancer patient's medical history. Breast cancer is one of the best examples of a malignancy for which a genetic predisposition influences clinical practice. The incidence of breast cancer may be double or more than double when one or more female relatives of a woman have suffered breast cancer. Hence, knowledge of a family's cancer history can help in planning early detection programs for high-risk subjects. The identification of two genes associated with an increased risk of breast cancer, ovarian cancer, and prostate cancer (BRCA1, BRCA2) has raised the possibility of testing for genetic susceptibility [66].

The most enduring hypothesis concerning the origin of cancer is that some genetic alteration, induced by elements in the environment, acts on a genetically determined predisposition and results in the unregulated proliferation of cells. One very exciting area of cancer research, which combines hereditary and environmental factors, is the study of oncogenes. It now appears that these genes are activated by radiation, chemicals, viruses, and other as yet undefined factors. These oncogenes then act as cellular transforming genes, causing uncontrolled proliferation of previously normal cells. Certain proteins produced by oncogenes have been identified, and in some cases the proteins form cell surface receptors for growth factors, intracellular signals that turn on or turn off cell growth, and factors that alter the expression of DNA. Our understanding of the biochemical mechanisms involved in cancer offers the potential for improved detection, prognosis, and treatment. Many of these oncogenes are silent until the gene moves or translocates from one chromosome to another. This chromosomal breakage and reunion is known to occur in several cancers, including chronic leukemia and lymphomas. Some genes suppress abnormal cell growth and when they are damaged or missing, cancer is more likely to develop. The best example of this type of gene is the Rb gene [67].

Oncogenes were first identified in viruses that cause cancer in animals, later it was learned that the viruses had captured a normal host gene that regulated stem cell proliferation. These oncogenic viruses caused cancer by activating that normal host gene inside a host cell. It is known that members of a group of small DNA viruses called papovaviruses cause a variety of animal tumors. Among them are the papilloma viruses, responsible for papillomas in rabbits [68] and the polyoma virus, which causes malignant tumors of the parotid gland [69], mammary gland [70], and kidney [71] as well as subcutaneous fibrosarcomas [72] when injected into mice. Also, ribonucleic acid (RNA) viruses have been shown to cause leukemia in chickens, mice [73], and cats [74], and mammary carcinomas in mice [75]. The human retrovirus T-cell lymphotropic virus (HTLV-1) has been recognized as the etiologic agent of the aggressive form of leukemia adult T-cell leukemia/lymphoma (ATLL) [76]. Also, in African Burkitt's lymphoma, a viral etiology seems possible. Generally, it occurs between the ages of 2 and 14, with a peak incidence at age 7. It is a cancer of the B-cell lymphocytes, and it is common in areas of the world where malaria is endemic. Viral involvement in Burkitt's lymphoma is difficult to discount because cells from nearly every biopsy of African Burkitt's lymphoma contain a herpes virus: the Epstein-Barr virus (EBV). EBV is also associated with carcinoma of the nasopharynx a common malignancy in Southern China, Malaysia, Indonesia, and parts of Africa. EBV has also been implicated in the etiology at Hodgkin's disease and in non-Hodgkin's lymphoma in patients who are immunosuppressed. Another factor implicating viruses in causing human cancers is that carcinomas of the cervix are more common after infection by the type II herpes virus [77]. Women who become sexually active at an early age and who have multiple partners are at greater than normal risk of developing cervical cancer directly correlated with HPV infection.

THERAPIES IN CANCER

Chemotherapy

The chemotherapy agents kill cancer cells by affecting DNA synthesis or function. Whereas surgery and radiation therapy are limited to treating cancers confined to specific areas, the major advantage of chemotherapy is its ability to treat widespread or metastatic cancer. The establishment that fast-growing cells would be more affected than the slow-growing ones constitutes the basis for many chemotherapy agents. Some chemotherapy agents may kill a cell only in one phase of the cycle and are called cell-cycle specific, whereas those that are active in all phases are cell-cycle nonspecific. As hair follicles, skin, and the cells that line the gastrointestinal tract are some of the fastest growing cells, therefore they are the most sensitive to the effects of chemotherapy. The way that most chemotherapy agents kill cancer cells is by affecting DNA synthesis or function. Chemotherapy agents are alkylating agents, antimetabolites, anthracyclines, plant alkaloids, antitumor antibiotics, taxanes, and platinums.

Alkylating Agents

These are the oldest class of anticancer drugs including active or latent nitrogen mustards. All share a common mechanism of action, but differ in their clinical activity. Alkylating agents work by attacking the negatively charged sites on the DNA (oxygen, nitrogen, phosphorous and sulphur atoms) by binding to the DNA [78]. This event permits duplication of the cell's genetic material altered and alkylation's DNA leads to DNA strand breaks and DNA strand cross-linking altering DNA, where cellular activity is stopped resulting in the death of the cell. This class of chemotherapy drugs is active in every phase of the cell cycle. As a result, alkylating agents are very powerful and are used in many types of cancer, including both solid tumors [79] and leukemia [80]. However, the prolonged use of these drugs will lead to decreased sperm production, cessation of menstruation, possibly permanent infertility and fetal malformations in the first trimester of pregnancy. It has been reported that secondary cancers such as leukemia (AML, or Acute Myeloid Leukemia) can occur years after therapy with an alkylating agent [60]. Some common drugs of this class are: Cyclophosphamide, Ifosfamide, Melphalan, Chlorambucil, BCNU, CCNU, Dacarbazine, Procarbazine, Busulfan, and Thiotepa.

Antimetabolites

The discovery by Dr. Sidney Farber (1948) [81] that in 10 out of the 16 childhood patients with leukemia treated with a folic acid analogue could induce remission, it took that to synthesize agents that either target naturally occurring compounds, inhibiting key enzymatic reactions in their biochemical pathways as those necessary for making new DNA. One of the most widely antimetabolite used in cancer therapy is Methotrexate, with activity against leukemia, and lymphoma [82], breast cancer [83], head and neck cancer [84], sarcomas [85], colon cancer [86], bladder cancer and [87], choriocarcinomas [88]. This drug inhibits the enzyme dihydrofolate reductase (DHFR) that participates in the conversion of dihydrofolate to the active tetrahydrofolate [89] form. Finally, folate is needed for purine base synthesis and Methotrexate, therefore, inhibits the synthesis of DNA, RNA, thymidylates, and proteins and therefore exerts its effect on the S phase of the cell cycle. Another widely antimetabolite used is 5-Fluorouracil (5-FU) which is metabolized in the body by dihydropyrimidine dehydrogenase (DPD). 5-FU has a wide range of activity including colon cancer [90], breast cancer [83], head and neck cancer [91], pancreatic cancer [92], gastric cancer [93], oesophageal cancer and hepatocarcinomas (primary liver tumor) [94]. The most important toxic effects include bone marrow suppression, severe GI toxicities, and neurotoxicities such as seizures and even coma. Other antimetabolites that inhibit DNA synthesis and DNA repair include: Cytarabine and Cladribine [95], Gemcitabine, 6-mercaptopurine [96] and Thioguanine [97], and Fludarabine [98].

Anthracyclines

Another source to develop effective anticancer drugs is the natural sources. Thus Daunorubicin was isolated from the soil-dwelling fungus *Streptomyces* and Doxorubicin which is more effective in the treatment of solid tumors was isolated from a mutated strain of the same fungus. Their mechanism of action is by the formation of free oxygen radicals that result in DNA strand breaks and subsequent inhibition of DNA synthesis and function. Anthracyclines, a class of chemotherapeutics not cell cycle specific, also affects the topoisomerase by forming a complex with the DNA that doesn't allow unwinding the DNA double strand helix for DNA repair, replication and transcription. One of the most important side effects of anthracyclines is the cardiac toxicity, because free radicals may damage the cells of the heart muscle [99]. Other commonly used drugs of this class are Idarubicin, Epirubicin, and Mitoxantrone.

Antitumor Antibiotics

This category includes Bleomycin, another anticancer drug isolated from *Streptomyces verticullus*. Its mechanism of action comprises formation of free oxygen radicals that result in DNA breaks leading to cancer cell death. Bleomycin commonly is used in conjunction with other chemotherapies. This drug is used in regimens for testicular cancer and Hodgkin's lymphoma and the most important side effect is lung toxicities due to oxygen free radical formation [100].

Plant Alkaloids

This group of chemotherapy agents is derived from plant materials and is used in many solid and liquid tumors. Plant alkaloids are cell-cycle specific, but the cycle affected varies from drug to drug. They comprise four groups: topoisomerase inhibitors, epipodophyllotoxins, taxanes and vinca alkaloids. Camptothecan analogs or topoisomerase I inhibitors include Irinotecan and Topotecan both of which are camptothecins. They act by forming a complex with topoisomerase and DNA resulting in the inhibition of DNA synthesis [101]. Camptothecan is a naturally occurring alkaloid found in the bark and wood of the Chinese tree *Camptotheca accuminata*. Etoposide and Teniposide are epipodophyllotoxin chemotherapy agents (also called topoisomerase II inhibitors) that work by similar mechanisms. They are isolated from the *May apple* plant and work in the late S and G2 phases [102]. Another chemotherapeutics of this class are Taxanes that include Paclitaxel and Docetaxel. Taxanes are specific for the M phase of the cell cycle where they bind with high affinity to the microtubules and inhibit their normal function [103]. These drugs are currently used in breast, lung, head and neck, ovarian [104], oesophageal, gastric [105], bladder [106] and prostate cancers [107]. The main side effect of these compounds is the lowering of the blood counts. Although Taxanes were first isolated from the bark of the Pacific yew tree *Taxus brevifolia* in 1963, it was not until 1971 that paclitaxel was identified as the active component and in 1993 it was available for medical use. Vinca alkaloids are extracted from the leaves of a periwinkle plant, *Vinca rosea* and are used in treating leukemia. Isolation and chemical characterization led to the widely used chemotherapy drugs: Vincristine, Vinblastine, and Vinorelbine. These compounds are active specifically during the M phase of the cell cycle by binding to the tubulin and lead to the disruption of the mitotic spindle apparatus [108]. They have a wide application to many different malignancies and the neurotoxicity is the most dose-limiting side effect.

Platinums

These are natural metal derivatives that work by cross-linking DNA subunits (between two strands or one strand of DNA). Resultant cross-link acts to inhibit DNA synthesis, transcription and finally the function [109]. These compounds can act in any cell cycle. Cisplatin is used commonly in lung cancer and testicular cancer [110] and the most important side effect is kidney damage. Carboplatin is a second generation platinum, which has fewer kidney side effects, and at times may be an appropriate substitute for regiments containing Cisplatinum. A third-generation platinum is Oxaliplatin active in colon cancer and without renal toxicity; however, it can produce severe neuropathies [111].

Other Metals

Metals and metal compounds have been used in medicine for several thousand years. These compounds comprise main-group metallic compounds of gallium, germanium, and bismuth, early-transition metal complexes of titanium, vanadium, rhodium, niobium, molybdenum, and rhenium, and late-transition metal complexes of ruthenium, iridium, copper, and gold [112-115]. Gallium has an anti-proliferative effect against certain human carcinomas and lymphomas, which could be related to its competition with the iron atom; the use of germanium has shown complete remission in pulmonary spindle cell carcinoma (SCC) a rare form of lung cancer [116]. Bismuth is used in gastric lymphoma and derivatives of titanium showed no evidence of nephrotoxicity or myelotoxicity; several derivatives of vanadium show anti-proliferative activity, but their toxicity must be overcome [117]. Niobium (niobocene complexes) has shown antitumor properties against Ehrlich ascites tumor in female CF1 mice [118]; whereas molybdenum was induced to decrease proliferation efficiency both in human leukemia cell lines HL-60 and K562 [119]. Rhenium is effective especially in patients with bone metastases [120] ruthenium in combination with photodynamic therapeutic treatment exhibited excellent phototoxicity toward human melanoma tumor cells [121] rhodium that belongs to the same group as platinum also presents important activity, but with the same nephrotoxicity. In 6 patients with angiosarcoma eyelid and periorbital region iridium resulting in partial regression and longer survival rates [122]; copper has shown to be important in human medulloblastoma [123] and finally, gold (I) and (III) compounds show anti-tumor activities, although toxicity remains high. Certain types of chemotherapies are orphan drugs, meaning there are no others like them. They include: L-asparaginase, Hydroxyurea, Thalidomide and Dactinomycin.

Radiation Therapy

Radiation therapy uses high energy X-rays to kill cancer cells, thereby damaging the DNA and although it also damages normal cells, they are able to repair this radiation damage because they grow slower than cancer cells.

In contrast to systemic therapies, such as chemotherapy, radiation therapy is a "local" therapy, meaning it treats a specific localized area of the body. There are two main types of radiation therapy: external radiation therapy, where a beam of radiation is directed from outside the body, and internal radiation therapy, also called brachytherapy or implant therapy, where a source of radioactivity is surgically placed inside the body near the tumor. External radiation is also called X-ray therapy, cobalt therapy, proton therapy, or intensity modulated radiation therapy (IMRT) and is administered using a linear accelerator. In order to avoid damage in normal organs located near the tumor it is possible to use a process known as 3D conformal radiotherapy. Computer software allows the beams of radiation to be adjusted to further optimize the dose to the tumor [124].

Internal radiation therapy places the source of the high-energy rays inside the body, as close as possible to the cancer cells by means of small pieces of the radioactive substance or by using an implanted reservoir, into which a liquid radioactive substance is injected. Radioactive substances used typically include radium, cesium, iodine, and phosphorus. However, others such as 99mTc-sestamibi for the identification of parathyroid adenomas or hyperplasia, or 111In-DTPA octreotide have been used for the identification of neuroendrocrine tumors [125]. The side effects are directly related to the area of the body being treated and the most common are: skin reaction as a sunburn, hair loss, nutritional problems, fatigue and neutropenia. Whereas in cases of long-term radiation, side effects may also include: memory impairment, confusion, personality changes, cataracts, dental problems, heart problems (high blood pressure, high cholesterol levels), infertility, hypothyroidism and development of another cancer as a result of damage to tissue [126].

Radiation Therapy Classification

Radiation therapy can be classified according to the various types of radiation particles or waves that are used to deliver the treatment, such as protons, photons, and electrons.

Protons vs X-rays

Protons are large particles with a positive charge that penetrate matter to a finite depth based on the energy of the beam, whereas X-rays are electromagnetic waves that have no mass or charge. X-rays are able to penetrate completely through tissue while losing some energy but depositing them in normal tissues beyond the tumor. An immediate consequence is the reduced toxicity by using protons and in respect are some reports of treatment for paediatric tumors mostly involving the central nervous system, the head, the orbit, and eye. Also the proton therapy has shown an increase in overall survival rates at 5-year for chondrosarcomas (100%) and chordomas (81%).

Photon Treatment

Photons can be used in different types of radiation therapy that include: orthovoltage radiation therapy, conventional radiation therapy, 3D conformational radiation therapy, intensity modulated radiation therapy (IMRT), brachytherapy, and stereotactic radiation therapy or stereotactic radio-surgery. Photon beams are the same type of beam used in diagnostic X-ray machines, but have much higher energy. Orthovoltage was commonly used before the development of linear accelerators. This class of radiation uses lower energy photons to treat skin tumors and other superficial lesions located on the skin or very close to them. Stereotactic radiotherapy involves delivering a high dose of radiation very precisely to a tumor from numerous different angles to focus the radiation at one small point, like a magnifying glass. The machines can be used to deliver stereotactic radiotherapy, including gamma knife machines. Due to the small focal spot of highly intense radiation used in stereotactic radiation, only lesions of about 3 cm or smaller are treatable with this technique specially tumors of the brain [127]. Brachytherapy involves the use of a radioactive source, which predominantly emits photons. There are two classes of sources; the first is implanted into the tumor (*interstitial brachytherapy).* Prostate seeds are an example, where radioactive seeds are placed directly into the prostate using needles [128]. The other source is implanted near the tumor, generally in a body cavity (*intracavitary brachytherapy)* such as in uterine cancer treated with a removable implant placed in the uterine cavity through the vagina [129]. The advantage of brachytherapy is that the amount of normal tissue affected by the radiation can be minimized, but this is not effective for treating large areas or deep tumors unless the source can be implanted correctly.

Electron Radiation

Although electrons constitute a different form of radiation than photons, they work the same as photons. The same linear accelerators that produce photons can also produce electrons. As electrons tend to release their energy close to the skin's surface, they are commonly used to treat superficial tumors, such as skin cancers and superficial lymph nodes which may be involved with tumors, for example in breast cancer [130].

OTHER THERAPIES

Biologic Therapy

Biologic therapies also called biologic agents, biologicals, biological response modifiers (BRMs), or immunotherapy help to reinforce the immune system in order to prevent disease. The goal of biologic therapy is to enhance its ability to fight cancer and help deal with the side effects of other treatments. This is possible by using substances that occur naturally in the body or are given back to the patient's body cells which are altered in the laboratory. There are so many ways to stimulate the immune system as there are different types of biologic therapies. Some of them: interferon, interleukin, colony stimulating factors, monoclonal antibodies, vaccines and gene therapy. Side effects of biologic therapies include fever, chills, body aches, nausea/vomiting, loss of appetite, fatigue, and depending on the doses and how the therapy is administered, patients may experience a decrease in their blood pressure and may develop a rash or swelling at the injection site.

The biologic therapies could be administered by different ways that include oral, intravenous, either under the skin (subcutaneous) or into a muscle (intramuscular). Also they may be inserted directly into a body cavity to treat a specific place, for example, gene therapy directed against meshotelioma (a type of pleural cancer) may be injected directly into the thoracic cavity [131].

Gene Therapy

Gene therapy could be applied by different ways in order to replace missing or non-functioning genes. For example, cells that are missing the tumor suppressor p53 or have a non-functioning copy due to a mutation may be solved by adding functioning copies of p53 to the cell. By stopping the function of oncogenes, the cancer and/or its metastases may be stopped. By means of the immune system inserting genes into cancer cells in order to turn them into foreign invaders, healthy cells are protected from the side effects of therapy. This creates genes that can enter cancer cells and cause them to self-destruct. By inserting genes into cancer cells, this makes them more susceptible to or prevents resistance to chemotherapy [132], radiation therapy, or hormone therapies. These genes can be used to prevent the blood vessels from forming the metastases.

Gene therapy is typically administered by means of viruses that are used as vectors. Cells with these viruses are matured *in vitro* and are then given back to the patient by intravenous infusion or are injected into a body cavity (i.e. the lung) or a tumor. Since gene therapy is still experimental, the technology to apply it is still developing.

The patient's immune system may react to the foreign vector, causing fever, severe chills (rigors), drop in blood pressure, nausea, vomiting, and headache, all of them symptoms that typically are gone within 24-48 hours of the infusion. However, the long term side effects are not clear. To date, gene therapy is generally given in conjunction with other therapies such chemotherapy.

Hormone Therapy

Hormones are chemical substances that are naturally produced by the endocrine system including the pancreas, pituitary, thyroid and adrenal glands. They include: oestrogen, testosterone, insulin, thyroid hormone, cortisol, and epinephrine.

Hormone therapy is most often used to treat cancer hormone dependents such as breast and prostate cancers, and it can be given in several ways: as oral medication, by subcutaneous or intramuscular injection, or by surgical intervention e.g. the removal of the ovaries in women or prostate gland in men to decrease the production of certain hormones.

Some examples of hormone therapies include: anti-estrogens, aromatase inhibitors, anti-androgens, and luteinizing hormone releasing the hormone agonist (LHRH Agonist).

(a) *Anti-Estrogens*. An antiestrogen or oestrogen blocker works by blocking oestrogen receptors in breast tissue, making the cancer cells that feed off oestrogen unable to survive [133]. The most common side effects include hot flashes, night sweats, weight gain, vaginal dryness and nausea and rarely blood clots can occur.

(b) *Aromatase Inhibitors*. In menopausal women, oestrogen is mainly produced by converting androgens into estrogens by means of the enzyme aromatase. Aromatase inhibitors block this conversion, decreasing the oestrogen in the body [134]. The side

effects are hot flashes, night sweats, headache, nausea, hair thinning, muscle aches, joint pain, and vaginal dryness.

(c) *Anti-Androgens.* Testosterone is an androgen produced by the testes and adrenal glands and its production can be stopped by surgically removing the testicles or through medication therapy. Anti-androgens work by blocking testosterone receptors, allowing the cancer cells to either grow slower, or to stop growing altogether [135]. The most common side effects include hot flashes, breast tenderness, nausea, loss of sex drive and impotence.

(d) *Luteinizing Hormone Releasing Hormone Agonist (LHRH Agonist).* Production of testosterone is stimulated by the luteinizing hormone, which is produced by the pituitary gland. LHRH agonists stop the production of the luteinizing hormone by the pituitary gland thus reducing the production of testosterone in men. The cancer cells may then grow slower or stop growing altogether [136]. Common side effects include tiredness, breast tenderness, nausea, loss of sex drive, and impotence.

Table 1. Tumor markers

Tumor	Tumor marker
Esophageal cancer	SCC
Lung cancer	CA-125, CEA, SLX, CYFRA, NSE, ProGRP
Squamous cell carcinoma	
Small cell carcinoma	
Lung cancer	AFP, PIVKA-II
Gallbladder cancer	CA 19-9, CEA
Prostate cancer	PSA
Germ cell tumor	NSE
Thyroid Medullary carcinoma	NSE
Breast cancer	CA-125, CEA,CA15-3, NCC-ST-439
Gastric cancer	CEA, STN
Pancreatic cancer	CA-125, CA 19-9, CEA- Elastase I, NCC-ST-439, STN
Colon cancer	CEA, NCC-ST-439, STN
Cervix cancer	βHCG, SCC, STN
Ovarian Cancer	βHCG, CA-125, STN, SLX

SCC: Squamous cell carcinoma antigen; **NSE**: Neuron-specific enolase; **CEA**: Carcinoembryonic antigen; **CYFRA**: Cytokeratin 19 fragment; **ProGRP**: Progastrin – releasing peptide; **AFP**: Alpha-fetoprotein; **PIVKA-II**: protein induced by vitamin K absence/antagonist-II; **PSA**: Prostate-specific antigen; **STN**: Sialyl-Tn; **βHCG**: Human chorionic gonadotropin beta; **SLX**: Sialyl; SSEA-1 antigen.
[Source: National Cancer Center (website). Center for Cancer Control and Information Services, META Corporation Japan. Available at: http://www.ncc.go.jp/index.html. Accessed on November 22, 2009].

In order to know the status of the cancer by the hormone therapy, it is necessary to carry out a follow-up of tumor markers. These are substances that are either produced by the tumor or by the body in response to the tumor. Some of these markers are specific to one cancer, while others are seen in several types of cancers. A good example of a tumor marker is the prostatic specific antigen (PSA) used to diagnose early prostate cancer. On the contrary, identification of abnormal (> or =5.0 ng/ml) pre- and post-operative serum carcino-embryonic antigen (CEA) levels may be useful in the auxiliary cancer prognosis or post-operative surveillance of patients with colon cancer recurrences [137]. (Table 1: Tumoral Markers).

Targeted Therapy

Targeted therapy is a medication or drug that targets a specific pathway in the growth and development of a tumor by attacking or blocking these targets or molecules that are known or suspected to play a role in cancer formation. There are several major classes of targeted therapies:

I) Tyrosine Kinase Receptor inhibitors

A tyrosine kinase receptor binds it with different substances such as hormones, antigens, drugs, or neurotransmitters triggering multiple reactions inside the cell. These reactions include cell multiplication, death, maturation, and migration that in tumor cells are critical for the cancer to survive, thrive, and spread all over the body. Different types of tyrosine kinase receptors include the human epidermal receptor family, or the HER family. The members of the family are: HER1 (Epidermal Growth Factor Receptor or EGFR), HER2 (ErbB2 or HER2/*neu*), HER3 (ErbB3), and HER4 (ErbB4) [138].

II) Angiogenesis Inhibitors

The new blood vessel formation or angiogenesis needs pro-angiogenic factors. The main pro-angiogenic factor is VEGF (Vascular Endothelial Growth Factor). This factor and other related proteins are important to stimulate new blood vessel growth. Tumors support and feed themselves, allowing them to grow. The angiogenesis inhibitors thwart this process and stop the tumor progression [139].

III) Proteasome Inhibitors

Proteasome is a cellular structure which breaks down proteins that have been labelled to undergo degradation and recycling. This event is important because it removes damaged or defective proteins in processes such as cellular growth, division, angiogenesis, death, etc. A drug by binding in a part of the proteasome can inhibit the breakdown of some proteins that have been marked for destruction, resulting in growth arrest or death of the cell, especially in cancer cells. NF-*k*B is a protein found in both normal and tumor cells. It is typically inactive, because it is bound by the *inhibitor* of *kappa* B (I*k*B*)-alpha*. When this inhibitor protein is broken down by proteasomes, the NF-*k*B is activated and can travel to the nucleus. Once there, the active NF-*k*B starts a chain of events that promote tumor growth and spreading. A drug that inhibits the proteosome can block the breakdown of I*k*B-*alpha,* and thus blocking activation of NF-*k*B. The result is a block of growth factors in the tumor cell [140].

IV) Immunotherapy

The immunotherapy agents are monoclonal antibodies that bind to their specific antigens of cancer cells, not to interfere with growth signals, but rather to trigger immune signals. Targeted immunotherapy agents can develop a series of anti-tumor immune reactions, ultimately causing the death of the tumor cell. When there is a radioisotope attached, these drugs are radio immune therapy agents.

Cancer Vaccines

Cancer vaccines are designed to spur the immune system into recognizing tumor cells as foreign invaders, since unlike the normal cells, the cancerous cells are not detected like infectious cells. Tumor cells often express distinct antigens known as tumor-associated antigens (TAAs); however, the most of TAAs are also present in normal cells. Because the immune system sees these antigens as self-antigens, no immune response is mounted and cross-reactivity can increase the toxicity of the treatment.

To date, cancer vaccines targeting cancers of the breast, prostate, liver, kidney, pancreas, and lung, as well as melanoma and certain types of leukemia and lymphomas are in clinical trials. Some cancers are associated with viral infections, thus human papilloma virus is known to cause cervical cancer or a certain type of liver cancer is associated with hepatitis B and C viruses. Vaccines that prevent infection from these viruses would help to prevent their associated cancers, but they are not cancer vaccines. Co-stimulation of the immune response must occur for there to be a vigorous immune response; however, a tumor can have different types of cells, each with different cell-surface antigens. This makes it difficult for the immune system to distinguish the cancer cells from normal cells, interfering with co-stimulation of the immune response. The immune response is often too weak for any significant effect on the tumor to occur. In order to solve this problem, cancer vaccines are often designed to provide co-stimulation in addition to the TAA with the intention of increasing the immune response. The immune response is dependent on the population of T-cells that was produced during childhood, becoming inactive in adults. A challenge of the cancer vaccines is inducing immune responses in a population of patients whose immune systems are naturally slowing down. Cancer cells can suppress the immune system in a number of ways. They can block co-stimulation, preventing a vigorous immune response. Cancer cells can inhibit the maturing or functioning of antigen presenting cells (APC), blocking the presentation of tumor-associated antigens to lymphocytes. In addition, cancer cells can directly block the activation of lymphocytes, preventing a response after the antigens have been presented. A number of different approaches have been used to introduce TAAs to the immune system and produce an adequate immune response to destroy the cancer cells.

Modified Tumor Cells as cancer Vaccines

The cancer vaccines like vaccines against infectious agents, usually utilize whole, inactivated tumor cells to generate the immune response. An advantage is that a number of antigens are presented so that the immune system can target; however, this compromises the specificity of the vaccine. This method has problems generating an aggressive immune response because of the lack of co-stimulatory molecules. This is the reason why a variety of cytokines and other co-stimulatory molecules are being concurrently administered.

Peptide Vaccines

A peptide is a fragment of a protein that can be used as the antigen in a cancer vaccine. By introducing the appropriate peptide directly to the APC, the vaccine can induce an immune response to cells producing that antigen. Often the peptide vaccine is given simultaneously with co-stimulatory signals (such as hapten) improving the immune response. The peptides can also be engineered by altering specific portions of the peptide that result in stronger immune reactions. Main disadvantages of the peptide vaccines include the need for the peptide to be accepted by the antigen presenting cells. If this does not occur, no immune response is seen. In addition, cells within a tumor are frequently changing and if the peptide that is used in the vaccine is not essential to the tumor, the cells can frequently stop making that protein and avoid detection by the immune system. Peptide vaccination has most commonly been studied in melanoma. Clinical trials have shown evidence of T-cell induction and response, though minimal. The concurrent administration of cytokines has been used to alter one or more amino acids in the antigen to improve the immunogenicity of the antigen. Another problem is that if the intact antigen does not appear, a population of cells T is not developed in order to be effective. Finally, tumor cells can avoid immune recognition by simply down sizing the antigen that the immune system is responding to. Especially if the antigen is not essential, this can be very easy for the tumor cells to accomplish [141].

Dendritic Cell-based Vaccines

Dendritic cells are important antigen presenting cells that seem to be essential in the propagation of the immune response, because of the many co-stimulatory molecules it releases inducing T-cell mediated immune responses. The development of cancer vaccines involves the manipulation of dendritic cells by different techniques. In animal models, vaccination with peptide-pulsed dendritic cells has shown to protect against later challenges with tumors bearing that antigen, whereas in patients with melanoma dendritic cells with whole tumor proteins has been attempted to induce a tumor-specific immunity vaccination resulted in the generation of peptide-specific cellular immune responses in most patients.

However, all of these methods are very expensive, making their widespread use difficult. Gene transfer methods using virus vectors or even retrovirus vectors have also been attempted. Again, there are limitations. With viral vectors, there is a risk of the dendritic cell expressing not only the desired antigen, but also the viral antigens, hence targeting itself for immune attack. With retroviral vectors, the retrovirus requires dividing cells for incorporation. Though this can be done with dendritic cells, the process is cumbersome and expensive. Another method involving dendritic cells includes creating hybrids of dendritic cells with tumor cells. This requires electrical or chemical fusion and remains a hopeful route of improving on cancer vaccines.

Viral Vector Vaccines

Viral vectors utilize a modified virus that remains mildly infectious. The gene that encodes the tumor-associated antigens is placed inside the virus, and when the virus infects a dendritic cell, it can induce the cell to produce large amounts of the antigen. This method has the advantage of being a much cheaper and easier way of introducing genes into dendritic cells than direct injection or electrical manipulation. The dendritic cells can be altered directly in the patient and do not need to first be removed from the patient and later reintroduced. In addition, current viral vaccines also include genes encoding co-stimulatory signals so that the dendritic cells will also produce these proteins, improving the immune response. However, one disadvantage of this system is the possibility of generating an immune response to the virus itself. If the viral antigens are recognized by the immune system, the virus can be cleared from the body before it has a chance to infect the dendritic cell. If the virus is cleared in a rapid way, no immune response against the cancer is mounted.

Heat Shock Protein Vaccines

Heat shock proteins (HSP) are produced by all the cells when they undergo environmental stress. When these proteins move outside of the cell, they act as stimulatory signals to the immune system and induce an immune response. Heat shock protein vaccines work by extracting HSPs directly from tumor cells. Heat shock proteins often contain tumor-specific antigens which are recognized by the immune system. When the HSPs are reintroduced to the patients, they both generate an immune response and direct that response to the specific antigens that they carry. However, a number of different HSPs can be produced by a tumor, and they can carry antigens that are found in normal tissue. In order for these vaccines to be clinically useful, only heat shock proteins that carry tumor-specific antigens can be used [142].

Gene Therapy Vaccines

Another approach in vaccine therapy is the use of genetic material, introduced into the antigen presenting cells as either naked DNA or as a viral vector, to encode the desired targeted tumor antigen. By introducing the DNA directly into the antigen presenting cells, the hope is that there would be a rapid and intense immune response. Preclinical investigations using naked DNA for this purpose has elicited only weak responses. Although the concurrent introduction of cytokines (to enhance the immune response) has had some success, overall this method is not being used in the clinic. The other way that DNA for gene therapy vaccines could be introduced is through viral vectors. This is using a modified virus, with the desired DNA contained within its genome to introduce the DNA. This approach is potentially limited by the generation of a host-immune response to the viral vector itself [143]. This could lead to a rapid clearance of the vector without much introduction of antigen. Ongoing work is focusing mainly on introducing cytokines or other co-stimulatory molecules along with the DNA to attempt to enhance the immune response.

Bone Marrow

Allogeneic Transplant (Bone Marrow & Stem Cell)

Bone marrow is made up of haematopoietic stem cells that mature to become white blood cells, red blood cells and platelets. Allogeneic transplanted cells come from a donor or the cells can even come from umbilical cord blood. If the cells come from an identical twin of the patient, the transplant is syngeneic and is essentially like an autologous transplant, because the cells are identical to those of the patient. The cells must be matched to the patient, which is done by human leukocyte antigen (HLA) testing. The HLA type is made up of 6 antigens, 3 are inherited from the mother, and 3 are inherited from the father. Siblings from the same parents have a 25% chance of matching each other, but if no siblings match, that patient's parents or children can be tested. Leukemia, lymphomas, multiple myeloma, severe aplastic anemia, and sickle cell disease, among others are treated with an allogeneic transplant. The patient can have side effects caused by the preparative regimen (chemotherapy and/or radiation) and they could include mucositis (sores in the mouth and throat), diarrhoea, nausea/vomiting, poor appetite, and fatigue. Still more complications because of the destruction of the bone marrow lead to low blood counts, low platelet counts, infections due to low white blood cell counts, and fatigue due to low red blood cell counts. In addition to these problems, there are complications specific to allogeneic transplants as graft versus host disease, graft rejection or failure, pulmonary (lung) complications, and liver problems (veno-occlusive disease of the liver) [144].

Autologous Stem Cell Transplant or Bone Marrow Transplant

In an autologous transplant, the patient donates his cells to himself. This class of transplants is used to treat leukemia, myelodysplastic syndrome, multiple myeloma [145], Hodgkin's disease, non-Hodgkin's lymphoma, testicular cancer, and neuroblastoma.

Novel Approaches to Therapy

Novel approaches to therapy for cancer include: antisense oligonucleotides; modulators of resistance-associated proteins; metabolic potentiators of conventional drugs; topoisomerase inhibitors; differentiating agents; apoptosis potentiators; modulators of signal transduction; targeted anti-neoplastic agents; anti-migration and/or adhesion agents and anti-angiogenic agents.

Conclusion

Several major cancers linked to chronic infectious conditions (including stomach and cervix) become less common as countries become economically developed, whereas cancers related to tobacco use and Western patterns of diet, physical inactivity, and reproduction (especially lung and bronchus, breast, and colorectal) increase with economic development. There has been significant progress in the development of drugs that specifically act on molecular abnormalities of certain tumors diminishing the damage to normal cells. On the other hand, the histological classification and the presence of more specific molecular markers in cancer cells could be determinants for individual treatments.

References

[1] Perkins, EA; Small, BJ; Balducci, L; Extermann, M; Robb, C; Haley, WE. Individual differences in well-being in older breast cancer survivors. *Crit Rev Oncol Hematol,* 2007 62, 74–83.

[2] Foulds, L. The experimental study of tumor progression: a review. *Cancer Res,* 1954 14, 327-339.

[3] Szymańska, K; Chen, JG; Cui, Y; Gong, YY; Turner, PC; Villar, S; Wild, CP; Parkin, DM; Hainaut, P. TP53 R249S mutations, exposure to aflatoxin, and occurrence of hepatocellular carcinoma in a cohort of chronic hepatitis B virus carriers from Qidong, China. *Cancer Epidemiol Biomarkers Prev,* 2009 18, 1638-1643.

[4] Ishiguro, S; Sasazuki, S; Inoue, M; Kurahashi, N; Iwasaki, M; Tsugane, S. Effect of alcohol consumption, cigarette smoking and flushing response on esophageal cancer risk: a population-based cohort study (JPHC study); JPHC Study Group. *Cancer Lett,* 2009 18, 240-246.

[5] Loeb, LA; Harris, CC. Advances in Chemical Carcinogenesis: A Historical Review and Prospective. *Cancer Res,* 2008 68, 6863-6582.

[6] Murth, NS; Aleyamma, M. Cancer epidemiology, prevention and control. *Current Science*, 2004 86(4), 518-527.

[7] Garcia, M; Jemal, A; Ward, EM; Center, MM; Hao, Y; Siegel, RL; Thun, MJ. Global Cancer Facts & Figures 2007. *American Cancer Society*, Atlanta, GA 2007, pp 1-52.

[8] NCI, National Cancer Institute [website]. Surveillance, Epidemiology, and End Results (SEER), Program of the National Cancer Institute. SEER Cancer Statistics Review 1975-2006. Available at: http://seer.cancer.gov/statfacts/html/all.html #ref10. Accessed on August 10, 2009.

[9] WHO, World Health Organization [website]. United Nations Media Center, Fact sheet N°297. Updated February 2009. Available at: http://www.who.int/media centre/factsheets/fs297/en/index.html. Accessed on August 10, 2009.

[10] Parkin, DM. The global health burden of infection-associated cancers in the year 2002. *Int J Cancer,* 2006 118, 3030-3044.

[11] WHO. The World Health Organization's Fight Against Cancer: Strategies That Prevent, Cure and Care. *WHO Library.* Cataloguing-in-Publication-Data. Switzerland, 2007.

[12] Armstrong, B; Doll, R. Environmental factors and cancer incidence in different countries, with special references to dietary practice. *Int J Cancer,* 1975 15, 617–631.

[13] Doll, R; Peto, R. The causes of cancer: quantitative estimates of avoidable risks of cancer in the United States today. *J Natl Cancer Inst,* 1981 66, 1191–1308.

[14] Kritchevsky, D. Diet and Cancer: what's next? *J Nutr,* 2003 133, 3827–3829.

[15] Bingham, SA; Day, NE; Luben, R; Ferrari, P; Slimani, N; Norat, T; Clavel-Chapelon, F; Kesse, E; Nieters, A; Boeing, H; Tjønneland, A; Overvad, K; Martinez, C; Dorronsoro, M; Gonzalez, CA; Key, TJ; Trichopoulou, A; Naska, A; Vineis, P; Tumino, R; Krogh, V; Bueno-de-Mesquita, HB; Peeters, PH; Berglund, G; Hallmans, G; Lund, E; Skeie, G; Kaaks, RM; Riboli, E. European Prospective Investigation into Cancer and Nutrition. Dietary fiber in food and protection against colorectal cancer in The European Prospective Investigation into Cancer and Nutrition (EPIC): an observational study. *Lancet,* 2003 361, 1496–1501.

[16] Shetty, K; Brown, J. Oral cancer risk factors among Mexican American Hispanic adolescents in South Texas. *J Dent Child (Chic),* 2009 76, 142-148.

[17] Benedetti, A; Parent, ME; Siemiatycki, J. Lifetime consumption of alcoholic beverages and risk of 13 types of cancer in men: results from a case-control study in Montreal. *Cancer Detect Prev,* 2009 32, 352-362.

[18] Lew, JQ; Freedman, ND; Leitzmann, MF; Brinton, LA; Hoover, RN; Hollenbeck, AR; Schatzkin, A; Park, Y. Alcohol and risk of breast cancer by histologic type and hormone receptor status in postmenopausal women: the NIH-AARP Diet and Health Study. *Am J Epidemiol,* 2009 170, 308-317.

[19] Sitas, F; Parkin, DM; Chirenje, M; Stein, L; Abratt, R; Wabinga, H.Part II: Cancer in Indigenous Africans--causes and control. *Lancet Oncol*, 2008 9, 786-95.

[20] de Sanjose, S; Mbisa, G; Perez-Alvarez, S; Benavente, Y; Sukvirach, S; Hieu, NT; Shin, HR, Anh, PT; Thomas, J; Lazcano, E; Matos, E; Herrero, R; Muñoz, N; Molano, M; Franceschi, S; Whitby, D. Geographic variation in the prevalence of Kaposi sarcoma-associated herpesvirus and risk factors for transmission. *J Infect Dis,* 2009 1991449-1456.

[21] Parkin, DM. Global cancer statistics, 2002. *CA Cancer J Clin,* 2005 55:74-108.

[22] Mackay, J, Jemal A; Lee, NC; Parkin, DM (Eds). The Cancer Atlas. *American Cancer Society*, Atlanta, 2006.

[23] Hawk, ET; Matrisian, LM; Nelson, WG; Dorfman, GS; Stevens, L; Kwok, J; Viner, J; Hautala, J; Grad, O. The Translational Research Working Group developmental pathways: introduction and overview. *Clin Cancer Res,* 2008 14, 5664-5671.

[24] Jacobs, JF; van Bokhoven, H; van Leeuwen, FN; Hulsbergen-van de Kaa, CA; de Vries, IJ; Adema, GJ; Hoogerbrugge, PM; de Brouwer, AP. Regulation of MYCN expression in human neuroblastoma cells. *BMC Cancer,* 2009 9, 239.

[25] Narter, KF; Ergen, A; Agaçhan, B; Görmüs, U; Timirci, O; Isbir, T. Bladder cancer and polymorphisms of DNA repair genes (XRCC1, XRCC3, XPD, XPG, APE1, hOGG1). *Anticancer Res,* 2009 29, 1389-1393.

[26] Koutros, S; Berndt, SI; Sinha, R; Ma, X; Chatterjee, N; Alavanja, MC; Zheng, T; Huang, WY; Hayes, RB; Cross, AJ. Xenobiotic metabolizing gene variants, dietary heterocyclic amine intake, and risk of prostate cancer. *Cancer Res,* 2009 69, 1877-1884.

[27] Mangala, LS; Zuzel, V; Schmandt, R; Leshane, ES; Halder, JB; Armaiz-Pena, GN; Spannuth, WA; Tanaka, T; Shahzad, MM; Lin, YG; Nick, AM; Danes, CG; Lee, JW; Jennings, NB; Vivas-Mejia, PE; Wolf, JK; Coleman, RL; Siddik, ZH; Lopez-Berestein, G; Lutsenko, S; Sood, AK. Therapeutic Targeting of ATP7B in Ovarian Carcinoma. *Clin Cancer Res*, 2009 15, 3770-3780.

[28] Pouyet, L; Carrier, A. Mutant mouse models of oxidative stress. *Transgenic Res*, 2009 (*In press).*

[29] Duong, YT; Jia, H; Lust, JA; Garcia, AD; Tiffany, AJ; Heneine, W; Switzer, WM. Short communication: Absence of evidence of HTLV-3 and HTLV-4 in patients with large granular lymphocyte (LGL) leukemia. *AIDS Res Hum Retroviruses*, 2008 24, 1503-1505.

[30] Mullenders, L; Atkinson, M; Paretzke, H; Sabatier, L; Bouffler, S. Assessing cancer risks of low-dose radiation. *Nat Rev Cancer,* 2009 9, 596-604.

[31] Amaral, AF; Cymbron, T; Gartner, F; Lima, M; Rodrigues, AS. Trace metals and over-expression of metallothioneins in bladder tumoral lesions: a case-control study. *BMC Vet Res,* 2009 5, 40.

[32] Kreuzer, M; Walsh, L; Schnelzer, M; Tschense, A; Grosche, B. Radon and risk of extrapulmonary cancers: results of the German uranium miners' cohort study, 1960-2003. *Br J Cancer,* 2008 99, 1946-1953.

[33] Mangano, JJ. A short latency between radiation exposure from nuclear plants and cancer in young children. *Int J Health Serv,* 2006 36, 113-135.

[34] Lynch, SM; Vrieling, A; Lubin, JH; Kraft, P; Mendelsohn, JB; Hartge, P; Canzian, F; Steplowski, E; Arslan, AA; Gross, M; Helzlsouer, K; Jacobs, EJ; LaCroix, A; Petersen, G; Zheng, W; Albanes, D; Amundadottir, L; Bingham, SA; Boffetta, P; Boutron-Ruault, MC; Chanock, SJ; Clipp, S; Hoover, RN; Jacobs, K; Johnson, KC; Kooperberg, C; Luo, J; Messina, C; Palli, D; Patel, AV; Riboli, E; Shu, XO; Rodriguez-Suarez, L; Thomas, G; Tjønneland, A; Tobias, GS; Tong, E; Trichopoulos, D; Virtamo, J; Ye, W; Yu, K; Zeleniuch-Jacquette, A; Bueno-de-Mesquita, HB; Stolzenberg-Solomon, RZ. Cigarette smoking and pancreatic cancer: a pooled analysis from the pancreatic cancer cohort consortium. *Am J Epidemiol,* 2009 170, 403-413.

[35] Ferguson, LR. Role of dietary mutagens in cancer and atherosclerosis. *Curr Opin Clin Nutr Metab Care,* 2009 12, 343-349.

[36] Levina, VV; Nolen, B; Su, Y; Godwin, AK; Fishman, D; Liu, J; Mor, G; Maxwell, LG; Herberman, RB; Szczepanski, MJ; Szajnik, ME; Gorelik, E; Lokshin, AE. Biological significance of prolactin in gynecologic cancers. *Cancer Res,* 2009 69, 5226-5233.

[37] Vogelstein, B; and Kinzler, KW. The Genetic Basis of Human Cancer (Ed) McGraw-Hill, New York 1998, 565-587.

[38] Caporaso, N; and Goldstein, A. Cancer genes: single and susceptibility: exposing the difference. *Pharmacogenetics,* 1995 5, 59–63.

[39] Sinha, R; Potter, JD. Diet, nutrition, and genetic susceptibility. *Cancer Epidemiol Biomark Prev,* 1997 6, 647–649.

[40] Ayesh, R; Idle, JR; Richie, JC; Crothers, MJ; Hetzel, MR. Metabolic oxidation phenotypes as markers for susceptibility to lung cancer. *Nature (Lond),* 1984 312, 169–170.

[41] Seidegard, J; Pero, RW; Miller, DG; Beattie, EJ. A glutathione transferase in human leukocytes as a marker for susceptibility to lung cancer. *Carcinogenesis,* 1986 7, 751–753.

[42] Sinha, R; Caporaso, N. Diet, Genetic Susceptibility and Human Cancer Etiology. Symposium: Interactions of Diet and Nutrition with Genetic Susceptibility in Cancer. Division of Cancer Epidemiology & Genetics, National Cancer Institute, National Institutes of Health, *J Nutr,* 1999 129, 556–559.

[43] Sorahan, T. Bladder cancer risks in workers manufacturing chemicals for the rubber industry. *Occup Med (Lond),* 2008 58, 496-501.

[44] Reger, RB; Morgan, WK. Respiratory cancers in mining. *Occup Med*, 1993 8, 185-204.

[45] d'Errico, A; Pasian, S; Baratti, A; Zanelli, R; Alfonzo, S; Gilardi, L; Beatrice, F; Bena, A; Costa. G. A case-control study on occupational risk factors for sino-nasal cancer. *Occup Environ Med*, 2009 66, 448-455.

[46] Costantini, AS; Benvenuto, A; Vineis, P; Kriebel, D; Tumino, R; Ramazzotti, V; Rodella, S; Stagnaro, E; Crosignani, P; Amadori, D; Mirabelli, D; Sommani, L; Belletti, I; Troschel, L; Romeo, L; Miceli, G; Tosí, GA; Mendico, I; Maltoni, SA; Miligi, L. Risk of leukemia and multiple myeloma associated with exposure to benzene and other organic solvents: evidence from the Italian Multicenter Case-control study. *Am J Ind Med,* 2008 51, 803-811.

[47] Roberts, HC; Patsios, DA; Paul, NS; DePerrot, M; Teel, W; Bayanati, H; Shepherd, F; Johnston, MR. Screening for malignant pleural mesothelioma and lung cancer in individuals with a history of asbestos exposure. *J Thorac Oncol,* 2009 4, 620-628.

[48] Seaberg, RM; Eski, S; Freeman, JL. Influence of previous radiation exposure on pathologic features and clinical outcome in patients with thyroid cancer. *Arch Otolaryngol Head Neck Surg*, 2009 135, 355-359.

[49] Nakanishi, M; Tanaka, K; Takahashi, T; Kyo, T; Dohy, H; Fujiwara, M; Kamada, N. Microsatellite instability in acute myelocytic leukemia developed from A-bomb survivors. *Int J Radiat Biol,* 2001 77, 687-694.

[50] Mould, RF. Depleted uranium and radiation-induced lung cancer and leukemia. *Br J Radiol,* 2001 74, 677-683.

[51] Anastasiou, I; Mygdalis, V; Mihalakis, A; Adamakis, I; Constantinides, C; Mitropoulos, D. Patient awareness of smoking as a risk factor for bladder cancer. *Int Urol Nephrol,* 2009 (*In Press).*

[52] Pöschl, G; Seitz, HK. Alcohol and cancer. *Alcohol Alcohol*, 2004 39, 155-165.

[53] Burkitt, DP. Dietary fiber and cancer. *J Nutr,* 1988 118, 531-513.

[54] Wild, CP; Montesano, R. A model of interaction: Aflatoxins and hepatitis viruses in liver cancer aetiology and prevention. *Cancer Lett, 2009* (*In Press*).

[55] Hede, K. Fat may fuel breast cancer growth. *J Natl Cancer Inst*, 2008 100(5), 298–299.

[56] Hursting, SD; Lashinger, LM; Wheatley, KW; et al. Reducing the weight of cancer: mechanistic targets for breaking the obesity-carcinogenesis link. *Best Practice and Research: Clinical Endocrinology and Metabolism*, 2008 22, 659–669.

[57] Cho, E; Hunter, DJ; Spiegelman, D; Albanes, D; Beeson, WL; van den Brandt, PA; Colditz, GA; Feskanich, D; Folsom, AR; Fraser, GE; Freudenheim, JL; Giovannucci, E; Goldbohm, RA; Graham, S; Miller, AB; Rohan, TE; Sellers, TA; Virtamo, J; Willett, WC; Smith-Warner, SA. Intakes of vitamins A, C and E and folate and multivitamins and lung cancer: a pooled analysis of 8 prospective studies. *Int J Cancer,* 2006 118, 970-978.

[58] Botelho, M; Ferreira, AC; Oliveira, MJ; Domingues, A; Machado, JC; da Costa, JM. Schistosoma haematobium total antigen induces increased proliferation, migration and invasion, and decreases apoptosis of normal epithelial cells. *Int J Parasitol*, 2009 39, 1083-1091.

[59] Radaelli, F; Onida, F; Rossi, FG; Zilioli, VR; Colombi, M; Usardi, P; Calori, R; Zanella, A. Second malignancies in essential thrombocythemia (ET): a retrospective analysis of 331 patients with long-term follow-up from a single institution. *Hematology,* 2008 13, 195-202.

[60] Kaatsch, P; Reinisch, I; Spix, C; Berthold, F; Janka-Schaub, G; Mergenthaler, A; Michaelis J; Blettner, M. Case-control study on the therapy of childhood cancer and the occurrence of second malignant neoplasms in Germany. *Cancer Causes Control,* 2009 20, 965-980.

[61] Abdelrahim, M; Ariazi, E; Kim, K; Khan, S; Barhoumi, R; Burghardt, R; Liu, S; Hill, D; Finnell, R; Wlodarczyk, B; Jordan, VC; Safe, S. 3-Methylcholanthrene and other aryl hydrocarbon receptor agonists directly activate estrogen receptor alpha. *Cancer Res,* 2006 66, 2459-2467.

[62] Martin, LJ; Minkin, S; Boyd, NF. Hormone therapy, mammographic density, and breast cancer risk. *Maturitas,* 2009 64, 20-26.

[63] Johnson, EB; Muto, MG; Yanushpolsky, EH; Mutter, GL. Phytoestrogen supplementation and endometrial cancer. *Obstet Gynecol,* 2001 98, 947-950.

[64] Giusti, RM; Iwamoto, K; Hatch, EE. Diethylstilbestrol revisited: a review of the long-term health effects. *Ann Intern Med,* 1995 122, 778-788.

[65] Sanada, N; Gotoh, Y; Shimazawa, R; Klinge, CM; Kizu, R. Repression of Activated Aryl Hydrocarbon Receptor–Induced Transcriptional Activation by 5α-Dihydrotestosterone in Human Prostate Cancer LNCaP and Human Breast Cancer T47D Cells. *J Pharmacol Sc,* 2009 109, 380-387.

[66] Euhus, D. Risk modeling in breast cancer. *Breast J,* 2004 10, 10-12.

[67] Peeper, DS. Ras and pRb: the relationship gets yet more intimate. *Cancer Cell,* 2009 15, 243-245.

[68] Cladel, NM; Hu, J; Balogh, K; Mejia, A; Christensen, ND. Wounding prior to challenge substantially improves infectivity of cottontail rabbit papillomavirus and allows for standardization of infection. *J Virol Methods,* 2008 148, 34-39.

[69] Ellies, LG. PyV-mT-induced parotid gland hyperplasia as detected by altered lectin reactivity is not modulated by inducible nitric oxide deficiency. *Arch Oral Biol,* 2003 48, 415-422.

[70] Landskroner-Eiger, S; Qian, B; Muise, ES; Nawrocki, AR; Berger, JP; Fine, EJ; Koba, W; Deng, Y; Pollard, JW; Scherer, PE. Proangiogenic contribution of adiponectin toward mammary tumor growth in vivo. *Clin Cancer Res,* 2009 15, 3265-3276.

[71] Baze, WB; Steinbach, TJ; Fleetwood, ML; Blanchard, TW; Barnhart, KF; McArthur, MJ. Karyomegaly and intranuclear inclusions in the renal tubules of sentinel ICR mice (mus musculus). *Comp Med,* 2006 56, 435-438.

[72] Kawabuchi, B; Nomura, K; Ohtake, K; Hino, O; Aizawa, S; Machinami, R; Kitagawa, T. Subcutaneous sarcomas of probable neuronal origin in a transgenic mouse strain containing an albumin promoter-fused simian virus 40 large T antigen gene. *Jpn J Cancer Res,* 1994 85, 601-609.

[73] Zeisig, BB; So, CW. Retroviral/Lentiviral transduction and transformation assay. *Methods Mol Biol,* 2009 538, 207-229.

[74] Levy, J; Crawford, C; Hartmann, K; Hofmann-Lehmann, R; Little, S; Sundahl, E; Thayer, V. American Association of Feline Practitioners' feline retrovirus management guidelines. *J Feline Med Surg,* 2008 10, 300-316.

[75] Fukuoka, H; Moriuchi, M; Yano, H; Nagayasu, T; Moriuchi, H. No association of mouse mammary tumor virus-related retrovirus with Japanese cases of breast cancer. *J Med Virol,* 2008 80, 1447-1451.

[76] Mahieux, R; Gessain, A. HTLV-1 and associated adult T-cell leukemia/ lymphoma. *Rev Clin Exp Hematol,* 2003 7, 336-361.

[77] Thorley-Lawson, DA; Allday, MJ. The curious case of the tumour virus: 50 years of Burkitt's lymphoma. *Nat Rev Microbiol,* 2008 6, 913-924.

[78] Mezencev, R; Kutschy, P; Salanova, A; Updegrove, T; McDonald, JF. The design, synthesis and anticancer activity of new nitrogen mustard derivatives of natural indole phytoalexin 1-methoxyspirobrassinol. *Neoplasma,* 2009 56, 321-330.

[79] Forouzesh, B; Hidalgo, M; Chu, Q; Mita, A; Mita, M; Schwartz, G; Jimeno, J; Gómez, J; Alfaro, V; Lebedinsky, C; Zintl, P; Rowinsky, EK. Phase I and pharmacokinetic study of trabectedin as a 1- or 3-hour infusion weekly in patients with advanced solid malignancies. *Clin Cancer Res,* 2009 15, 3591-3599.

[80] Masiello, D; Tulpule, A. Bendamustine therapy in chronic lymphocytic leukemia. *Expert Opin Pharmacother,* 2009 10, 1687-1698.

[81] Farber, S; Diamond, LK. Temporary remissions in acute leukemia. in children produced by folic acid antagonist, 4-aminopteroyl-glutamic acid. *N Engl J Med,* 1948 238, 787-793.

[82] Kang, MH; Harutyunyan, N; Hall, CP; Papa, RA; Lock, RB. Methotrexate and aminopterin exhibit similar in vitro and in vivo preclinical activity against acute lymphoblastic leukemia and lymphoma. *Br J Haematol,* 2009 145, 389-393.

[83] Das, JR; Fryar-Tita, EB; Zhou, Y; Green, S; Southerland, WM; Bowen, D. Sequence-dependent administration of 5-fluorouracil maintains methotrexate antineoplastic activity in human estrogen-negative breast cancer and protects against methotrexate cytotoxicity in human bone marrow. *Anticancer Res,* 2007 27, 3791-3799.

[84] Chen, G; Wright, JE; Rosowsky, A. Dihydrofolate reductase binding and cellular uptake of nonpolyglutamatable antifolates: correlates of cytotoxicity toward methotrexate-sensitive and -resistant human head and neck squamous carcinoma cells. *Mol Pharmacol,* 1995 48, 758-765.

[85] Pasello, M; Hattinger, CM; Stoico, G; Manara, MC; Benini, S; Geroni, C; Mercuri, M; Scotlandi, K; Picci, P; Serra, M. 4-Demethoxy-3'-deamino-3'-aziridinyl-4'-methylsulphonyl-daunorubicin (PNU-159548): a promising new candidate for chemotherapeutic treatment of osteosarcoma patients. *Eur J Cancer,* 2005 41, 2184-2195.

[86] Peñuelas, S; Noé, V; Ciudad, CJ. Modulation of IMPDH2, survivin, topoisomerase I and vimentin increases sensitivity to methotrexate in HT29 human colon cancer cells. *FEBS J,* 2005 272, 696-710.

[87] Bolling, C; Graefe, T; Lübbing, C; Jankevicius, F; Uktveris, S; Cesas, A; Meyer-Moldenhauer, WH; Starkmann, H; Weigel, M; Burk, K; Hanauske, AR. Phase II study of MTX-HSA in combination with cisplatin as first line treatment in patients with advanced or metastatic transitional cell carcinoma. *Invest New Drugs,* 2006 24, 521-527.

[88] Hatse, S; Naesens, L; Degrève, B; Vandeputte, M; Waer, M; De Clercq, E; Balzarini, J. In vitro and in vivo inhibitory activity of the differentiation-inducing agent 9-(2-phosphonylmethoxyethyl) adenine (PMEA) against rat choriocarcinoma. *Adv Exp Med Biol* 1998 431, 605-609.

[89] Cronstein BN. Molecular mechanism of methotrexate action in inflammation. *Inflammation,* 1992 16, 411–423.

[90] Torigoe, S; Ogata, Y; Matono, K; Shirouzu, K. Molecular mechanisms of sequence-dependent antitumor effects of SN-38 and 5-fluorouracil combination therapy against colon cancer cells. *Anticancer Res,* 2009 29, 2083-2089.

[91] Yasumatsu, R; Nakashima, T; Uryu, H; Masuda, M; Hirakawa, N; Shiratsuchi, H; Tomita, K; Fukushima, M; Komune, S. The role of dihydropyrimidine dehydrogenase expression in resistance to 5-fluorouracil in head and neck squamous cell carcinoma cells. *Oral Oncol,* 2009 45, 141-147.

[92] Ikeda, M; Okada, S; Ueno, H; Okusaka, T; Tanaka, N; Kuriyama, H; Yoshimori, M. A phase II study of sequential methotrexate and 5-fluorouracil in metastatic pancreatic cancer. *Hepatogastroenterology,* 2000 47, 862-865.

[93] Neri, B; Pantaleo, P; Giommoni, E; Grifoni, R; Paoletti, C; Rotella, V; Pantalone, D; Taddei, A; Mercatelli, A; Tonelli, P. Oxaliplatin, 5-fluorouracil/leucovorin and epirubicin as first-line treatment in advanced gastric carcinoma: a phase II study. *Br J Cancer,* 2007 96, 1043-1046.

[94] Morise, Z; Sugioka, A; Fujita, J; Hoshimoto, S; Kato, T; Ikeda, M. S-1 plus cisplatin combination therapy for the patients with primary liver carcinomas. *Hepatogastroenterology,* 2007 54, 2315-2318.

[95] Rubnitz, JE; Crews, KR; Pounds, S; Yang, S; Campana, D; Gandhi, VV; Raimondi, SC; Downing, JR; Razzouk, BI; Pui, CH; Ribeiro, RC. Combination of cladribine and cytarabine is effective for childhood acute myeloid leukemia: results of the St Jude AML97 trial. *Leukemia,* 2009 23, 1410-1416.

[96] Parsels, LA; Morgan, MA; Tanska, DM; Parsels, JD; Palmer, BD; Booth, RJ; Denny, WA; Canman, CE; Kraker, AJ; Lawrence, TS; Maybaum, J. Gemcitabine sensitization by checkpoint kinase 1 inhibition correlates with inhibition of a Rad51 DNA damage response in pancreatic cancer cells. *Mol Cancer Ther,* 2009 8, 45-54.

[97] Hogarth, LA; Redfern, CP; Teodoridis, JM; Hall, AG; Anderson, H; Case, MC; Coulthard, SA. The effect of thiopurine drugs on DNA methylation in relation to TPMT expression. *Biochem Pharmacol* 2008 76, 1024-1035.

[98] Zhenchuk, A; Lotfi, K; Juliusson, G; Albertioni, F. Mechanisms of anti-cancer action and pharmacology of clofarabine. *Biochem Pharmacol,* 2009 *(In press).*

[99] Lyu, YL; Kerrigan, JE; Lin, CP; Azarova, AM; Tsai, YC; Ban, Y; Liu, LF. Topoisomerase IIbeta mediated DNA double-strand breaks: implications in doxorubicin cardiotoxicity and prevention by dexrazoxane. *Cancer Res,* 2007 67, 8839-8846.

[100] de Azambuja, E; Fleck, JF; Barreto, SS; Cunha, RD. Pulmonary epithelial permeability in patients treated with bleomycin containing chemotherapy detected by technetium-99m diethylene triamine penta-acetic acid aerosol (99mTc-DTPA) scintigraphy. *Ann Nucl Med,* 2005 19, 131-135.

[101] Mathijssen, RH; Loos, WJ; Verweij, J; Sparreboom, A. Pharmacology of topoisomerase I inhibitors irinotecan (CPT-11) and topotecan. *Curr Cancer Drug Targets,* 2002 2, 103-123.

[102] Morgan, SE; Cadena, RS; Raimondi, SC; Beck, WT. Selection of human leukemic CEM cells for resistance to the DNA topoisomerase II catalytic inhibitor ICRF-187 results in increased levels of topoisomerase IIalpha and altered G(2)/M checkpoint and apoptotic responses. *Mol Pharmacol,* 2000 57, 296-307.

[103] Fu, Y; Li, S; Zu, Y; Yang, G; Yang, Z; Luo, M; Jiang, S; Wink, M; Efferth, T. Medicinal Chemistry of Paclitaxel and its Analogues. *Curr Med Chem,* 2009 *(In press).*

[104] De Ligio, JT; Velkova, A; Zorio, DA; Monteiro, AN. Can the status of the breast and ovarian cancer susceptibility gene 1 product (BRCA1) predict response to taxane-based cancer therapy? *Anticancer Agents Med Chem,* 2009 5, 543-549.

[105] Sun, Q; Liu, C; Zhong, H; Zhong, B; Xu; Shen, W; Wang, D. Multi-center phase II trial of weekly paclitaxel plus cisplatin combination chemotherapy in patients with advanced gastric and gastro-esophageal cancer. *Jpn J Clin Oncol,* 2009 39, 237-243.

[106] Smaldone, MC; Gayed, BA; Tomaszewski, JJ; Gingrich, JR. Strategies to enhance the efficacy of intravescical therapy for non-muscle invasive bladder cancer. *Minerva Urol Nefrol,* 2009 61, 71-89.

[107] Bode, C; Trojan, L; Weiss, C; Kraenzlin, B; Michaelis, U; Teifel, M; Alken, P; Michel, MS. Paclitaxel encapsulated in cationic liposomes: a new option for neovascular targeting for the treatment of prostate cancer. *Oncol Rep,* 2009 22, 321-326.

[108] McGrogan, BT; Gilmartin, B; Carney, DN; McCann, A. Taxanes, microtubules and chemoresistant breast cancer. *Biochim Biophys,* 2008, 1785, 96–132.

[109] Wagner, JM; Karnitz, LM. Cisplatin-induced DNA damage activates replication checkpoint signaling components that differentially affect tumor cell survival. *Mol Pharmacol,* 2009 76, 208-214.

[110] Boeck, S; Metzeler, KH; Hausmann, A; Baumann, A; Gallmeier, E; Parhofer, KG; Stemmler, HJ. Cisplatin-based chemotherapy for pulmonary metastasized germ cell tumors of the testis--be aware of acute respiratory distress syndrome. *Onkologie,* 2009, 32, 125-128.

[111] Leonard, GD; Wagner, MR; Quinn, MG; Grem, JL. Severe disabling sensory-motor polyneuropathy during oxaliplatin-based chemotherapy. *Anticancer Drugs,* 2004, 15, 733-735.

[112] Desoize, B. Metals and metal compounds in cancer treatment. *Anticancer Res,* 2004 24, 1529-1544.

[113] Ott I, Gust R. Non platinum metal complexes as anti-cancer drugs. *Arch Pharm* (Weinheim), 2007, 340, 117-126

[114] Köpf-Maier, P. Complexes of metals other than platinum as antitumour agents. *Eur J Clin Pharmacol,* 1994 47, 1-16.

[115] Zhang, CX; Lippard, SJ. New metal complexes as potential therapeutics. *Curr Opin Chem Biol* 2003 7, 481-489.

[116] Mainwaring, MG; Poor, C; Zander, DS; Harman, E. Complete remission of pulmonary spindle cell carcinoma after treatment with oral germanium sesquioxide. *Chest* 2000 117, 591-593.

[117] Etcheverry, SB; Ferrer, EG; Naso, L; Rivadeneira, J; Salinas, V; Williams, PA. Antioxidant effects of the VO (IV) hesperidin complex and its role in cancer chemoprevention. *J Biol Inorg Chem,* 2008 13, 435-447.

[118] Köpf-Maier, P; Klapötke, T. Antitumor activity of ionic niobocene and molybdenocene complexes in high oxidation states. *J Cancer Res Clin Oncol,* 1992 118, 216-221.

[119] Thomadaki, H; Karaliota, A; Litos, C; Scorilas, A. Enhanced antileukemic activity of the novel complex 2,5-dihydroxybenzoate molybdenum(VI) against 2,5-dihydroxybenzoate, polyoxometalate of Mo(VI), and tetraphenylphosphonium in the human HL-60 and K562 leukemic cell lines. *J Med Chem,* 2007 50, 1316-1321.

[120] Koutsikos, J; Leondi, A. Re-186 HEDP treatment in breast cancer patients with bone metastases. *J Natl Med Assoc,* 2008 100, 447.

[121] Schmitt, F; Govindaswamy, P; Zava, O; Süss-Fink, G; Juillerat-Jeanneret, L; Therrien, B. Combined arene ruthenium porphyrins as chemotherapeutics and photosensitizers for cancer therapy. *J Biol Inorg Chem*, 2009 14, 101-119.

[122] de Keizer RJ, de Wolff-Rouendaal D, Nooy MA. Angiosarcoma of the eyelid and periorbital region. Experience in Leiden with iridium192 brachytherapy and low-dose doxorubicin chemotherapy. *Orbit,* 2008 27, 5-12.

[123] Mejia, C; Ruiz-Azuara, L. Casiopeinas IIgly and IIIia induce apoptosis in medulloblastoma cells. Pathology and Oncology Research, 2008 14, 467-472.

[124] Viswanathan, AN; Erickson, BA. Three-Dimensional Imaging in Gynecologic Brachytherapy: A Survey of the American Brachytherapy Society. *Int J Radiat Oncol Biol Phys,* 2009 (*In press*).

[125] Bitencourt, AG; Lima, EN; Pinto, PN; Martins, EB; Chojniak, R. New applications of radioguided surgery in oncology. *Clinics (Sao Paulo),* 2009 64, 397-402.

[126] Habrand, JL; Schneider, R; Alapetite, C; Feuvret, L; Petras, S; Datchary, J; Grill, J; Noel, G; Helfre, S; Ferrand, R; Bolle, S; Sainte-Rose, C. Proton therapy in pediatric skull base and cervical canal low-grade bone malignancies. *Int J Radiat Oncol Biol Phys,* 2008 71, 672-675.

[127] Schwer, AL; Kavanagh, BD; McCammon, R; Gaspar, LE; Kleinschmidt-De Masters, BK; Stuhr, K; Chen, C. Radiographic and histopathologic observations after combined EGFR inhibition and hypofractionated stereotactic radiosurgery in patients with recurrent malignant gliomas. *Int J Radiat Oncol Biol Phys,* 2009 73, 1352-1357.

[128] Pieters, BR; de Back, DZ; Koning, CC; Zwinderman, AH. Comparison of three radiotherapy modalities on biochemical control and overall survival for the treatment of prostate cancer: A systematic review. *Radiother Oncol,*. 2009 *(In Press*).

[129] Cameron, AL; Cornes, P; Al-Booz, H. Brachytherapy in endometrial cancer: quantification of air gaps around a vaginal cylinder. *Brachytherapy,* 2008 7, 355-358.

[130] Ludwig, MS; McNeese, MD; Buchholz, TA; Perkins, GH; Strom, EA. The Lateral Decubitus Breast Boost: Description, Rationale, and Efficacy. *Int J Radiat Oncol Biol Phys,* 2009 (*In press*).

[131] Su, S. Mesothelioma: path to multimodality treatment. *Semin Thorac Cardiovasc Surg,* 2009 21, 125-131.

[132] Abuzeid, WM; Jiang, X; Shi, G; Wang, H; Paulson, D; Araki, K; Jungreis, D; Carney, J; O'Malley, BW Jr; Li, D. Molecular disruption of RAD50 sensitizes human tumor cells to cisplatin-based chemotherapy. *J Clin Invest,* 2009 119, 1974-1985.

[133] Wang, T; You, Q; Huang, FS; Xiang, H. Recent advances in selective estrogen receptor modulators for breast cancer. *Mini Rev Med Chem* 2009 9, 1191-1201.

[134] Freedman, OC; Amir E, Hanna W, Kahn H, O'Malley F, Dranitsaris G, Cole DE, Verma S, Folkerd E, Dowsett M, Clemons M. A randomized trial exploring the biomarker effects of neoadjuvant sequential treatment with exemestane and anastrozole in post-menopausal women with hormone receptor-positive breast cancer. *Breast Cancer Res Treat,* 2009 (*In press*).

[135] Chen, Y; Clegg, NJ; Scher, HI. Anti-androgens and androgen-depleting therapies in prostate cancer: new agents for an established target. *Lancet Oncol,* 2009 10, 981-91.

[136] Gulley JL, Aragon-Ching JB, Steinberg SM, Hussain MH, Sartor O, Higano CS, Petrylak DP, Chatta GS, Arlen PM, Figg WD, Dahut WL. Kinetics of serum androgen normalization and factors associated with testosterone reserve after limited androgen deprivation therapy for nonmetastatic prostate cancer. *J Urol,* 2008, 180, 1432-1437.

[137] Wang, JY; Lu, CY; Chu, KS; Ma, CJ; Wu, DC; Tsai, HL; Yu, FJ; Hsieh, JS. Prognostic significance of pre- and postoperative serum carcinoembryonic antigen levels in patients with colorectal cancer. *Eur Surg Res,* 2007 39, 245-250.

[138] Löbke, C; Laible, M; Rappl, C; Ruschhaupt, M; Sahin, O; Arlt, D; Wiemann, S; Poustka, A; Sültmann, H; Korf, U. Contact spotting of protein microarrays coupled with spike-in of normalizer protein permits time-resolved analysis of ERBB receptor signaling. *Proteomics,* 2008 8, 1586-1594.

[139] Evensen, L; Micklem, DR; Link, W; Lorens JB.A novel imaging-based high-throughput screening approach to anti-angiogenic drug discovery. *Cytometry A,* 2009 (*In press*).

[140] Kandel, ES. NFkappaB inhibition and more: a side-by-side comparison of the inhibitors of IKK and proteasome. *Cell Cycle,* 2009 8, 1819-1820.

[141] Pilla, L; Rivoltini, L; Patuzzo, R; Marrari, A; Valdagni, R; Parmiani G. Multipeptide vaccination in cancer patients. *Expert Opin Biol Ther,* 2009 9, 1043-1055.

[142] Shumway, NM; Ibrahim, N; Ponniah, S; Peoples, GE; Murray, JL. Therapeutic breast cancer vaccines: a new strategy for early-stage disease. *BioDrugs,* 2009 23, 277-287.

[143] Chung, YS; Miyatake, S; Miyamoto, A; Miyamoto, Y; Dohi, T; Tanigawa, N. Oncolytic recombinant herpes simplex virus for treatment of orthotopic liver tumors in nude mice. *Int J Oncol,* 2006 28, 793-798.

[144] Cooper, LJ. New approaches to allogeneic hematopoietic stem cell transplantation in pediatric cancers. *Curr Oncol Rep,* 2009 11, 423-430.

[145] Louw, VJ; Louw, HM; Webb, MJ. Autologous stem-cell transplantation for multiple myeloma. *N Engl J Med,* 2009 361, 1118-1119.

In: New Approaches in the Treatment of Cancer
Editors: Carmen Mejia Vazquez et al. pp.33-42
ISBN 978-1-62100-067-9

Chapter II

BIOLOGICAL THERAPY OF CANCER

J. Alberto Serrano-Olvera[*]
Instituto Nacional de Cancerología y Servicio de Oncología Médica, México D.F.

ABSTRACT

Those agents who are able to exert a therapeutic effect on a specific target constitute the biological therapy; they could modify the routes and stimulating proteins of the cellular growth, the apoptosis or their surface markers. Monoclonal antibodies, tyrosine-kinases and proteasome inhibitors, antisense and epigenetic therapy are the main targets. For optimizing the efficiency of these types of therapies, it is preferable to have a marker able to predict the agent's activity. The security profile of biologic agents is lower than traditional cytotoxic drugs, but some adverse effects can be observed and affect the quality of life of the patients, and others could produce severe and dangerous toxicities.

INTRODUCTION

From the understanding of the normal cellular cycle, multiple elements that participate in the regulation of their functions generating an ample and better knowledge of the processes and alterations that appear in the malignant cells have been identified. This accumulation of knowledge has allowed development of new drugs of chemotherapy and a novel form of pharmacological treatment for cancer, biological therapy. The term "biological therapy" commonly is used to designate those agents that are able to exert a therapeutic effect on a specific target [1].

Recently numerous drugs have been developed that could modify the routes and stimulating proteins of the cellular growth, the apoptosis or their surface markers. Some of them already have proven their therapeutic effectiveness and others are still in the

[*] Correspondence concerning this article should be addressed to: J. Alberto Serrano-Olvera, Instituto Nacional de Cancerología Av. San Fernando No. 22, Col. Sección XVI, Delegación Tlalpan, C.P. 14080 México, D.F. Tel.: 5628-0400/ 5655-1055; E-mail: serranoolvera@yahoo.com.mx.

investigation process. In this chapter we review the groups of biological agents designed and approved for their clinical use in the last 15 years. They will be grouped regarding their structure and action site.

Monoclonal Antibodies

The monoclonal antibodies can affect the tumor cells through several mechanisms: when forming complexes with the respective ligands of the growth factor's receptors; when blocking or stimulating to the receptors; when exerting a direct toxic effect or by indirect immunological effects. These drugs can be divided into chimerical, humanized, and recombinant groups, which imply different possibilities to activate secondary reactions mainly of hypersensitivity reactions. Until now, the available antibodies have been focused on inhibiting the activity of the receptors for the following growth factors: receptor of the epidermal growth factor [EGFR-1 (HER1)] (Cetuximab, Panitumumab) [2,3], HER2 - Trastuzumab - implied in the routes of MAPK and PI3K and increase in the PTEN gene suppressor activity [4,5], and Bevacizumab, that can inhibit the receptor of the vascular endothelial growth factor (VEGFR) [6,7].

Rituximab and Alemtuzumab are monoclonal antibodies (chimerical and humanized, respectively) that are directed against elements expressed in the cellular surface, CD20 and CD52 [8,9]. Now, other drugs are under investigation These drugs are directed to block the platelet-derived growth factor (PDGF), the receptor of the insulin-like growth factor-1 (IGF-1), as well as to block the tumor necrosis factor (TNF) related to apoptosis-inducing ligand (Apo-2L) or the integrins systems related to the development of metastasis, growth and angiogenesis [10].

Inhibitors of Tyrosine-kinases

Many of the signalling pathways are mediated by tyrosine-kinases (TK), enzymes that catalyze the phosphorylation of tyrosine residues in a protein which is able to control the growth, survival, proliferation, differentiation, and cellular apoptosis. These TK integrate two great groups: those with and without receptors [11]. There are two mechanisms by which the effects of the TK can be inhibited: first by means of monoclonal antibodies (Bevacizumab, Cetuximab) that affect the extracellular dominion of the TK receptor or through molecules that prevent the phosphorylation of the residues of intracellular tyrosine, located in the receptor (Erlotinib and Gefitinb) [12,13] or in cytosol (Imatinib) [14,15]. These molecules can block specific oncoproteins, an important gene suppressor or simultaneously block several signalling pathways, among them Ras-MEK-ERK (Sunitinib, Sorafenib) [16-18] or m-TOR (Temsirolimus) [19].

Proteasome Inhibitors

The natural route of degradation of cellular proteins is implied in the processes of the cellular regulation. The route ubiquitine-proteasome degrades proteins through its union to the ubiquitine - helped by different enzymes (E1, E2 and E3) - allowing the proteasome 26S - complex of proteases - using ATP, to digest proteins and release short peptides of aminoacids and intact ubiquitinazed units to be reused. The inhibition of this route generates cellular death by an increased apoptotic activity, or increased expression of cyclines A, B, D, or E, as well as transcription factors as in the case of the agent Bortezomib [20,21].

Antisense Oligonucleotides

The anterograde sense of the duplication of the desoxyrribonucleic acid (DNA) implies that the ribonucleic acid (RNA) messenger copies the nucleic acid sequence that will be translated by ribosomas within a specific protein. That protein can be responsible for the growth of a neoplasm. These proteins are represented mainly by bcl-2 and Raf-1. Therefore, the antisense therapy has the intention of blocking the process by incorporating oligonucleotides, phosphorothioates being the most frequent [22,23].

Epigenetic Therapy

The epigenetic changes are alterations in the genes' expression that are not accompanied by modifications in the sequence of DNA. This implies that these alterations can be transferred from cell to cell, but can be reverted through inducing the correct expression of a gene or protein. The silencing of genes or proteins is a key factor for the cellular operation. The two most understood epigenetic mechanisms today are the DNA methylation and the histones acetylating; in the first, the methylation works like a protector of genetic silencing and with the second, modifications in the chromatin structure are induced [24,25]. Currently, drugs are under investigations which are able to inhibit the DNA methylation and suppress the deacetylation of histones [26,27].

Effectiveness of the Biological Therapy

The overall survival rate is the main parameter to estimate the effectiveness of antineoplastic drugs. Nevertheless, in the metastatic stage of cancer other variables have gained acceptance like effective subsidiaries, among them; progression free-survival as well as the capacity to reduce the tumoral volume, which is known as the objective response rate. On the other hand, the disease free-survival rate is important when talking about the early phases attended by adjuvant therapy. Examples of the obtained effectiveness (objective response rate) when using only a biological agent for a cancer in metastatic stage, previously treated with chemotherapy or immunotherapy are: Imatinib [28], Erlotinib [29], Sorafenib [30], Sunitinb [31], Panitumumab [32], Vorinostat [33].These are used in the treatment of the gastrointestinal stromal tumors, pulmonary, renal, colorectal cancer and cutaneous T cell lymphoma. These clinical trials have been able to induce the reduction of the tumor size in 20% to 45% of the cases, in spite of being different diseases. In other cases, such as multiple myeloma, the use of Bortezomib has increased the time of progression [33], as the monoclonal antibody Panitumumab has done in pre-treated metastatic colon cancer [32]. The overall survival rate also has improved in hepatocarcinoma, where the survival time was of 10.7 months in patients treated with Sorafenib and 7,9 months in patients who received placebo [34] as well as in those with renal cancer treated with Temsirolimus [35].

The therapeutic success of these agents has taken some of them to be used in the secondary prevention of the development of neoplasms, as is the case of the Trastuzumab that until now is the unique biological agent used like adjuvant treatment for the early phases of positive HER2 3^+ mammary cancer. Four randomized studies have shown that this one drug increases the free survival rate of the diseased and reduces the risk of recurrence in 50% [4,5,36].

The effectiveness of the biological agents has been an attractive reason why clinical studies have been designed where the traditional drugs of chemotherapy and biological agents combine in order to improve the survival rate, progression time and overall survival. The combination of these therapeutic modalities has shown to increase the parameters of effectiveness in different cancers, among them: breast cancer, colon, lung, head and neck, non-Hodgkin lymphoma, etc; mainly with the use of the monoclonal antibodies. Radiotherapy and Cetuximab, in head and neck cancer, increase the objective response rate (74% vs. 64%), the time of progression of disease (24.4 vs. 14.9 months) and the overall survival rate (49 vs. 29.3 months) in comparison with radiation alone [37]. Rituximab associated with the CHOP scheme has improved the survival rate [HR: 0.65 (C95% 0.54-0.78)] and objective response rate [RR: 1.21 (IC95% 1.16-1.27)] of follicular and the mantle lymphomas [38]. Cetuximab associated with Irinotecan increased the objective response rate (22.9 vs. 10.8%), the time of progression of the disease (4.1 vs. 1.5 months) and the overall survival rate (8.6 vs. 6.9 months) in patients previously treated with Irinotecan [39]. Bevacizumab and FOLFOX4 compared with FOLFOX4 alone have increased the objective response (22.2% vs. 8%) the time of progression (7.5 vs. 4.5 months) and the overall survival rate (13 vs 10.8 months) in previously treated metastatic colon cancer patients [40]. Also, Bevacizumab, combined with Paclitaxel and Carboplatino, has produced similar effects in non-small cell lung cancer [41], as well as in breast cancer when it is combined with Paclitaxel or Capecitabine [42,43].

Nevertheless, it is not always successful to combine chemotherapy and biological therapy as is demonstrated by the results of some clinical trials with Genitifib [44,45] or Erlotinib [46,47] in lung cancer. In order to optimize the effectiveness of these types of therapies, it is preferable to have a marker able to predict the agent activity, as is HER2 3^+ in breast cancer, C-KIT in gastrointestinal stromal tumors, CD20 in non-Hodgkin lymphomas, EGFR in pulmonary cancer or K-Ras in colorectal cancer.

Table 1. Biological agents for cancer treatment approved by the Food & Drug Administration

Agent	Type	Affected *via*	Target	Indications
Trastuzumab	Monoclonal antibody, humanized, IgG1	Epidermal Growth Factor	HER-2	Metastatic breast cancer Adjuvant in early HER2 (overexpressed or amplified), breast cancer
Bevacizumab	Monoclonal antibody, humanized, recombinant, IgG1	Vascular Endothelial Growth Factor	VEGF-r	Metastatic breast cancer NSCLC Metastatic colorectal cancer
Cetuximab	Monoclonal antibody, chimeric, mouse-human, IgG1	Epidermal Growth Factor	EGF-r	Head & neck cancer Colorectal cancer NSCLC
Rituximab	Monoclonal antibody, chimeric IgG1	Apoptosis – Caspases	CD20	Non- Hodgkin lymphoma $CD20^{+}$
Panitumumab	Monoclonal antibody, humanized – IgG2	ERK1 and ERK2 PI3K-akt JaK2/STAT3	EGF-r FNT-α	Metastatic colorectal cancer
Alemtuzumab	Monoclonal antibody, humanized IgG1	Epidermal Growth Factor	CD52	Chronical lymphocitic leukemia
Lapatininb	Dual Inhibitor of TK	Epidermal Growth Factor	HER1 and HER2	Metastatic breast cancer refractory or resistant to Trastuzumab
Gefitinib	TK Inhibitor	Epidermal Growth Factor	EGF-r	Metastatic NSCLC
Erlotinib	TK Inhibitor	Epidermal Growth Factor	EGF-r	Metastatic NSCLC
Imatinib	TK Inhibitor	ABL C-KIT FCDP	Bcr-abl	GIST Chronic myeloid leukemia
Sorafenib	TK Inhibitor	Ras/Raf/MEK/ERK	Raf-1 EGF-r VEGF-r PDGF -r	Metastatic renal cancer Hepatocarcinoma
Sunitinib	TK Inhibitor	Ras/Raf/ mitogens	VEGF-r KIT-r Flt3-r PDGF -r	Metastatic renal cancer
Bortezomib	Proteasome Inhibitor	Ubiquitine-proteasome		Second line therapy in multiple myeloma
Temsirulimus	m-TOR Inhibitor	PI3K-akt	VEGF	Metastatic renal cancer
Vorinostat	Histones deacetylation inhibitor	Histones deacetylation		Cutaneous T cell lymphoma

EGF-r: epidermal growth factor receptor. VEGF-r: vascular endothelial growth factor receptor. PDGF: platelet-derived growth factor. TK: tyrosine-kinases. TNF-α: tumoral necrosis factor alpha. GIST: gastrointestinal stromal tumor. NSCLC: non-small cell lung cancer.

Toxic Effects of the Biological Therapy

The evaluation of the associated toxicity, as in all drugs, is required for the biological agents. The toxic effects of these new drugs are smaller in frequency and intensity, compared with chemotherapy; they are mainly cutaneous erythema, diarrhoea, anorexia, fatigue, nausea, infections, mucositis, pruritus, dry skin, conjunctivitis. Other effects can be added and affect the patient's quality of life, among these are: hand-foot syndrome, arthralgias and myalgias as well as arterial hypertension. Some of the biological agents can produce toxicities that acquire major relevance since they put in danger the life of the patient, for example; cardiotoxicity, haemorrhage, respiratory insufficiency, anaphylactic reaction and intestinal perforation.

Other toxicities can go unnoticed and if they are detected would not bring fatal consequences, such as the hypomagnesaemia, proteinury, and infection by cytomegalovirus. In spite of the ample margin of security associated with the biological agents, it is necessary to remember that very frequently they are used in combination with traditional drugs of chemotherapy, which can increase the frequency and intensity of their toxic effects.

Future of Biological Therapy

Actually, the most of the available biological drugs exert their effects on a specific target; however, we have learned and understood that when modifying the behaviour of a specific site, sometimes is possible to inactivate a series of essential steps for the optimal operation of the malignant cells. Lapatinib and Pertuzumab [48-50], until now, are the unique drugs that have been developed and approved in order to block the activity of two or three targets simultaneously: HER1, HER2, and HER3. A new generation of biological agents with capacity to block 2, 3 or more routes of signalling simultaneously will be arriving in the next 5 years [50-51]. These can improve the therapeutic effectiveness and provide drugs to treat the resistance to its predecessors; nevertheless, we must wait for the results of the clinical tests that are being developed to know if the toxic effects also increase.

Conclusion

Cancer's biological therapy offers different new agents with selective capacity to block or to modulate one or more critical sites in the growth and survival of the malignant cells. The valuation of its therapeutic effects and toxicity profile must still be analyzed in a greater number of clinical studies. New approaches have been oriented to optimize the results induced from this therapeutic modality. The investigation in oncologic therapy will be dominated in the following years by the biological agents.

REFERENCES

[1] Druker, BJ. Presente y futuro del tratamiento de blancos moleculares. In *Oncología Clínica*. Abeloff, MD; Armitage, JO; Niederhuber, JE; Kastan, MB; McKenna, WG. Elseiver, Madrid, España. 3ª edición. Pp: 623-638.

[2] Non-Authors. Cetuximab approved by FDA for treatment of head and neck squamous cell cancer. *Cancer Biol Ther,* 2006, 5, 339-348.

[3] Giusti, RM; Shastri, KA; Cohen, MH; et al. FDA drug approval summary: Panitumumab (Vectibix ®). *The Oncologist*, 2007, 12, 577-583.

[4] Hudis, CA. Trastuzumab – mechanism of action and use in clinical practice. *N Engl J Med*, 2007, 357, 39-51.

[5] Robert, NJ; Favret, AN. HER2-positive advanced breast cancer. *Hematol Oncol Clin N Am*, 2007, 297-302.

[6] Cohen, MH; Gootenberg, J; Keegan, P; Pazdur, R. FDA drug approval summary: Bevacizumab plus FOLFOX4 as second line treatment of colon cancer. *The Oncologist,* 2007, 12, 356-361.

[7] Cohen, MH; Gootenberg, J; Keegan, P; Pazdur, R. FDA drug approval summary: Bevacizumab (Avastin®) plus carboplatin and paclitaxel as first line treatment of advanced/metastatic recurrent non-squamous non-small cell lung cancer. *The Oncologist*, 2007, 12, 713-718.

[8] Leget, GA; Czuczman, MS. Use of rituximab, the new FDA-approved antibody. *Curr Opinion Oncol,* 1998, 10, 548-551.

[9] Demko, S; Summers, J; Keegan, P; Pazdur, R. FDA drug approval summary; Alemtuzumab as single agent treatment for B-cell chronic lymphocytic leukemia. *The Oncologist,* 2008, 13, 167-174.

[10] Cohen, SJ; Cohen, RB; Meropol, NJ. Targeting signal transduction with antibobies. In DeVita, VT-Jr; Lawrence, TS; Rosemberg, SA. *Cancer: principles & practice of oncology*. Wolters Kluwer/Lippincott Williams & Wilkins. 8Th Edition, 2008; Philadelphia, USA, pp: 469-477.

[11] LoRusso, PM; Ryan, AJ; Boerner, SA; Herbst, RS. Small-molecule tyrosine kinase inhibitors. In DeVita, VT-Jr; Lawrence, TS; Rosemberg, SA. *Cancer: principles & practice of oncology*. Wolters Kluwer/Lippincott Williams & Wilkins. 8Th Edition, 2008; Philadelphia, USA, pp: 457-468.

[12] Cohen, MH; Johnson, JR; Chen, YF; et al. FDA drug approval summary: Erlotinib (Tarceva ®) tablets. *The Oncologist,* 2005, 10, 461-466.

[13] Cohen, MH; Williams, GA; Sridhara, R; et al. FDA drug approval summary: Gefitinib (ZD1839) (Iressa ®) tablets. *The Oncologist*, 2003, 8, 303-306.

[14] Dagher, R; Chen, M; Williams, G; et al. Approval summary: Imatinib mesylate in the treatment of metastatic and or unresectable malignant gastrointestinal stromal tumors. *Clin Cancer Res*, 2002, 8, 3034-3038.

[15] Johnson, JR; Bross, P; Cohen, M; et al. Approval summary: Imatinib mesylate capsules for treatment of adult patients with newly diagnosed Philadelphia chromosome positive chronic myelogenous leukemia in chronic phase. *Clin Cancer Res,* 2003, 9, 1972-1979.

[16] Goodman, VL; Rock, EP; Dagher, R; et al. Approval summary: sunitinib for the treatment imatinib refractory or intolerant gastrointestinal stromal tumors and advanced renal cell carcinoma. *Clin Cancer Res,* 2007, 13, 1367-1373.

[17] Kane, RC; Farrell, AT; Saber, H; et al. Sorafenib for the treatment of advanced renal cell carcinoma. *Clin Cancer Res*, 2006, 12, 7271-7278.

[18] Lang, L. FDA approves Sorafenib for patients with inoperable liver cancer. *Gastroenterology*, 2008, 134, 379

[19] Gore, ME. Temsirolimus in the treatment of advanced renal cell carcinoma. *Ann Oncol,* 2007, 18(suppl 9), b87-b88.

[20] Molineaux, CJ; Crews, CM. Proteasome inhibitors. In DeVita, VT-Jr; Lawrence, TS; Rosemberg, SA. *Cancer: principles & practice of oncology*. Wolters Kluwer/Lippincott Williams & Wilkins. 8Th Edition, 2008; Philadelphia, USA, pp: 486-490.

[21] Kane, RC; Farrell, AT; Sridhara, R; Pazdur, R. United States Food and Drug Administration Approval summary: Bortezomib for the treatment of the progressive multiple myeloma after one prior therapy. *Clin Cancer Res*, 2006, 12, 2955-2960.

[22] Stein, CA; Benimetskaya, L; Kornblum, N; Mani, S. Antisense agents. In DeVita, VT-Jr; Lawrence, TS; Rosemberg, SA. *Cancer: principles & practice of oncology*. Wolters Kluwer/Lippincott Williams & Wilkins. 8Th Edition, 2008; Philadelphia, USA, pp: 522-527.

[23] Zhang, C; Pei, J; Kumar, D, et al. Antisense oligonucleotides: Target validation and development of systematically delivered therapeutic nanoparticles. *Methods Mol Biol,* 2007, 361, 163-185.

[24] Gore, SD; Baylin, SB; Herman, JG. Histone deacetylase inhibitors and demethylating agents. In DeVita, VT-Jr; Lawrence, TS; Rosemberg, SA. *Cancer: principles & practice of oncology*. Wolters Kluwer/Lippincott Williams & Wilkins. 8Th Edition, 2008; Philadelphia, USA, 477-485.

[25] Esteller, M, Epigenetics in cancer. *N Engl J Med*, 2008, 358, 1148-1159.

[26] Candelaria, M; Gallardo-Rincón, D; Arce, C; et al. A phase II study of epigenetic therapy with hydralazine and magnesium valproate to overcome chemotherapy resistance in refractory solid tumors. *Ann Oncol,* 2007, 18, 1529-1538.

[27] Mann, BS; Jonson, JR; He, K; et al. Vorinostat for treatment cutaneous manifestations of advanced primary cutaneous T-cell lymphoma. *Clin Cancer Res*, 2007, 13, 2318-2322.

[28] Blanke, CD; Rankin, C; Demetri, GD; et al. Phase III randomized, intergroup trial assessing imatinib mesylate at two dose level in patients with unresectable or metastatic gastrointestinal stromal tumor expressing the KIT receptor tyrosine kinase: S0033. *J Clin Oncol*, 2008, 26, 626-632.

[29] Bareschino, MA; Schettino, C; Troiani, T; et al. Erlotinib in cancer treatment. *Ann Oncol*, 2007, 18 (supl 6), vi35-41.

[30] Escudier, B; Eisen, T; Stadler, WM; et al. Sorafenib in advanced clear cell renal cell carcinoma. *N Engl J Med*, 2007, 356, 125-134.

[31] Motzer, RJ; Hutson, TE; Tomczak, P; et al. Sunitinib versus interferon alpha in metastatic renal cell carcinoma. *N Engl J Med*, 2007, 356, 115-124.

[32] Van Cutsem, E; Peeters, M; Siena, S; et al. Open-label phase III trial of panitumumab plus best supportive care compared with best supportive care alone in patients with

chemotherapy-refractory metastatic colorectal cancer. *J Clin Oncol*, 2007, 25, 1658-1664.

[33] Olsen, EA; Kim, YH; Kuzel, TM; et al. Phase IIB multicenter trial of vorinostat in patients withpersisten, progressive, or treatment reafractory cutaneous T cell lymphoma. *J Clin Oncol*, 2007, 25, 3109-3015.

[34] Llovet, JM; Ricci, S; Mazzaferro, V; et al. Sorafenib in advanced hepatocellular carcinoma. *N Engl J Med*, 2008, 359, 378-390.

[35] Hudes, G; Carducci, M; Tomczak, P; et al. Temsirolimus, interferon alpha or both for advanced renal-cell carcinoma. *N Engl J Med*, 2007, 356, 2271-2281.

[36] Stuart, NS; Bishop, J; Bale, C. Trastuzumab for early breast cancer. *Lancet*, 2006, 367(9505), 107-108.

[37] Bonner, JA; Harari, PM; Giralt, J; et al. Radiotherapy plus cetuximab for squamous cell carcinoma of the head and neck. *N Engl J Med*, 2006, 354, 567-578.

[38] Schulz, H; Bohlius, J; Skoetz, N; et al. Chemotherapy plus rituximab versus chemotherapy alone for B-cell non-Hodgkin´s lymphoma. *Cochrane Database Syst Rev*, 2007, Oct 17 (4), CD003805.

[39] Cunningham, D; Humblet, Y; Siena, S; et al. Cetuximab monotherapy and cetuximab plus irinotecan in irinotecan refractory metastatic colon cancer. *N Engl J Med*, 2004, 351, 337-345.

[40] Giantonio, BJ; Catalano, PJ; Meropol, JN; et al. Bevacizumab in combination with oxaliplatin, fluorouracil, and leucovorin (FOLFOX4) for previously untreated metastatic colorectal cancer: results from the Eastern Cooperative Oncology Group Study E3200. *J Clin Oncol*, 2007, 25, 1539-1544.

[41] Sandler, A; Gray, R; Perry, MC; et al. Paclitaxel-Carboplatine alone or with bevacizumab for non-small cell lung cancer. *N Eng J Med*, 2006, 355, 2542-2550.

[42] Miller, KD; Chap, LI; Holmes, FA; et al. Randomized phase III trial of capecitabine compared with bevacizumab plus capecitabine in patients with previusly treated metastatic breast cancer. *J Clin Oncol*, 2005, 23, 792-799.

[43] Miller, K; Wang, M; Gralow, J; et al. Paclitaxel plus bevacizumab versus paclitaxel alone for metastatic breast cancer. *N Engl J Med*, 2007, 357, 2666-2676.

[44] Giaccone, G; Herbst, RS; Manegold, C; et al. Gefitinib in combination with gemcitabine and cisplatin in advanced non-small cell lung cancer: A phase III trial – INTAC 1. *J Clin Oncol*, 2004, 22, 777-784.

[45] Herbst, RS; Giaccone, G; Schiller, JH; et al. Gefitinib in combination with paclitaxel and carboplatin in advanced non-small cell lung cancer: A phase III trial – INTAC 2. *J Clin Oncol*, 2004, 22, 785-794.

[46] Herbst, RS; Prager, D; Hermann, R; et al. TRIBUTE: a phase III trial of erlotinib dehydrocloride (OSI-774) combined with carboplatin and paclitaxel in advanced non-small cell lung cancer. *J Clin Oncol*, 2005, 23, 5892-5899.

[47] Gatzemeier, U; Pluzanska, A; Szczesna, A; et al. Phase III study or erlotinib in combination with cisplatin and gemcitabine in advanced non-small cell lung cancer. The Tarceva Lung Cancer Investigation Trial. *J Clin Oncol*, 2007, 25, 1545-1552.

[48] Bilancia, D; Rosatin, G; Dinota, A; et al. Lapatinib in breast cancer. *Ann Oncol*, 2007, 18 (supl 6), vi26-30.

[49] Cameron, D; Casey, M; Press, M; et al. A phase III randomized comparison of lapatinibe plus capecitabine versus capecitabine alone in women with advanced breast

cancer that has progressed on tratuzumab: update efficacy and biomarker analyses. *Breast Cancer Res Treat,* 2008.

[50] Reid, A; Vidal, L; Shaw, H; et al. Dual inhibition of ErbB1 (EGFR/HER1) and ErbB2 (HER2/neu). *Eur J Cancer*, 2007, 43, 481-489.

[51] Wheeler, D; Huang, S; Kruser, TJ; et al. Mechanisms of acquired resistance of cetuximab: role of HER2 (ErbB) family members. *Oncogene*, 2008, 27, 3944-3956.

In: New Approaches in the Treatment of Cancer
Editors: Carmen Meija Vazquez et al. pp.43-69
ISBN 978-1-62100-067-9

Chapter III

MOLECULAR-GUIDED THERAPY OF NEUROBLASTOMA

Eva Villamón[1], Marta Piqueras[1], Elena Grau[2], Adela Cañete[2], Victoria Castel[2] and Rosa Noguera[1,*,#]

[1]University of Valencia, Spain
[2]Hospital La Fe, Valencia, Spain

ABSTRACT

Combination therapy has improved outcome for some malignancies such as neuroblastoma (NB), the most common pediatric solid tumor. Despite this advance, progression-free survival for children with advanced disease is 45% at best, even with double autologous stem cell transplantation. For those children whose disease is cured, morbidity from intensive chemotherapy is significant. New approaches to the treatment of this malignancy are needed. At a time when promising approaches to NB treatment have already reached clinical testing or have proved to be successful in preclinical models of the disease, and an extraordinary number of small molecules are in development, the rational selection of compounds for clinical testing becomes even more important. In the current review we focus on genetic abnormalities, neural differentiation, apoptosis, immunomodulation, angiogenesis and gene expression profiling as tools for generating novel molecular-guided therapeutic approaches. The developments of all these approaches to facilitate combination therapy have opened up new avenues in NB treatment.

* Correspondence concerning this article should be addressed to: Rosa Noguera, Department of Pathology, Medical School, University of Valencia, Avda. Blasco Ibáñez 17, Valencia 46010, Spain. E-mail: rosa.noguera@uv.es.

Grant sponsors: Instituto de Salud Carlos III (Acción Transversal del Cáncer nº20080143; FIS PI06/1576; RETICS RD06/0020/01022010102), Fundación Asociación Española Contra el Cáncer and Conselleria de Sanitat AP046/09..

Introduction

Neuroblastoma (NB) is a childhood neoplasm that arises from neural crest cells and is most commonly located in the adrenal medulla or paraspinal sympathetic ganglia [1,2] Patient prognosis is classified as favourable or unfavourable depending on the degree of neuroblast differentiation, Schwannian stroma content, and mitosis-karyorrhexis index, patient age and clinical stage at the time of diagnosis [3]. In addition, amplification of the *MYCN* oncogene is strongly associated with unfavourable prognosis [4,5]. NB accounts for more than 15% of cancer-related deaths in early childhood [6]. Thus, new drugs are needed for the treatment of this disease.

The natural history and tumor biology of NB could be considered as a model for tumor cell maturation processes in general, and human sympathetic differentiation in particular [7]. NB cells are typically undifferentiated, round and small with scant cytoplasm. However, many tumors contain differentiated cells with larger nuclei and cytoplasm, being classified as ganglioneuroblastoma. Some tumors exclusively contain ganglion-like cells; these benign tumors are termed ganglioneuromas. The International Neuroblastoma Pathological Classification (INPC) soon revealed that high differentiation stage correlates to favourable prognosis, and confirmed by subsequent differentiation marker studies [8,9].

NB can present at birth and throughout early childhood with only occasional cases diagnosed after 10 years of age. NB is clinically classified into five stages, ranging from the localized stage 1 tumors to stage 4 cases with extensive tumor dissemination [1]. Children with stage 1 and 2 tumors are basically treated with surgery alone, whereas children with stage 4 tumors receive intensive chemotherapy and radiation. Some tumors fall within the intriguing stage 4s category [1]. This stage is characterized by localized primary tumors and dissemination limited to liver, skin and/or bone marrow. The tumors occur in infants, and can regress spontaneously [10,11]. Despite their sometimes extensively disseminated disease, the overall survival (OS) rate of stage 4s patients is approximately 80%, contrasting the close to 20% survival rate of stage 4 patients older than 1 year [6]. Furthermore, it is noteworthy that the OS of stage 4 patients has increased only slightly in the last 20 years in spite of the efforts to improve the therapeutic approach [12,13].

These discouraging results emphasize the limits of conventional anti-neoplastic treatments, i.e. chemotherapy, radiotherapy and surgery, in poor prognosis neuroblastic tumors. Therefore, the search for alternative therapeutic strategies is warranted and represents the objective of many investigators. To this end, the study of tumor cell genetics and biology is of pivotal importance to identify the right targets for innovative treatments. Here we will review the most advanced therapeutic strategies that have been already tested in preclinical models or in preliminary clinical trials.

Genetic Abnormalities Guides Therapeutic Decision

The amplification of *MYCN* oncogene was first described in NB cell lines and human tumors in 1983 by Schwab *et al.* [14]. Subsequent studies by Brodeur [15] and Seeger [16] demonstrated the relationship of rapid tumor progression and poor prognosis with the presence of *MYCN* amplification. Since then the detection of *MYCN* amplification has been included in protocols to decide therapeutic strategy because it distinguishes between favorable and unfavorable outcomes in NB patients [17,18]. The SIOP-Europe Neuroblastoma (SIOPEN) has studied the treatment of localized (stage 1 and 2) NB based on *MYCN* gene status. Patients with localized, resectable and *MYCN* non-amplified tumors were treated with surgery only and survival results were excellent, whereas patients with localized, but *MYCN* amplified tumors had a high risk of relapse [19,20]. Multi-agent myeloablative regimens are widely used as consolidation therapy for children with stage 4 disease, and in those with other disease stages when the *MYCN* gene copy number in tumor cells is amplified [21]. On the other hand, survival of infants with unresected localized NB without *MYCN* amplification is excellent, and is no different from patients treated with surgery or chemotherapy. A wait-and-see strategy is justified in this case because spontaneous regression is regularly seen in these patients and is not limited to the first year of life [22].

MYCN has a very restricted expression pattern: it is mainly expressed during embryonic development but then becomes downregulated, while in adults it is usually detected in B-cell development. Identification of selective inhibitors of *MYCN* and its mRNA and protein could be important for development of effective and less toxic therapeutic agents for NB. Antisense oligodeoxynucleotides inhibit *MYCN* production and have anti-tumor activity *in vitro* and *in vivo* for NB. Peptide nucleic acids (PNA), the most recent generation of nucleic acid therapeutics, form stable duplexes with DNA and RNA and are resistant to degradation. Encouraging results have been reported using a PNA-based antisense strategy for inhibition of *MYCN* expression in NB [23]. *MYCN* is also a potential target for cancer immunotherapy due to its overexpression in human malignancies, whereas undetectable expression of *MYCN* gene in normal tissues avoids immune cross reactions. Himoudi *et al.* [24] suggest epitope sequences from *MYCN* with high affinity for HLA-2A could be used as cancer vaccines.

It has recently been suggested that *MYCN* acts as a regulator of microRNAs (miRNAs) [25]. miRNAs are non-protein-coding, small RNAs that play an important role in normal cellular function. Emerging evidence suggests that miRNAs play also an important role in the pathogenesis of human cancers, controlling cell differentiation and apoptosis, or targeting cancer oncogenes and/or tumor suppressors [26]. Loss in 1p is closely associated to *MYCN* amplified tumors [27]. Due to this frequent association, Wei *et al.* [28] examined the role of microRNAs that map to the commonly deleted region of 1p36 and hypothesized that the loss of one or more of theses microRNAs contributes to a malignant phenotype of *MYCN*-amplified tumors. They demonstrated that miR-34a directly inhibits MYCN protein, and can suppress cell cycle genes and induces a neural phenotype. In addition, E2F3, another direct target of miR-34a, can directly regulate *MYCN* transcription. So, a small non-coding microRNA in 1p36 region can exert potential tumor suppressor effects through direct modulation of MYCN protein levels as well as of other multiple genes and pathways not directly related to *MYCN* [29].

MYCN amplification is detected in approximately 20% of primary NBs [30,31]. One third of high-risk (HR) patients have amplified *MYCN,* but the outcome of the non-amplified is also poor, so there must be other unfavorable molecular alterations playing a role in survival [32]. There are several chromosomal alterations with known prognostic value, such as 3p, 11q and 17q [27,33-39]. New prospective trials that include some of these alterations are currently ongoing to confirm their therapeutic utility [40]. Some of 29 recently-published new human miRNA sequences are found within regions of chromosomal rearrangements associated with

NB, for instance, miRNAs located on 3p, 9p21, 11q32 or 17q [41]. So, microRNAs have significant potential as therapeutic targets in NB [26].

Recently, DNA copy number changes have been considered useful to predict outcome more accurately than specific alterations [42-44]. Several clinical trials performed by cooperative groups, like the Pediatric Oncology Group (POG) and Children's Oncology Group (COG), have analyzed the clinical significance of *MYCN* amplification and ploidy. Survival of patients whose tumors were *MYCN* non-amplified and hyperploid was excellent, even in children 12 to 18 months old with metastatic NB with high-dose therapy, and suggests therapy reduction [45,46]. In contrast, patients with non-amplified *MYCN* and diploid tumors presented improved free event survival after more intensive therapy [45]. In favorable-stage patients, those whose tumors were *MYCN* amplified and diploid had more reduced survival compared to those whose tumors were amplified but hyperploid [47].

Recently, gain of function mutations or amplification of *ALK* was shown to be associated with hereditary forms of NB and occur also in a substantial fraction of sporadic cases [48]. *ALK* gene is expressed in the neural system and is located in 2p23. It encodes a tyrosine kinase transmembrane receptor. Its expression is restricted to the developing nervous system and has a possible role in the regulation of neuronal differentiation [49]. Recent data suggest that *ALK* may contribute to tumor development, so mutations affecting critical domains of this gene must be studied to validate their potential as therapeutic targets [50,51]. Caren *et al.* [50] detected *ALK* alterations (amplifications or rearrangements) and mutations in sporadic NB tumors of all clinical stages analyzed by CGH-array. In a group of 50 sporadic NBs analyzed by FISH, we observed a tendency of synchronic copy number aberrations of *ALK* and *MYCN* genes in 51% of tumors [52]. However, in our study, *MYCN* alterations were also seen in tumors without *ALK* aberrations. In addition, we could not observe a correlation between *ALK* aberrations and alterations of 11q, 17q and 1p36. Several pharmacological antagonists of *ALK* are under development for specific targeted cancer therapy because activation of *ALK* is the genetic base of sensitization to *ALK* kinase inhibition [53,54]. George *et al.* [51] studied the effect of TAE684, an *ALK* small-molecule inhibitor, in NB cell lines with activating *ALK* mutations. Thus, it will be important to test the ability of each mutant *ALK* protein to confer sensitivity to *ALK* inhibitory drugs as they move into therapeutic trials.

Differentiation and Apoptotic Therapy

Differentiation to a neuronal cell phenotype is one plausible way to inhibit NB [55-57], another potentially useful strategy is selective activation of apoptotic pathways that ultimately lead to death of NB cells [58]. Differentiation studies have utilized *in vitro* models in which NB cell lines have been induced to differentiate in the presence of various agents and growth factors. Since the first report [55], a number of NB differentiation protocols have been published employing among others retinoids and growth factors. These observations fostered a hope that patients with advanced NB might successfully be treated by inducing their tumor cells to differentiate [55]. It turned out that naturally occurring and synthetic retinoids have so far had the greatest clinical impact and usage as differentiation inducers, although the action mechanism of retinoids in NB patients with residual disease is not fully known [56].

The effects of retinoids are mediated by two classes of non-steroid nuclear hormone receptors, the retinoic acid (RAR α, β, γ) and the retinoic X (RXR α, β, γ) receptors [59]. The naturally occurring all-*trans*-retinoic acid (ATRA) and 9-*cis*-retinoic acid (9-*cis*-RA), and the synthetic 13-*cis*-retinoic acid (13-*cis*-RA) are examples of retinoids studied in NB. It was soon established that ATRA stimulation of NB cells results in growth inhibition, decreased anchorage-independent growth, and neuronal differentiation as indicated by morphology, increased NSE (neuron-specific enolase) activity, a slight accumulation of norepinephrine, and upregulated expression of *GAP43* coding for growth associated protein 43, an important protein important in axonal growth [60,61]. Later, downregulation of the proto-oncogenes *MYCN*, *MYB*, *HRAS* was shown to precede the morphological differentiation, followed by changes in the expression of a set of other proto-oncogenes [62,63]. Even though ATRA-induced differentiation appears to be neuronal, the outcome differs depending on the NB cell line studied. While some cell lines develop a sympathetic noradrenergic phenotype, a cholinergic switch has been suggested in other cell lines [64-66]. Similar results are obtained when NB cell lines are treated *in vitro* with the 13-*cis*-RA, although the latter molecule proves to be more potent [67]. A major difference between ATRA and 13-*cis*-RA lies in their pharmacokinetics [56].

As a therapeutic tool, 13-*cis*-RA, administered as a high dose pulse treatment, is beneficial for patients with minimal residual disease (MRD) [56]. In a clinical setting, the induction of neurotrophin receptor expression and neurotrophin responsiveness by retinoids might be important mechanisms contributing to the improved outcome of NB patients [68]. It has been shown that immunomodulatory functions of retinoids inducing immunoproteasome formation and up-regulation of HLA class I expression on the surface of human NB cell lines [56]. Gangliosides are a group of glycosphingolipids found principally in the surface membrane of nerve cells. Disialoganglioside (GD2) is part of this family, with the particularity that it is expressed on the surface of all NB cells and rarely in normal tissue. The COG and the SIOPEN are testing the association of 13-*cis*-RA with the anti-GD2 chimeric antibody ch14.18 (see below), as protocols for stage 4 HR-NB patients, based upon preliminary results showing synergistic effects of these agents *in vitro* on human NB cell lines. A further promising approach is the use of anti-GD2-targeted immunoliposomes loaded with synthetic retinoids such as N-(4-hydroxyphenyl) retinamide (HPR), also known as fenretinide [69]. NB xenografts treated with anti-GD2 liposomal HPR showed complete inhibition of growth and spread. Recently, it has been demonstrated that HPR exerts antiangiogenic effects related to both direct effects on endothelial cell proliferation and inhibition of the response of endothelial cells to the proliferative stimuli imparted by angiogenic growth factors [70].

Apoptosis of NB cells can take place *in vivo* [71] or be induced through different *in vitro* mechanisms, such as engagement of neurotrophin receptors, RA receptors, TRAIL and CD95 [71]. *In vitro* as well as clinical data indicate that HPR might also prove valuable in cells resistant to RA. The effect seems independent of retinoid receptors and appears not to involve differentiation, but induction of apoptosis as well as necrosis [56,72-74]. Because the effects of retinoids are mediated by nuclear receptors in the absence of a ligand, these receptors act as transcriptional repressors due to the binding of coexpressor complexes that contain histone deacetylases (HDAC). Ligand binding allows the release of coexpressors and facilitates the ordered recruitment of coactivator complexes, some of which possess histone acetylase activity, that cause transcriptional stimulation [75]. HDAC inhibitors (HDACi) produce extensive apoptotic cell death in NB cell lines. The combination of ATRA with HDACi results in improved antitumorigenic activity *in vitro*. The effects of combination therapy are synergistic with respect to inhibition of cellular viability and induction of apoptosis [76,77]. Recently, vitamin E analogues, epitomized by α-tocopheryl succinate (α-TOS), have been proposed as a potential therapy because they also selectively induce apoptosis in NB cells [78].

Retinoids (ATRA, 9-*cis*-RA, 13-*cis*-RA and HPR) have diverse effects on NB cells including inhibition of malignant neuroblast proliferation, differentiation and/or apoptosis. Furthermore, some retinoids can increase the immunogenicity of human NB cells and mediate antiangiogenic activity. Thus, these drugs have great potentiality when administered in combination with chemotherapy, hematopoietic stem cell transplantation and immunotherapy. In addition, clinical data suggest that differentiation therapy may play a complementary role in the treatment of NB when used in combination with other therapies [70,77]. Because differentiation is aberrant in this malignancy, compounds that modulate transcription, such as HDACi, are of particular interest and reinforce the idea that combination therapy could be useful to inhibit tumor growth.

Immunotherapy

Achieving a cure for metastatic NB remains a challenge despite its sensitivity to chemotherapy and radiotherapy. Most patients achieve remission, but a failure to eliminate minimal residual disease (MRD) often leads to relapse. Immunotherapy is potentially useful for chemotherapy-resistant disease and may be particularly effective for low levels of MRD that are below the threshold for detection by routine radiological and histological methods. GD2 is ubiquitous and abundant on NB cells and is an ideal target for immunotherapy. Taking GD2 as antigen, different monoclonal antibodies (mAbs) have been developed, both murine and humanized [79-82]. The mechanisms whereby anti-GD2 mAbs kill tumor cells are likely related to complement activation and antibody mediated cell cytotoxicity. Anti-GD2 mAbs currently form the mainstay of NB immunotherapy and their safety profile has been well-established. Although responses in patients with gross disease have been observed infrequently, histologic responses of bone marrow disease are consistently achieved in >75% of patients with primary refractory NB [79,82,83].

Two murine mAbs, 3F8 and 14G2a, and one human-mouse chimeric mAb, ch14.18 has been used in relapsed /refractory NB. In phase I trials they were used alone, but in some of the phase II trials, anti-GD2 mAbs were used in combination with granulocyte-macrophage colony stimulating factor (GM-CSF) and interleukin-2 (IL-2). The results of these studies showed that all three had therapeutic efficacy for NB, with bone marrow disease being the most responsive, and refractory disease more responsive than relapses. They share dose-dependent similar side effects, although 3F8 appears the most toxic. The major side effects are neuropathic pain, fever, tachycardia, hyper or hypotension and decreased K and Na. These side effects are usually reversible within a few hours of administration [79,82,83].

A phase I study conducted by COG, determined the maximum tolerated dose (MTD) of the ch14.18 mAb in combination with a standard dose of GM-CSF for patients with NB who recently completed stem-cell transplantation and to determine the toxicities in this setting.

They concluded that ch14.18 mAb can be administered with GM-CSF in patients with NB with manageable toxicities. The MTD was 40 mg/m2/d for 4 days [84,85]. These findings provided the scientific rationale for the concept of conducting Phase III clinical trials with the mAb in NB patients. The COG is currently conducting the study ANBL0032 to determine whether addition of immunotherapy (consisting of ch14.18 mAb given with GM-CSF or IL-2) to 13-*cis*-RA therapy improves the outcome for HR-NB patients who have undergone an autologous bone marrow transplant. The patients are randomized to receive immunotherapy plus *cis*-RA or *cis*-RA alone. The study is ongoing [86].

In preparation for a European phase III clinical trial (HR-NBL-1/ESIOP), the cell line used for production of ch14.18 mAb was changed. Specifically, the plasmid encoding for ch14.18 mAb was re-cloned into CHO cells. Identical binding of ch14.18/CHO to the nominal antigen GD2 *in vitro* compared to ch14.18/SP2/0 and ch14.18/NS0 was demonstrated. Binding was GD2-specific, since all precursor- and metabolite-gangliosides of GD2 tested were not recognized by ch14.18/CHO. Second, the functional properties of ch14.18/CHO were determined in complement-dependent cytotoxicity (CDC) and antibody-dependent cellular cytotoxicity (ADCC) reactions against GD2 positive neuroectodermal tumor cell lines *in vitro*. There was no difference in CDC-mediated specific tumor cell lysis among the three different ch14.18 mAb preparations. Interestingly, ch14.18/CHO showed superior ADCC activity at low antibody concentrations. Third, the efficacy of ch14.18/CHO was evaluated in the NXS2 NB model *in vivo*. Importantly, the ch14.18/CHO preparation was effective in suppression of experimental liver metastasis in this model. *In vivo* depletion of NK-cells completely abrogated this effect, suggesting that the mechanism involved in the ch14.18/CHO-induced anti-NB effect is mediated by NK-dependent ADCC [87]. javascript:AL_get(this, 'ptyp', 'Research Support, Non-U.S. Gov\'t');The SIOPEN is conducting a trial in HR-NB patients, HR-NBL-1, that randomizes patients in the last part of the study to receive ch14.18/CHO antibody plus 13-*cis*-RA or RA alone [87].

Anti-idiotype antibody, 1A7, functionally mimics the tumor-associated antigen GD2, which is overexpressed on the surface of a number of neuroectodermal tumors such as melanoma, NB, soft tissue sarcoma, and small cell carcinoma of the lung. Immunization of mice with 1A7 generated the production of anti-GD2 antibodies. In a phase I clinical trial, immunization of patients with 1A7, mixed with the adjuvant QS21, demonstrated that 1A7 could act as a surrogate antigen for GD2 and induce strong humoral immune responses in advanced stage melanoma patients [88].

IL-2 is a potent stimulator of T and NK cell proliferation, as well as of their cytotoxic activity. A small clinical trial with IL-2 and "lymphokine activated killer" (LAK) cells was carried out in stage 4 NB patients [89], and more recently recombinant (r)IL-2 has been administered to relapsed NB patients. In both studies some response was observed, but the toxicity was remarkable [89,90]. The role of cytokine therapy remains limited; however, the association with anti-GD2 antibodies is being clinically evaluated. A fusion protein, including IL-2 and anti-GD2 has demonstrated good anti-NB activity in animal models and is now being tested in phase II clinical studies [91]. DNA vaccines have recently been shown to invoke humoral as well as cellular responses in injected hosts against the transgenic product and are a promise for the future [92-94].

ANGIOGENESIS AS TARGET FOR TREATMENT

Angiogenesis is a well-known and complex phenomenon in cancer. First described by Jude Folkman in 1962 [95], it has been studied in-depth in almost all malignant tumors in adults[95]. HR-NB represents the paradigm of malignant diseases, with an aggressive clinical course and dismal prognosis worldwide [13,30] in spite of intensified treatment, which combines all therapeutic strategies (induction chemotherapy, delayed surgery, high-dose megatherapy with stem cell rescue, local radiotherapy and biological treatment, either with retinoids or immunotherapy) [13,30]. This section summarizes the new aspects of anti-angiogenesis therapy in NB; it is not a review of angiogenesis or its prognosis [96,97] in NB [96,97]. However, it briefly describes those biological aspects related with new antiangiogenic therapies.

The origin of neo-vessels within the expanding NB is the result of at least four different mechanisms: 1) Sprouting [95] of new blood microvessels from pre-existing capillaries under the influence of pro-angiogenic growth factor expression, such as vascular endothelial growth factor–A (VEGF-A), basic fibroblast growth factor (bFGF) and angiopoietin (Ang) [95]. 2) Mobilisation and functional incorporation of endothelial progenitor cells (EPC) that originate from bone marrow migrate and are arrested at local sites being involved in the generation of new vessels [98]. 3) By co-option [99]: endothelialization of adjacent and pre-existing blood vasculature [99]. 4) Through "vasculogenic mimicry" [100], a phenomenon that describes the ability of tumor cells to mimic and transform themselves into vascular cells [100].

Most malignant NB cells are potently angiogenic as a result of an increased secretion of angiogenic stimulators (pro-angiogenic phenotype in HR tumors [101]) and a decreased production of inhibitors. Nevertheless, other mechanisms appear to play a role in the complex regulation of angiogenesis in NB. 1) Oncogene *MYCN* is frequently amplified in HR-NB. The suppressed expression of three angiogenesis inhibitors in these tumors, such as activin A [102], interleukin-6 and leukaemia inhibitory factor (LIF) has recently been described [103,104]. 2) Schwann cells produce anti-proliferative and differentiation-inducing factors, and also, several inhibitors of angiogenesis including tissue inhibitor of metalloproteinases (TIMP2) [105], pigment epithelial-derived growth factor (PEDGF) [106] and secreted protein acidic and rich in cysteine (SPARC) [107]. 3) Hypoxia leads to rapid response mechanisms that ensure adaptive strategies for cellular survival, including angiogenesis. The initial vasculature is insufficient to cope with the high-index proliferation of NB cells, leading to areas of low oxygen supply. This has been clearly shown *in vitro* [108]. The hypoxia-inducible transcription factors, HIF-1α and HIF-2α, are critical for this adaptive response being differentially regulated in NB [109]. HIF-2α a promotes an aggressive phenotype and high levels of HIF-2α highlight an immature neural crest-like NB cell cohort located in a perivascular niche [110].

Targeting tumor vasculature represents a promising new tool for cancer therapy and is commonly used in adult oncology. There are several strategies [101] which could be used to treat NB with new antiangiogenic compounds[101]. a) In parallel with standard chemotherapy: this is mostly used in several adult cancers. However, recent studies suggest that concomitant administration of both might actually causes vascular rebound with endothelial cell recovery during rest periods, a process that could counteract the anti-cancer effect of chemotherapy. b) Administration before chemotherapy could increase the efficacy of chemotherapy via normalization of the tumor vasculature. It would also apply to radiotherapy by improving oxygen supply. c) Administration after chemotherapy could have an effect on EPC mobilised during bone marrow recovery. d) Administration of protracted low doses of chemotherapeutic agents (metronomic chemotherapy) in addition to antiangiogenic drugs in order to treat MRD.

The preclinical and clinical studies with antiangiogenic drugs in NB described up to now are:

- Alpha-Iinterferon alfa, described by Folkman [111], this was the first antiangiogenic drug to be used [111].
- Retinoids [112]: Although well-known as inductors of NB differentiation, they have been shown in experimental models to inhibit angiogenesis by the inhibition of endothelial migration along with the production of inhibitors such as thrombospondin [112].
- TNP-470 [113]: This was one of the first drugs studied in experimental models in NB, suggesting a synergistic action in combination with cisplatin, paclitaxel or cyclophosphamide[113].
- Endostatin [114], a 20 kDa C-terminal fragment of collagen XVIII, inhibits endothelial proliferation *in vitro* and tumor growth *in vivo* when given systemically. Two preclinical studies have been performed in NB, one of them showing a "deceleration" in tumor growth [114].
- Angiostatin is a 38 Kda circulating endogenous protein that mediates its anti-angiogenic activity through binding ATP synthetase on the surface of human endothelial cells. As a result, it causes tumor cell apoptosis and inhibition of endothelial cell migration and tubule formation. Preclinical testing in NB has been evaluated in a gene therapy approach using a recombinant adenovirus encoding the human angiostatin kringle 1-3 directly fused to human serum albumin (HAS) (AdK3-HAS) [115].
- Thrombospondin-1 (TSP-1) is a glycoprotein capable of inhibiting endothelial cell proliferation and migration. ABT-510 is a peptide derived from TSP-1 that more effectively inhibits the growth of small NB xenografts. It has also been combined with valproic acid as an effective antiangiogenesis strategy [116].
- Monoclonal VEGF-A antibody and monoclonal antibodies against VEGF receptors have been developed and studied in different preclinical NB models, either alone or in combination with low-dose vinblastine [117].
- Bevacizumab deserves a special mention since it has been shown to suppress NB progression in the setting of MRD [118,119].
- Small molecules as inhibitors of VEGF receptors such as Sugen 5416 are of special interest, but data concerning their use in NB have not yet been published.
- Clinical-grade vasculature-targeted liposomal doxorubicin [120]. This is a novel drug developed by Italian investigators who, in a preclinical setting, have shown statistically significant reductions in cell proliferation, blood vessel density and microvessel area, with increased tumor cell apoptosis.
- Zoledronic acid [121], a bisphosphonate that reduces experimental NB growth by interfering with tumor angiogenesis [121].
- Low-dose daily irinotecan [122] has been shown to inhibit angiogenesis in NB [122]. In a very elegant preclinical model, investigators from Japan have shown that low-dose daily irinotecan inhibits tumor-growth, but could not completely abolish it. Diminished VEGF

gene and protein expression is closely correlated with tumor growth inhibition and inhibition of angiogenesis by CPT-11 in NB xenografts, but a persistent blocker of stroma-derived VEGF will need to be combined with CPT-11 to completely inhibit the growth of chemosensitive NB.

- HDACIs [123] in combination with other anticancer drugs may play a role in NB. Trichostatin A (TSA) and alpha-interferon were the most effective combination across a range of different cancer cell lines, including NB [123].
- Bortezomid [124,125] inhibits angiogenesis and reduces tumor burden in a murine model of NB [124,125]. The results of these studies warrant the beginning of clinical studies by different cooperative groups.
- Combined effect of vinblastine and rapamycin [126].
- VEGFR inhibitor, AZD2171 [127] is in a pediatric preclinical testing program (PPTP), this is a potent VEGFR inhibitor, orally bioavailable that has shown *in vitro* and *in vivo* activities in the PPTP in 5 out of 6 NB xenografts [127].

It is important to emphasize that all these trials must be carried out in the setting of well-controlled, cooperative studies among the different POGs (COG, SIOPEN, Japan etc.) involved in NB. Severe toxicity in the adult population treated with antiangiogenic drugs such as bevacizumab has been described (proteinuria, hypertension, bleeding, gastrointestinal perforation, delayed wound healing). Angiogenesis is also a physiological phenomenon in growth and an important feature in childhood that could be disturbed by long and protracted antiangiogenic treatment in children.

Gene Therapy

Although gene therapy is a promising treatment option for a number of diseases (including inherited disorders, some types of cancer, and certain viral infections), the technique remains risky and is still under study to ensure its safety and efficacy. Gene therapy is currently only being tested for the treatment of diseases that have no other cures, and is being developed for the treatment of a number of different cancers. At present many clinical trials are taking place, using a wide variety of different types of gene therapy for many different types of cancer. Nearly all these studies are at a very early stage. In the future, this technique may allow doctors to treat a disorder by inserting a gene into a patient's cells instead of using drugs or surgery. Researchers are testing several approaches to gene therapy, including: replacing a mutated gene that causes disease with a healthy copy of the gene; inactivating, or "knocking out," a mutated gene that is functioning improperly; introducing a new gene into the body to help fight a disease.

In the case of NB, the few clinical studies carried out have made use of autologous or allogeneic malignant cells engineered to express cytokine and/or chemokine genes in order to increase the level of recognition of tumor cells by the patient's immune system.

Brenner and coworkers pioneered gene therapy in NB using tumor cells transfected with viral vectors, selected *in vitro* and reinfused *in vivo* as vaccines. The authors investigated the effects of transferring the IL-2 gene to malignant neuroblast in children with advanced disease., Iin this study the authors found evidence of a systemic antitumor immune response that involved both helper and cytotoxic T lymphocytes and was associated with systemic antitumor reduction. These results suggest that IL-2 transduction of neuroblast provides an immunotherapeutic stimulus and that adenoviral vectors are useful for this clinical approach; however, the study elicited only limited local antitumor response and essentially no systemic antitumor immunity [128,129]. Recently, this group studied the frequency of associated immune changes when patients with HR-NB are vaccinating with autologous NB tumor cells modified to secrete IL-2. The results showed that the vaccine was well tolerated. Injection site biopsies revealed increased cellularity caused by infiltration of CD4 and CD8 lymphocytes, eosinophils, and dendritic cells. Enzyme-linked immunosorbent spot assays for interferon-gamma and IL-15 demonstrated that vaccination produced a rise in circulating CD4 and CD8 T cells [90]. Other cytokines such as IL-12, IL-21, IL-27 have been studied in murine models showing different protective effects [130-132].

Different studies have demonstrated the synergistic potential of chemokine-cytokine combinations in different cancer types [133,134]. The apparently beneficial interaction between IL-2 and lymphotactin (Lptn) in enhancing lymphocyte attraction and expansion in NB murine models prompted a second evaluation in patients with advanced NB to determine whether a combination of individual molecules acting at different phases of the immune response may produce a more potent immune response to an otherwise weakly immunogenic tumor. Allogeneic tumor cell vaccines combining transgenic Lptn with IL-2 appeared to have little toxicity in humans and can induce an antitumor immune response, although the immune response was insufficient to overcome active recurrent NB [91,135].

An interesting approach to tumor gene therapy is the production of chimeric T cells. A common strategy has been to introduce a synthetic receptor with an antigen-binding domain from an antibody coupled to a signal-transducing endodomain derived from the native T cell receptor into activated T cells. These chimeric antigen receptors thus have the specificity of an antibody coupled to the cytotoxic effector mechanisms of the T cell. The NB pilot study showed that the persistence of cytolytic T lymphocyte clones in circulation is short in patients with massive disease [136]. Recently, Epstein-Barr virus-specific cytotoxic T lymphocytes to express a chimeric antigen receptor directed to the GD2, which is present on the tumor cells of most individuals with NB, have been engineered. These virus-specific cytotoxic T lymphocytes persist in higher numbers and for longer times after administration to individuals with NB than do activated T cells expressing the same receptor but lacking viral specificity [53].

The identification of cancer-associated molecules and/or genes holds promise for the development of novel therapeutic strategies that selectively target tumor cells. Among these strategies, antisense oligonucleotides can be used to decrease tumor-associated gene expression, resulting in specific anticancer effects and minimal damage to normal tissues. In addition to their direct effects on gene expression, antisense oligonucleotides can have antitumor effects via indirect, immune-stimulatory mechanisms, if they are designed to contain unmethylated cytosine-guanine (CpG) motifs. These motifs present potent immunostimulating effects mediated by macrophages, dendritic cells, B cells and NK cells [137,138]. These features make CpG-containing antisense oligonucleotides potentially useful as immune adjuvants.

Although antisense oligonucleotides, with or without CpG motifs, show promise as therapeutic agents for direct or indirect tumor cell killing, there are a number of problems associated with their clinical use. Indeed, liposome encapsulation of antisense oligonucleotides specific for the *raf* oncogene lead to increased levels of antisense oligonucleotides in plasma and tissues and improved antitumor effects relative to the free oligonucleotides [139]. Liposomes have been found to facilitate the delivery of antisense oligonucleotides targeting the *Bcl-2*, *MDR1*, or *c-myc* genes *in vivo* [140-142]. A CpG oligonucleotide has been reported to inhibit the *in vivo* growth of the murine NB cell line Neuro-2a in syngeneic A/J mice [143].

The *c-myb* proto-oncogene is the best characterized member of the *myb* family of transcription factor genes. Expression of *c-myb* has been detected in several solid tumors of different origin, including NB, and is linked to cell proliferation and/or differentiation [144, 145]. Studies show that *c-myb* antisense oligonucleotide entrapped in GD2-targeted liposomes inhibits NB growth *in vitro* by specifically reducing c-myb protein expression and increasing the survival of mice grafted with human NB [146,147].

Gene Expression Profile as "Signature" of Therapeutic Targets

Clusters of differentially-expressed genes, associated with a peculiar phenotype are assumed as a "signature" of the cancer cell. By combining the results of gene expression profiling with the data obtained from the unveiling of the human genome it is possible to identify specific genes that are associated with tumor progression and response to drug treatment. Recently, the cDNA microarray method has been applied to comprehensively demonstrate the expression profiles of primary NB and cell lines (Table 1). The first microarray-based gene expression profiling study of NB was reported by Khan *et al.* [148] who demonstrated that the small, round blue-cell tumors (SRBCTs), including NB, could be distinguished on the basis of their patterns of gene expression using artificial neural networks (ANNs).

Further microarray studies on NB tumor samples propose group discriminations by known clinical or biological factors. Thus, subsequent microarray studies have facilitated class separation of differentiating NB (dNB) tumors from poorly differentiated tumors (pdNB), and of HR-tumors from low risk tumors. For example, Yamanaka *et al.* [149] examined 14 NB by 23,040 cDNAs microarray, and identified 78 genes whose expression levels were significantly different between dNB and pdNB. In expression profiling by microarray studies it is important to take into account the fact that NB tumors are highly complex biological tissues represented by a mixture of cell types. Accordingly, Albino *et al.* [150] reported a genome-wide expression analysis of whole tumors and microdissected NB and Schwannian stromal cells, and found 16 common genes driving the separation between stroma-rich and stroma-poor neuroblastic tumors.

On the other hand, other studies have focussed on certain genomic aberrations and the corresponding gene expression profiles in prognosis prediction and survival associations. McArdle *et al.* [154] identified transcripts that were differentially expressed in the 11q loss, *MYCN* non amplified and hyperdiploid subtypes of NB. Janoueix-Lerosey *et al.* [155] compared the expression profiles between the tumors with 1p loss and those with normal 1p status and identified the genes with decreased expression in NB with 1p deletion. An increasing amount of information is now available on genes that can distinguish prognosis for

Table 1. Differentially expressed genes identified by gene expression profiling using microarray. (Adapted from Ohira *et al.* [163])

	Genes identified	Genes on microarray	Sample number	Category
			NB diagnosis	
Khan *et al.* [148]	15 genes	6567 cDNAs	16 NB	*DPYSL4, CDH2, AF1Q, CRMP1, KIF3C, GAP43, MAP1B, RCV1, SFRP1, GATA2, PFN2, FHL1* (highly and specifically expressed in NB)
			Expression profiling	
Yamanaka *et al.* [149]	78 genes	23040 cDNAs	14 NB	dNB vs. pdNB: *ITGE, SYP, OLIG2, MADH2, DFFB, CASP8, CASP9* (upregulated in dNB) *CLDN5, CCND1, NFKBIL2* (up-regulated in pdNB)
Berwanger *et al.* [151]	36 genes	4608 cDNAs	90 NB	Stage 1 vs. stage 4 *MYCN* non-amplified: *FYN, AFAP, CTNNA1, NRCAM,* tropomodulin, *MARCKS* (down-regulated in advanced stage NB)
Takita *et al.* [152]	3 genes	1700 genes	20 NB	Stage 1 vs. stage 4: BIRC3, CDKN2D (up-regulated in the early-stage group) SMARCD3 (down-regulated in the early-stage group)
Hiyama *et al.* [153]	123 genes	6272 cDNAs	20 NB	Unfavourable (uf) vs. favourable (f) 43 genes including *MYCN, hTERT, NME1, CCND1, CCNE1, E1, BIRC5, BIRC1* (up-regulated in ufNB). 80 genes (up-regulated in fNB): *CD44, IGF2, TRKA, ANK1* (highly expressed in maturing NB) and *CASP8, CASP9, TNFSF10, NGFA, GDF10* (highly expressed in regressing NB)
McArdle *et al.* [154]		14500 genes	20 NB	Differentially expressed in the 11q-, *MYCN* non-amplified and hyperdiploid subtypes of NB
Janoueix-Lerosey *et al.* [155]		320genes on 1p35-36	43 NB	1p loss vs. 1p normal *CDC42, VAMP3, CLSTN1, GNB1, STMN1, RPA2, RBAF600, FBXO6, MAD2L2* (decreased expression in NB with 1p deletion)
Alaminos *et al.* [156]	222 genes	62839 cDNAs	40 NB 12 cell lines	*MYCN* highly expressed vs. *MYCN* normal expression. Differentially expressed genes were strongly associated with *MYCN* expression.
Fischer *et al.* [157]	18 genes	213235 SAGE tags	76 NB	Stage 4S vs. Stage 4 *A2BP1, CHRNA7, DST, CNR1, IGSF4, MEIS1, ROBO1, TFAP2B, DMC1, PCBP4, RBM5, Scotin, CADPS, CLSTN3, MAP7, SNAP91, SYN3, PRAME* genes differentially expressed
Wang *et al.* [158]		12625 genes	101 NB	Differentially expressed in the 1p36 loss and *MYCN* amplified and 11q loss subtypes of NB
Oberthuer *et al.* [159]		42578 cDNA	49 NB	144-gene predictor constructed to risk estimation in divergent clinical NB
Cheung *et al.* [160]	34 genes		48 NB 9 remission BM	MRD markers differentially expressed in stage 4 NB: *CCND1, CRMP1, DDC, GABRB3, ISL1, KIF1A, PHOX2B, TACC2.*
			Prognosis prediction	
Wei *et al.* [161]	19 genes	42578 cDNA	56 NB	To develop an accurate predictor of survival for patient with NB. *DLK1, PRSS3, ARC, SLIT3, MYCN, JPH1* (up-regulated in poor-outcome NB); *ARHI, CNR1, CD44, ROBO2, BTBD3, KLRC3* (down-regulated in poor-outcome NB)
Ohira *et al.* [162]	70 genes	5340 cDNA	136 NB	To develop an accurate predictor of survival for patient with NB

the NB patient as described above. These data need to be integrated and organized to construct a simple prediction system for clinical practice. Such efforts are now ongoing, although alternative technologies to cDNA microarrays such as Multiplex real-time PCR

(Taqman Low Density Arrays) are also available that might be a promising approach to reduce the complexity of information obtained from whole-genome array experiments [164].

Microarray technology can also be used for signal transduction pathway analysis and pharmacogenomics in cell culture models in NB. Yuza *et al.* [165] used expression profiling as an approach to monitor the differentiating effects of 13-*cis*-RA treatment in SK-N-SH and CHP-134 NB cell lines. In this model, during differentiation of NB cells, several genes, including *MYCN*, *cyclin D3* and *Wnt10B,* were down-regulated, whereas *RB1* and related genes (*p107*, *RB2/p130*, *p300/CBP*, *E2F-1*, *DP-1*) were up-regulated. Vitali *et al.* [166] evaluated the effect of imatinib mesylate on invasion, and analyzed the genes modulated by imatinib mesylate treatment in NB cells. *Slug* (*SNAI2*) gene was down-regulated by imatinib mesylate. *Slug* down-regulation facilitates apoptosis induced by proapoptotic drugs in NB cells and decreases their invasion capability *in vitro* and *in vivo*. *Slug* inhibition, possibly combined with imatinib mesylate, may represent a novel strategy for treatment of metastatic NB.

Recently, in addition to gene expression profiling, other genome aberrations as well as epigenetic alterations have been reported to be strongly related to patient prognosis with NB. Abe *et al.* [167] indicated that HR-NB showed increased methylation, and that the methylation of certain CpG islands, such as the Protocadherin beta family, can predict poor prognosis in NB with high sensitivity. In the near future a "poor signature" will be used to guide the administration of adjuvant therapies.

Conclusion

The hallmark of NB is its heterogeneity in clinical presentation as well as in tumor phenotype. Age at diagnosis, stage of disease, *MYCN* status, tumor histopathology and DNA content are different prognostic markers used to predict clinical behaviour and decide on treatment strategy. Genetic studies show also the existence of tumor heterogeneity and the utility of tumor biologic data to predict patient outcome and determine possible candidate molecular targets. In spite of the high rate of clinical response to first-line therapy in NB, complete eradication of NB cells is rarely achieved. As a consequence, the majority of patients with advanced NB undergo relapse, which is often resistant to conventional therapy. Thus, after initial apparent remission, new therapeutic strategies are needed to try to eradicate the surviving NB cells and to prevent relapse. Using the innovative approaches to NB therapy described in this chapter, it will soon be possible to complement the traditional anti-neoplastic treatment of this disease.

References

[1] Brodeur, GM; Pritchard, J; Berthold, F; Carlsen, NL; Castel, V; Castelberry, RP; De Bernardi, B; Evans, AE; Favrot, M; Hedborg, F;et al. Revisions of the international criteria for neuroblastoma diagnosis, staging, and response to treatment. *J Clin Oncol,* 1993 11, 1466-1477.

[2] Evans, AE. Neuroblastoma: a historical perspective 1864-1998. In: Brodeur G.M., Sawada T., Tsuchida Y., Voute P.A. (ed). *Neuroblastoma*. Elsevier: Amsterdam, 2000, pp 1-6.

[3] Burgues, O; Navarro, S; Noguera, R; Pellin, A; Ruiz, A; Castel, V; Llombart-Bosch, A. Prognostic value of the International Neuroblastoma Pathology Classification in Neuroblastoma (Schwannian stroma-poor) and comparison with other prognostic factors: a study of 182 cases from the Spanish Neuroblastoma Registry. *Virchows Arch,* 2006 449, 410-420.

[4] Maris, JM; Matthay, KK. Molecular biology of neuroblastoma. *J Clin Oncol,* 1999 17, 2264-2279.

[5] Weinstein, JL; Katzenstein, HM;Cohn, SL. Advances in the diagnosis and treatment of neuroblastoma. *Oncologist,* 2003 8, 278-292.

[6] Brodeur, GM. Neuroblastoma: biological insights into a clinical enigma. *Nat Rev Cancer,* 2003 3, 203-216.

[7] Patterson, PH. Control of cell fate in a vertebrate neurogenic lineage. *Cell,* 1990 62, 1035-1038.

[8] Shimada, H; Umehara, S; Monobe, Y; Hachitanda, Y; Nakagawa, A; Goto, S; Gerbing, RB; Stram, DO; Lukens, JN; Matthay, KK. International neuroblastoma pathology classification for prognostic evaluation of patients with peripheral neuroblastic tumors: a report from the Children's Cancer Group. *Cancer,* 2001 92, 2451-2461.

[9] Navarro, S; Amann, G; Beiske, K; Cullinane, CJ; d'Amore, ES; Gambini, C; Mosseri, V; De Bernardi, B; Michon, J; Peuchmaur, M. Prognostic value of International Neuroblastoma Pathology Classification in localized resectable peripheral neuroblastic tumors: a histopathologic study of localized neuroblastoma European Study Group 94.01 Trial and Protocol. *J Clin Oncol,* 2006 24, 695-699.

[10] D'Angio, GJ; Evans, AE; Koop, CE. Special pattern of widespread neuroblastoma with a favourable prognosis. *Lancet,* 1971 1, 1046-1049.

[11] Noguera, R; Canete, A; Pellin, A; Ruiz, A; Tasso, M; Navarro, S; Castel, V; Llombart-Bosch, A. MYCN gain and MYCN amplification in a stage 4S neuroblastoma. *Cancer Genet Cytogenet,* 2003 140, 157-161.

[12] Olshan AF, BG. Epidemiology of Neuroblastoma. In: Brodeur G.M., Sawada T., Tsuchida Y., Voute P.A. (ed). *Neuroblastoma*. Elsevier: Amsterdam, 2000, pp 33-37.

[13] Castel, V; Canete, A; Navarro, S; Garcia-Miguel, P; Melero, C; Acha, T; Navajas, A; Badal, MD. Outcome of high-risk neuroblastoma using a dose intensity approach: improvement in initial but not in long-term results. *Med Pediatr Oncol,* 2001 37, 537-542.

[14] Schwab, M; Alitalo, K; Klempnauer, KH; Varmus, HE; Bishop, JM; Gilbert, F; Brodeur, G; Goldstein, M; Trent, J. Amplified DNA with limited homology to myc cellular oncogene is shared by human neuroblastoma cell lines and a neuroblastoma tumour. *Nature,* 1983 305, 245-248.

[15] Brodeur, GM; Seeger, RC; Schwab, M; Varmus, HE; Bishop, JM. Amplification of N-myc in untreated human neuroblastomas correlates with advanced disease stage. *Science,* 1984 224, 1121-1124.

[16] Seeger, RC; Brodeur, GM; Sather, H; Dalton, A; Siegel, SE; Wong, KY; Hammond, D. Association of multiple copies of the N-myc oncogene with rapid progression of neuroblastomas. *N Engl J Med,* 1985 313, 1111-1116.

[17] Maris, JM. How does MYCN amplification make neuroblastomas behave aggressively? Still more questions than answers. *Pediatr Blood Cancer,* 2005 45, 869-870.

[18] Spitz, R; Hero, B; Skowron, M; Ernestus, K;Berthold, F. MYCN-status in neuroblastoma: characteristics of tumours showing amplification, gain, and non-amplification. *Eur J Cancer,* 2004 40, 2753-2759.

[19] De Bernardi, B; Mosseri, V; Rubie, H; Castel, V; Foot, A; Ladenstein, R; Laureys, G; Beck-Popovic, M; de Lacerda, AF; Pearson, AD; De Kraker, J; Ambros, PF; de Rycke, Y; Conte, M; Bruzzi, P; Michon, J. Treatment of localised resectable neuroblastoma. Results of the LNESG1 study by the SIOP Europe Neuroblastoma Group. *Br J Cancer,* 2008 99, 1027-1033.

[20] Mejia, C; Navarro, S; Pellin, A; Ruiz, A; Castel, V; Llombart-Bosch, A. Prognostic significance of cell proliferation in human neuroblastoma: comparison with other prognostic factors. *Oncol Rep,* 2003 10, 243-247.

[21] Pritchard, J; Cotterill, SJ; Germond, SM; Imeson, J; de Kraker, J;Jones, DR. High dose melphalan in the treatment of advanced neuroblastoma: results of a randomised trial (ENSG-1) by the European Neuroblastoma Study Group. *Pediatr Blood Cancer,* 2005 44, 348-357.

[22] Hero, B; Simon, T; Spitz, R; Ernestus, K; Gnekow, AK; Scheel-Walter, HG; Schwabe, D; Schilling, FH; Benz-Bohm, G; Berthold, F. Localized infant neuroblastomas often show spontaneous regression: results of the prospective trials NB95-S and NB97. *J Clin Oncol,* 2008 26, 1504-1510.

[23] Pession, A; Tonelli, R. The MYCN oncogene as a specific and selective drug target for peripheral and central nervous system tumors. *Curr Cancer Drug Targets,* 2005 5, 273-283.

[24] Himoudi, N; Yan, M; Papanastasiou, A; Anderson, J. MYCN as a target for cancer immunotherapy. *Cancer Immunol Immunother,* 2008 57, 693-700.

[25] Schulte, JH; Horn, S; Otto, T; Samans, B; Heukamp, LC; Eilers, UC; Krause, M; Astrahantseff, K; Klein-Hitpass, L; Buettner, R; Schramm, A; Christiansen, H; Eilers, M; Eggert, A; Berwanger, B. MYCN regulates oncogenic MicroRNAs in neuroblastoma. *Int J Cancer,* 2008 122, 699-704.

[26] Zhang, B; Pan, X; Cobb, GP; Anderson, TA. microRNAs as oncogenes and tumor suppressors. *Dev Biol,* 2007 302, 1-12.

[27] Spitz, R; Hero, B; Ernestus, K; Berthold, F. FISH analyses for alterations in chromosomes 1, 2, 3, and 11 define high-risk groups in neuroblastoma. *Med Pediatr Oncol,* 2003 41, 30-35.

[28] Wei, JS; Song, YK; Durinck, S; Chen, QR; Cheuk, AT; Tsang, P; Zhang, Q; Thiele, CJ; Slack, A; Shohet, J; Khan, J. The MYCN oncogene is a direct target of miR-34a. *Oncogene,* 2008 27, 5204-5213.

[29] Noguera, R; Piqueras, M; Subramaniam, M; Cruz, J; Canete, A; Bosch, AL; Navarro, S. Immunohistochemical evaluation of a novel clone of monoclonal anti-MYCN antibody B8.4B in neuroblastic tumours: a correlation with MYCN gene status. *Virchows Arch,* 2006 449, 277-278.

[30] Maris, JM; Hogarty, MD; Bagatell, R;Cohn, SL. Neuroblastoma. *Lancet,* 2007 369, 2106-2120.

[31] Ambros, IM; Benard, J; Boavida, M; Bown, N; Caron, H; Combaret, V; Couturier, J; Darnfors, C; Delattre, O; Freeman-Edward, J; Gambini, C; Gross, N; Hattinger, CM;

Luegmayr, A; Lunec, J; Martinsson, T; Mazzocco, K; Navarro, S; Noguera, R; O'Neill, S; Potschger, U; Rumpler, S; Speleman, F; Tonini, GP; Valent, A; Van Roy, N; Amann, G; De Bernardi, B; Kogner, P; Ladenstein, R; Michon, J; Pearson, AD; Ambros, PF. Quality assessment of genetic markers used for therapy stratification. *J Clin Oncol,* 2003 21, 2077-2084.

[32] Cohn, SL; Tweddle, DA. MYCN amplification remains prognostically strong 20 years after its "clinical debut". *Eur J Cancer,* 2004 40, 2639-2642.

[33] Spitz, R; Hero, B; Ernestus, K; Berthold, F. Deletions in chromosome arms 3p and 11q are new prognostic markers in localized and 4s neuroblastoma. *Clin Cancer Res,* 2003 9, 52-58.

[34] Attiyeh, EF; London, WB; Mosse, YP; Wang, Q; Winter, C; Khazi, D; McGrady, PW; Seeger, RC; Look, AT; Shimada, H; Brodeur, GM; Cohn, SL; Matthay, KK;Maris, JM. Chromosome 1p and 11q deletions and outcome in neuroblastoma. *N Engl J Med,* 2005 353, 2243-2253.

[35] Spitz, R; Hero, B; Simon, T; Berthold, F. Loss in chromosome 11q identifies tumors with increased risk for metastatic relapses in localized and 4S neuroblastoma. *Clin Cancer Res,* 2006 12, 3368-3373.

[36] Brinkschmidt, C; Christiansen, H; Terpe, HJ; Simon, R; Lampert, F; Boecker, W; Dockhorn-Dworniczak, B. Distal chromosome 17 gains in neuroblastomas detected by comparative genomic hybridization (CGH) are associated with a poor clinical outcome. *Med Pediatr Oncol,* 2001 36, 11-13.

[37] Bown, N; Lastowska, M; Cotterill, S; O'Neill, S; Ellershaw, C; Roberts, P; Lewis, I; Pearson, AD. 17q gain in neuroblastoma predicts adverse clinical outcome. U.K. Cancer Cytogenetics Group and the U.K. Children's Cancer Study Group. *Med Pediatr Oncol,* 2001 36, 14-19.

[38] Piqueras, M; Navarro, S; Castel, V; Canete, A; Llombart-Bosch, A;Noguera, R. Analysis of biological prognostic factors using tissue microarrays in neuroblastic tumors. *Pediatr Blood Cancer,* 2008 52, 209-214.

[39] Villamón, E; Piqueras, M; Mackintosh, C; Alonso, J; de Alava, E; Navarro, S; Noguera, R. Comparison of different techniques for the detection of genetic risk-identifying chromosomal gains and losses in neuroblastoma. *Virchows Arch,* 2008 453, 47-55.

[40] Simon, T; Spitz, R; Hero, B; Berthold, F; Faldum, A. Risk estimation in localized unresectable single copy MYCN neuroblastoma by the status of chromosomes 1p and 11q. *Cancer Lett,* 2006 237, 215-222.

[41] Afanasyeva, EA; Hotz-Wagenblatt, A; Glatting, KH; Westermann, F. New miRNAs cloned from neuroblastoma. *BMC Genomics,* 2008 9, 52.

[42] Spitz, R; Oberthuer, A; Zapatka, M; Brors, B; Hero, B; Ernestus, K; Oestreich, J; Fischer, M; Simon, T; Berthold, F. Oligonucleotide array-based comparative genomic hybridization (aCGH) of 90 neuroblastomas reveals aberration patterns closely associated with relapse pattern and outcome. *Genes Chromosomes Cancer,* 2006 45, 1130-1142.

[43] Schleiermacher, G; Michon, J; Huon, I; d'Enghien, CD; Klijanienko, J; Brisse, H; Ribeiro, A; Mosseri, V; Rubie, H; Munzer, C; Thomas, C; Valteau-Couanet, D; Auvrignon, A; Plantaz, D; Delattre, O;Couturier, J. Chromosomal CGH identifies patients with a higher risk of relapse in neuroblastoma without MYCN amplification. *Br J Cancer,* 2007 97, 238-246.

[44] Mosse, YP; Diskin, SJ; Wasserman, N; Rinaldi, K; Attiyeh, EF; Cole, K; Jagannathan, J; Bhambhani, K; Winter, C; Maris, JM. Neuroblastomas have distinct genomic DNA profiles that predict clinical phenotype and regional gene expression. *Genes Chromosomes Cancer,* 2007 46, 936-949.

[45] Bagatell, R; Rumcheva, P; London, WB; Cohn, SL; Look, AT; Brodeur, GM; Frantz, C; Joshi, V; Thorner, P; Rao, PV; Castleberry, R; Bowman, LC. Outcomes of children with intermediate-risk neuroblastoma after treatment stratified by MYCN status and tumor cell ploidy. *J Clin Oncol,* 2005 23, 8819-8827.

[46] George, RE; London, WB; Cohn, SL; Maris, JM; Kretschmar, C; Diller, L; Brodeur, GM; Castleberry, RP; Look, AT. Hyperdiploidy plus nonamplified MYCN confers a favorable prognosis in children 12 to 18 months old with disseminated neuroblastoma: a Pediatric Oncology Group study. *J Clin Oncol,* 2005 23, 6466-6473.

[47] Schneiderman, J; London, WB; Brodeur, GM; Castleberry, RP; Look, AT; Cohn, SL. Clinical significance of MYCN amplification and ploidy in favorable-stage neuroblastoma: a report from the Children's Oncology Group. *J Clin Oncol,* 2008 26, 913-918.

[48] Mosse, YP; Laudenslager, M; Longo, L; Cole, KA; Wood, A; Attiyeh, EF; Laquaglia, MJ; Sennett, R; Lynch, JE; Perri, P; Laureys, G; Speleman, F; Kim, C; Hou, C; Hakonarson, H; Torkamani, A; Schork, NJ; Brodeur, GM; Tonini, GP; Rappaport, E; Devoto, M; Maris, JM. Identification of ALK as a major familial neuroblastoma predisposition gene. *Nature,* 2008 455, 930-935.

[49] Iwahara, T; Fujimoto, J; Wen, D; Cupples, R; Bucay, N; Arakawa, T; Mori, S; Ratzkin, B; Yamamoto, T. Molecular characterization of ALK, a receptor tyrosine kinase expressed specifically in the nervous system. *Oncogene,* 1997 14, 439-449.

[50] Caren, H; Abel, F; Kogner, P; Martinsson, T. High incidence of DNA mutations and gene amplifications of the ALK gene in advanced sporadic neuroblastoma tumours. *Biochem J,* 2008 416, 153-159.

[51] George, RE; Sanda, T; Hanna, M; Frohling, S; Luther, W, 2nd; Zhang, J; Ahn, Y; Zhou, W; London, WB; McGrady, P; Xue, L; Zozulya, S; Gregor, VE; Webb, TR; Gray, NS; Gilliland, DG; Diller, L; Greulich, H; Morris, SW; Meyerson, M; Look, AT. Activating mutations in ALK provide a therapeutic target in neuroblastoma. *Nature,* 2008 455, 975-978.

[52] Subramaniam, MM; Piqueras, M; Navarro, S; Noguera, R. Aberrant copy numbers of ALK gene is a frequent genetic alteration in neuroblastomas. *British Journal of Cancer,* 2009 in press.

[53] Pule, MA; Savoldo, B; Myers, GD; Rossig, C; Russell, HV; Dotti, G; Huls, MH; Liu, E; Gee, AP; Mei, Z; Yvon, E; Weiss, HL; Liu, H; Rooney, CM; Heslop, HE;Brenner, MK. Virus-specific T cells engineered to coexpress tumor-specific receptors: persistence and antitumor activity in individuals with neuroblastoma. *Nat Med,* 2008 14, 1264-1270.

[54] McDermott, U; Iafrate, AJ; Gray, NS; Shioda, T; Classon, M; Maheswaran, S; Zhou, W; Choi, HG; Smith, SL; Dowell, L; Ulkus, LE; Kuhlmann, G; Greninger, P; Christensen, JG; Haber, DA;Settleman, J. Genomic alterations of anaplastic lymphoma kinase may sensitize tumors to anaplastic lymphoma kinase inhibitors. *Cancer Res,* 2008 68, 3389-3395.

[55] Pahlman, S; Odelstad, L; Larsson, E; Grotte, G; Nilsson, K. Phenotypic changes of human neuroblastoma cells in culture induced by 12-O-tetradecanoyl-phorbol-13-acetate. *Int J Cancer,* 1981 28, 583-589.

[56] Reynolds, CP; Matthay, KK; Villablanca, JG; Maurer, BJ. Retinoid therapy of high-risk neuroblastoma. *Cancer Lett,* 2003 197, 185-192.

[57] Navarro, S; Noguera, R; Pellin, A; Mejia, C; Ruiz, A; Llombart-Bosch, A. Pleomorphic anaplastic neuroblastoma. *Med Pediatr Oncol,* 2000 35, 498-502.

[58] Fulda, S; Debatin, KM. Apoptosis pathways in neuroblastoma therapy. *Cancer Lett,* 2003 197, 131-135.

[59] Rastinejad, F. Retinoid X receptor and its partners in the nuclear receptor family. *Curr Opin Struct Biol,* 2001 11, 33-38.

[60] Sidell, N. Retinoic acid-induced growth inhibition and morphologic differentiation of human neuroblastoma cells in vitro. *J Natl Cancer Inst,* 1982 68, 589-596.

[61] Pahlman, S; Ruusala, AI; Abrahamsson, L; Mattsson, ME; Esscher, T. Retinoic acid-induced differentiation of cultured human neuroblastoma cells: a comparison with phorbolester-induced differentiation. *Cell Differ,* 1984 14, 135-144.

[62] Thiele, CJ; Deutsch, LA;Israel, MA. The expression of multiple proto-oncogenes is differentially regulated during retinoic acid induced maturation of human neuroblastoma cell lines. *Oncogene,* 1988 3, 281-288.

[63] Thiele, CJ; Reynolds, CP;Israel, MA. Decreased expression of N-myc precedes retinoic acid-induced morphological differentiation of human neuroblastoma. *Nature,* 1985 313, 404-406.

[64] Hill, DP; Robertson, KA. Characterization of the cholinergic neuronal differentiation of the human neuroblastoma cell line LA-N-5 after treatment with retinoic acid. *Brain Res Dev Brain Res,* 1997 102, 53-67.

[65] Handler, A; Lobo, MD; Alonso, FJ; Paino, CL;Mena, MA. Functional implications of the noradrenergic-cholinergic switch induced by retinoic acid in NB69 neuroblastoma cells. *J Neurosci Res,* 2000 60, 311-320.

[66] Edsjo, A; Lavenius, E; Nilsson, H; Hoehner, JC; Simonsson, P; Culp, LA; Martinsson, T; Larsson, C; Pahlman, S. Expression of trkB in human neuroblastoma in relation to MYCN expression and retinoic acid treatment. *Lab Invest,* 2003 83, 813-823.

[67] Chu, PW; Cheung, WM; Kwong, YL. Differential effects of 9-cis, 13-cis and all-trans retinoic acids on the neuronal differentiation of human neuroblastoma cells. *Neuroreport,* 2003 14, 1935-1939.

[68] Santos, A; Calvet, L; Terrier-Lacombe, MJ; Larsen, A; Benard, J; Pondarre, C; Aubert, G; Morizet, J; Lavelle, F; Vassal, G. In vivo treatment with CPT-11 leads to differentiation of neuroblastoma xenografts and topoisomerase I alterations. *Cancer Res,* 2004 64, 3223-3229.

[69] Raffaghello, L; Pagnan, G; Pastorino, F; Cosimo, E; Brignole, C; Marimpietri, D; Montaldo, PG; Gambini, C; Allen, TM; Bogenmann, E; Ponzoni, M. In vitro and in vivo antitumor activity of liposomal Fenretinide targeted to human neuroblastoma. *Int J Cancer,* 2003 104, 559-567.

[70] Matthay, KK; Villablanca, JG; Seeger, RC; Stram, DO; Harris, RE; Ramsay, NK; Swift, P; Shimada, H; Black, CT; Brodeur, GM; Gerbing, RB; Reynolds, CP. Treatment of high-risk neuroblastoma with intensive chemotherapy, radiotherapy, autologous bone

marrow transplantation, and 13-cis-retinoic acid. Children's Cancer Group. *N Engl J Med,* 1999 341, 1165-1173.

[71] Tonini, GP; Mazzocco, K; di Vinci, A; Geido, E; de Bernardi, B; Giaretti, W. Evidence of apoptosis in neuroblastoma at onset and relapse. An analysis of a large series of tumors. *J Neurooncol,* 1997 31, 209-215.

[72] Garaventa, A; Luksch, R; Lo Piccolo, MS; Cavadini, E; Montaldo, PG; Pizzitola, MR; Boni, L; Ponzoni, M; Decensi, A; De Bernardi, B; Bellani, FF; Formelli, F. Phase I trial and pharmacokinetics of fenretinide in children with neuroblastoma. *Clin Cancer Res,* 2003 9, 2032-2039.

[73] Ponthan, F; Lindskog, M; Karnehed, N; Castro, J; Kogner, P. Evaluation of anti-tumour effects of oral fenretinide (4-HPR) in rats with human neuroblastoma xenografts. *Oncol Rep,* 2003 10, 1587-1592.

[74] Ponzoni, M; Bocca, P; Chiesa, V; Decensi, A; Pistoia, V; Raffaghello, L; Rozzo, C; Montaldo, PG. Differential effects of N-(4-hydroxyphenyl) retinamide and retinoic acid on neuroblastoma cells: apoptosis versus differentiation. *Cancer Res,* 1995 55, 853-861.

[75] Aranda, A; Pascual, A. Nuclear hormone receptors and gene expression. *Physiol Rev,* 2001 81, 1269-1304.

[76] De los Santos, M; Zambrano, A; Aranda, A. Combined effects of retinoic acid and histone deacetylase inhibitors on human neuroblastoma SH-SY5Y cells. *Mol Cancer Ther,* 2007 6, 1425-1432.

[77] Hahn, CK; Ross, KN; Warrington, IM; Mazitschek, R; Kanegai, CM; Wright, RD; Kung, AL; Golub, TR; Stegmaier, K. Expression-based screening identifies the combination of histone deacetylase inhibitors and retinoids for neuroblastoma differentiation. *Proc Natl Acad Sci U S A,* 2008 105, 9751-9756.

[78] Swettenham, E; Witting, PK; Salvatore, BA;Neuzil, J. Alpha-tocopheryl succinate selectively induces apoptosis in neuroblastoma cells: potential therapy of malignancies of the nervous system? *J Neurochem,* 2005 94, 1448-1456.

[79] Cheung, NK; Kushner, BH; LaQuaglia, M; Kramer, K; Gollamudi, S; Heller, G; Gerald, W; Yeh, S; Finn, R; Larson, SM; Wuest, D; Byrnes, M; Dantis, E; Mora, J; Cheung, IY; Rosenfield, N; Abramson, S; O'Reilly, RJ. N7: a novel multi-modality therapy of high risk neuroblastoma (NB) in children diagnosed over 1 year of age. *Med Pediatr Oncol,* 2001 36, 227-230.

[80] Modak, S; Cheung, NK. Disialoganglioside directed immunotherapy of neuroblastoma. *Cancer Invest,* 2007 25, 67-77.

[81] Nakamura, K; Tanaka, Y; Shitara, K; Hanai, N. Construction of humanized anti-ganglioside monoclonal antibodies with potent immune effector functions. *Cancer Immunol Immunother,* 2001 50, 275-284.

[82] Simon, T; Hero, B; Faldum, A; Handgretinger, R; Schrappe, M; Niethammer, D; Berthold, F. Consolidation treatment with chimeric anti-GD2-antibody ch14.18 in children older than 1 year with metastatic neuroblastoma. *J Clin Oncol,* 2004 22, 3549-3557.

[83] Cheung, N-KV, Yu, A.L. Immunotherapy of neuroblastoma. In: Brodeur GM, Sawada T., Tsuchida Y., Voute P.A. (ed). *Neuroblastoma.* Elsevier: Amsterdam, 2000, pp 541-549.

[84] Osenga, KL; Hank, JA; Albertini, MR; Gan, J; Sternberg, AG; Eickhoff, J; Seeger, RC; Matthay, KK; Reynolds, CP; Twist, C; Krailo, M; Adamson, PC; Reisfeld, RA; Gillies,

SD; Sondel, PM. A phase I clinical trial of the hu14.18-IL2 (EMD 273063) as a treatment for children with refractory or recurrent neuroblastoma and melanoma: a study of the Children's Oncology Group. *Clin Cancer Res,* 2006 12, 1750-1759.

[85] Ozkaynak, MF; Sondel, PM; Krailo, MD; Gan, J; Javorsky, B; Reisfeld, RA; Matthay, KK; Reaman, GH; Seeger, RC. Phase I study of chimeric human/murine anti-ganglioside G(D2) monoclonal antibody (ch14.18) with granulocyte-macrophage colony-stimulating factor in children with neuroblastoma immediately after hematopoietic stem-cell transplantation: a Children's Cancer Group Study. *J Clin Oncol,* 2000 18, 4077-4085.

[86] Yu, AL, Batova, A., Gribi, R., Diccianni, M., Bridgeman, L., Geske, D., London, W., Gilman, A., Ozkaynak, F. Antibody-dependent cellular cytotoxicity (ADCC) in COG ANBL0032: A phase III randomized trial of chimeric anti-GD2 and GM-CSF/IL2 in high-risk neuroblastoma following myeloablative therapy and autologous stem cell transplant (ASCT). *Journal Clinical Oncology* (Meeting Abstract); 2004. p 22:2582.

[87] Fest, S; Huebener, N; Weixler, S; Bleeke, M; Zeng, Y; Strandsby, A; Volkmer-Engert, R; Landgraf, C; Gaedicke, G; Riemer, AB; Michalsky, E; Jaeger, IS; Preissner, R; Forster-Wald, E; Jensen-Jarolim, E; Lode, HN. Characterization of GD2 peptide mimotope DNA vaccines effective against spontaneous neuroblastoma metastases. *Cancer Res,* 2006 66, 10567-10575.

[88] Zeytin, HE; Tripathi, PK; Bhattacharya-Chatterjee, M; Foon, KA; Chatterjee, SK. Construction and characterization of DNA vaccines encoding the single-chain variable fragment of the anti-idiotype antibody 1A7 mimicking the tumor-associated antigen disialoganglioside GD2. *Cancer Gene Ther,* 2000 7, 1426-1436.

[89] Schwinger, W; Klass, V; Benesch, M; Lackner, H; Dornbusch, HJ; Sovinz, P; Moser, A; Schwantzer, G; Urban, C. Feasibility of high-dose interleukin-2 in heavily pretreated pediatric cancer patients. *Ann Oncol,* 2005 16, 1199-1206.

[90] Russell, HV; Strother, D; Mei, Z; Rill, D; Popek, E; Biagi, E; Yvon, E; Brenner, M; Rousseau, R. A phase 1/2 study of autologous neuroblastoma tumor cells genetically modified to secrete IL-2 in patients with high-risk neuroblastoma. *J Immunother,* 2008 31, 812-819.

[91] Russell, HV; Strother, D; Mei, Z; Rill, D; Popek, E; Biagi, E; Yvon, E; Brenner, M; Rousseau, R. Phase I trial of vaccination with autologous neuroblastoma tumor cells genetically modified to secrete IL-2 and lymphotactin. *J Immunother,* 2007 30, 227-233.

[92] Kowalczyk, A; Wierzbicki, A; Gil, M; Bambach, B; Kaneko, Y; Rokita, H; Repasky, E; Fenstermaker, R; Brecher, M; Ciesielski, M; Kozbor, D. Induction of protective immune responses against NXS2 neuroblastoma challenge in mice by immunotherapy with GD2 mimotope vaccine and IL-15 and IL-21 gene delivery. *Cancer Immunol Immunother,* 2007 56, 1443-1458.

[93] Uttenreuther-Fischer, MM; Kruger, JA; Fischer, P. Molecular characterization of the anti-idiotypic immune response of a relapse-free neuroblastoma patient following antibody therapy: a possible vaccine against tumors of neuroectodermal origin? *J Immunol,* 2006 176, 7775-7786.

[94] Yan, X; Johnson, BD; Orentas, RJ. Induction of a VLA-2 (CD49b)-expressing effector T cell population by a cell-based neuroblastoma vaccine expressing CD137L. *J Immunol,* 2008 181, 4621-4631.

[95] Folkman, MJ; Long, DM, Jr.; Becker, FF. Tumor growth in organ culture. *Surg Forum,* 1962 13, 81-83.

[96] Canete, A; Navarro, S; Bermudez, J; Pellin, A; Castel, V; Llombart-Bosch, A. Angiogenesis in neuroblastoma: relationship to survival and other prognostic factors in a cohort of neuroblastoma patients. *J Clin Oncol,* 2000 18, 27-34.

[97] Meitar, D; Crawford, SE; Rademaker, AW; Cohn, SL. Tumor angiogenesis correlates with metastatic disease, N-myc amplification, and poor outcome in human neuroblastoma. *J Clin Oncol,* 1996 14, 405-414.

[98] Asahara, T; Masuda, H; Takahashi, T; Kalka, C; Pastore, C; Silver, M; Kearne, M; Magner, M; Isner, JM. Bone marrow origin of endothelial progenitor cells responsible for postnatal vasculogenesis in physiological and pathological neovascularization. *Circ Res,* 1999 85, 221-228.

[99] Holash, J; Maisonpierre, PC; Compton, D; Boland, P; Alexander, CR; Zagzag, D; Yancopoulos, GD; Wiegand, SJ. Vessel cooption, regression, and growth in tumors mediated by angiopoietins and VEGF. *Science,* 1999 284, 1994-1998.

[100] Sood, AK; Fletcher, MS; Hendrix, MJ. The embryonic-like properties of aggressive human tumor cells. *J Soc Gynecol Investig,* 2002 9, 2-9.

[101] Rossler, J; Taylor, M; Geoerger, B; Farace, F; Lagodny, J; Peschka-Suss, R; Niemeyer, CM; Vassal, G. Angiogenesis as a target in neuroblastoma. *Eur J Cancer,* 2008 44, 1645-1656.

[102] Breit, S; Ashman, K; Wilting, J; Rossler, J; Hatzi, E; Fotsis, T; Schweigerer, L. The N-myc oncogene in human neuroblastoma cells: down-regulation of an angiogenesis inhibitor identified as activin A. *Cancer Res,* 2000 60, 4596-4601.

[103] Fotsis, T; Breit, S; Lutz, W; Rossler, J; Hatzi, E; Schwab, M; Schweigerer, L. Down-regulation of endothelial cell growth inhibitors by enhanced MYCN oncogene expression in human neuroblastoma cells. *Eur J Biochem,* 1999 263, 757-764.

[104] Hatzi, E; Murphy, C; Zoephel, A; Ahorn, H; Tontsch, U; Bamberger, AM; Yamauchi-Takihara, K; Schweigerer, L; Fotsis, T. N-myc oncogene overexpression down-regulates leukemia inhibitory factor in neuroblastoma. *Eur J Biochem,* 2002 269, 3732-3741.

[105] Huang, D; Rutkowski, JL; Brodeur, GM; Chou, PM; Kwiatkowski, JL; Babbo, A; Cohn, SL. Schwann cell-conditioned medium inhibits angiogenesis. *Cancer Res,* 2000 60, 5966-5971.

[106] Crawford, SE; Stellmach, V; Ranalli, M; Huang, X; Huang, L; Volpert, O; De Vries, GH; Abramson, LP; Bouck, N. Pigment epithelium-derived factor (PEDF) in neuroblastoma: a multifunctional mediator of Schwann cell antitumor activity. *J Cell Sci,* 2001 114, 4421-4428.

[107] Chlenski, A; Liu, S; Crawford, SE; Volpert, OV; DeVries, GH; Evangelista, A; Yang, Q; Salwen, HR; Farrer, R; Bray, J; Cohn, SL. SPARC is a key Schwannian-derived inhibitor controlling neuroblastoma tumor angiogenesis. *Cancer Res,* 2002 62, 7357-7363.

[108] Semenza, GL. HIF-1 and tumor progression: pathophysiology and therapeutics. *Trends Mol Med,* 2002 8, S62-67.

[109] Holmquist-Mengelbier, L; Fredlund, E; Lofstedt, T; Noguera, R; Navarro, S; Nilsson, H; Pietras, A; Vallon-Christersson, J; Borg, A; Gradin, K; Poellinger, L; Pahlman, S. Recruitment of HIF-1alpha and HIF-2alpha to common target genes is differentially

regulated in neuroblastoma: HIF-2alpha promotes an aggressive phenotype. *Cancer Cell,* 2006 10, 413-423.

[110] Pietras, A; Gisselsson, D; Ora, I; Noguera, R; Beckman, S; Navarro, S; Pahlman, S. High levels of HIF-2alpha highlight an immature neural crest-like neuroblastoma cell cohort located in a perivascular niche. *J Pathol,* 2008 214, 482-488.

[111] Folkman, J. Tumor angiogenesis: therapeutic implications. *N Engl J Med,* 1971 285, 1182-1186.

[112] Weninger, W; Rendl, M; Mildner, M; Tschachler, E. Retinoids downregulate vascular endothelial growth factor/vascular permeability factor production by normal human keratinocytes. *J Invest Dermatol,* 1998 111, 907-911.

[113] Wassberg, E; Pahlman, S; Westlin, JE; Christofferson, R. The angiogenesis inhibitor TNP-470 reduces the growth rate of human neuroblastoma in nude rats. *Pediatr Res,* 1997 41, 327-333.

[114] Kuroiwa, M; Takeuchi, T; Lee, JH; Yoshizawa, J; Hirato, J; Kaneko, S; Choi, SH; Suzuki, N; Ikeda, H; Tsuchida, Y. Continuous versus intermittent administration of human endostatin in xenografted human neuroblastoma. *J Pediatr Surg,* 2003 38, 1499-1505.

[115] Joseph, JM; Bouquet, C; Opolon, P; Morizet, J; Aubert, G; Rossler, J; Gross, N; Griscelli, F; Perricaudet, M; Vassal, G. High level of stabilized angiostatin mediated by adenovirus delivery does not impair the growth of human neuroblastoma xenografts. *Cancer Gene Ther,* 2003 10, 859-866.

[116] Yang, Q; Tian, Y; Liu, S; Zeine, R; Chlenski, A; Salwen, HR; Henkin, J; Cohn, SL. Thrombospondin-1 peptide ABT-510 combined with valproic acid is an effective antiangiogenesis strategy in neuroblastoma. *Cancer Res,* 2007 67, 1716-1724.

[117] Klement, G; Baruchel, S; Rak, J; Man, S; Clark, K; Hicklin, DJ; Bohlen, P; Kerbel, RS. Continuous low-dose therapy with vinblastine and VEGF receptor-2 antibody induces sustained tumor regression without overt toxicity. *J Clin Invest,* 2000 105, R15-24.

[118] Segerstrom, L; Fuchs, D; Backman, U; Holmquist, K; Christofferson, R; Azarbayjani, F. The anti-VEGF antibody bevacizumab potently reduces the growth rate of high-risk neuroblastoma xenografts. *Pediatr Res,* 2006 60, 576-581.

[119] Sims, TL; Williams, RF; Ng, CY; Rosati, SF; Spence, Y;Davidoff, AM. Bevacizumab suppresses neuroblastoma progression in the setting of minimal disease. *Surgery,* 2008 144, 269-275.

[120] Pastorino, F; Di Paolo, D; Piccardi, F; Nico, B; Ribatti, D; Daga, A; Baio, G; Neumaier, CE; Brignole, C; Loi, M; Marimpietri, D; Pagnan, G; Cilli, M; Lepekhin, EA; Garde, SV; Longhi, R; Corti, A; Allen, TM; Wu, JJ; Ponzoni, M. Enhanced antitumor efficacy of clinical-grade vasculature-targeted liposomal doxorubicin. *Clin Cancer Res,* 2008 14, 7320-7329.

[121] Backman, U; Svensson, A; Christofferson, RH; Azarbayjani, F. The bisphosphonate, zoledronic acid reduces experimental neuroblastoma growth by interfering with tumor angiogenesis. *Anticancer Res,* 2008 28, 1551-1557.

[122] Kaneko, S; Ishibashi, M; Kaneko, M. Vascular endothelial growth factor expression is closely related to irinotecan-mediated inhibition of tumor growth and angiogenesis in neuroblastoma xenografts. *Cancer Sci,* 2008 99, 1209-1217.

[123] Kuljaca, S; Liu, T; Tee, AE; Haber, M; Norris, MD; Dwarte, T; Marshall, GM. Enhancing the anti-angiogenic action of histone deacetylase inhibitors. *Mol Cancer,* 2007 6, 68.

[124] Hamner, JB; Dickson, PV; Sims, TL; Zhou, J; Spence, Y; Ng, CY; Davidoff, AM. Bortezomib inhibits angiogenesis and reduces tumor burden in a murine model of neuroblastoma. *Surgery,* 2007 142, 185-191.

[125] Brignole, C; Marimpietri, D; Pastorino, F; Nico, B; Di Paolo, D; Cioni, M; Piccardi, F; Cilli, M; Pezzolo, A; Corrias, MV; Pistoia, V; Ribatti, D; Pagnan, G; Ponzoni, M. Effect of bortezomib on human neuroblastoma cell growth, apoptosis, and angiogenesis. *J Natl Cancer Inst,* 2006 98, 1142-1157.

[126] Marimpietri, D; Brignole, C; Nico, B; Pastorino, F; Pezzolo, A; Piccardi, F; Cilli, M; Di Paolo, D; Pagnan, G; Longo, L; Perri, P; Ribatti, D; Ponzoni, M. Combined therapeutic effects of vinblastine and rapamycin on human neuroblastoma growth, apoptosis, and angiogenesis. *Clin Cancer Res,* 2007 13, 3977-3988.

[127] Maris, JM; Courtright, J; Houghton, PJ; Morton, CL; Gorlick, R; Kolb, EA; Lock, R; Tajbakhsh, M; Reynolds, CP; Keir, ST; Wu, J; Smith, MA. Initial testing of the VEGFR inhibitor AZD2171 by the pediatric preclinical testing program. *Pediatr Blood Cancer,* 2008 50, 581-587.

[128] Bowman, L; Grossmann, M; Rill, D; Brown, M; Zhong, WY; Alexander, B; Leimig, T; Coustan-Smith, E; Campana, D; Jenkins, J; Woods, D; Kitchingman, G; Vanin, E; Brenner, M. IL-2 adenovector-transduced autologous tumor cells induce antitumor immune responses in patients with neuroblastoma. *Blood,* 1998 92, 1941-1949.

[129] Bowman, LC; Grossmann, M; Rill, D; Brown, M; Zhong, WY; Alexander, B; Leimig, T; Coustan-Smith, E; Campana, D; Jenkins, J; Woods, D; Brenner, M. Interleukin-2 gene-modified allogeneic tumor cells for treatment of relapsed neuroblastoma. *Hum Gene Ther,* 1998 9, 1303-1311.

[130] Croce, M; Meazza, R; Orengo, AM; Fabbi, M; Borghi, M; Ribatti, D; Nico, B; Carlini, B; Pistoia, V; Corrias, MV;Ferrini, S. Immunotherapy of neuroblastoma by an Interleukin-21-secreting cell vaccine involves survivin as antigen. *Cancer Immunol Immunother,* 2008 57, 1625-1634.

[131] Pertl, U; Luster, AD; Varki, NM; Homann, D; Gaedicke, G; Reisfeld, RA; Lode, HN. IFN-gamma-inducible protein-10 is essential for the generation of a protective tumor-specific CD8 T cell response induced by single-chain IL-12 gene therapy. *J Immunol,* 2001 166, 6944-6951.

[132] Salcedo, R; Stauffer, JK; Lincoln, E; Back, TC; Hixon, JA; Hahn, C; Shafer-Weaver, K; Malyguine, A; Kastelein, R; Wigginton, JM. IL-27 mediates complete regression of orthotopic primary and metastatic murine neuroblastoma tumors: role for CD8+ T cells. *J Immunol,* 2004 173, 7170-7182.

[133] Emtage, PC; Wan, Y; Hitt, M; Graham, FL; Muller, WJ; Zlotnik, A; Gauldie, J. Adenoviral vectors expressing lymphotactin and interleukin 2 or lymphotactin and interleukin 12 synergize to facilitate tumor regression in murine breast cancer models. *Hum Gene Ther,* 1999 10, 697-709.

[134] Xia, DJ; Zhang, WP; Zheng, S; Wang, J; Pan, JP; Wang, Q; Zhang, LH; Hamada, H; Cao, X. Lymphotactin cotransfection enhances the therapeutic efficacy of dendritic cells genetically modified with melanoma antigen gp100. *Gene Ther,* 2002 9, 592-601.

[135] Rousseau, RF; Haight, AE; Hirschmann-Jax, C; Yvon, ES; Rill, DR; Mei, Z; Smith, SC; Inman, S; Cooper, K; Alcoser, P; Grilley, B; Gee, A; Popek, E; Davidoff, A; Bowman, LC; Brenner, MK; Strother, D. Local and systemic effects of an allogeneic tumor cell vaccine combining transgenic human lymphotactin with interleukin-2 in patients with advanced or refractory neuroblastoma. *Blood,* 2003 101, 1718-1726.

[136] Park, JR; Digiusto, DL; Slovak, M; Wright, C; Naranjo, A; Wagner, J; Meechoovet, HB; Bautista, C; Chang, WC; Ostberg, JR; Jensen, MC. Adoptive transfer of chimeric antigen receptor re-directed cytolytic T lymphocyte clones in patients with neuroblastoma. *Mol Ther,* 2007 15, 825-833.

[137] Hartmann, G; Weeratna, RD; Ballas, ZK; Payette, P; Blackwell, S; Suparto, I; Rasmussen, WL; Waldschmidt, M; Sajuthi, D; Purcell, RH; Davis, HL; Krieg, AM. Delineation of a CpG phosphorothioate oligodeoxynucleotide for activating primate immune responses in vitro and in vivo. *J Immunol,* 2000 164, 1617-1624.

[138] Tamm, I; Dorken, B; Hartmann, G. Antisense therapy in oncology: new hope for an old idea? *Lancet,* 2001 358, 489-497.

[139] Gokhale, PC; Soldatenkov, V; Wang, FH; Rahman, A; Dritschilo, A; Kasid, U. Antisense raf oligodeoxyribonucleotide is protected by liposomal encapsulation and inhibits Raf-1 protein expression in vitro and in vivo: implication for gene therapy of radioresistant cancer. *Gene Ther,* 1997 4, 1289-1299.

[140] Gutierrez-Puente, Y; Tari, AM; Stephens, C; Rosenblum, M; Guerra, RT; Lopez-Berestein, G. Safety, pharmacokinetics, and tissue distribution of liposomal P-ethoxy antisense oligonucleotides targeted to Bcl-2. *J Pharmacol Exp Ther,* 1999 291, 865-869.

[141] Pastorino, F; Brignole, C; Marimpietri, D; Pagnan, G; Morando, A; Ribatti, D; Semple, SC; Gambini, C; Allen, TM; Ponzoni, M. Targeted liposomal c-myc antisense oligodeoxynucleotides induce apoptosis and inhibit tumor growth and metastases in human melanoma models. *Clin Cancer Res,* 2003 9, 4595-4605.

[142] Stuart, DD; Kao, GY; Allen, TM. A novel, long-circulating, and functional liposomal formulation of antisense oligodeoxynucleotides targeted against MDR1. *Cancer Gene Ther,* 2000 7, 466-475.

[143] Weiss, WA; Aldape, K; Mohapatra, G; Feuerstein, BG; Bishop, JM. Targeted expression of MYCN causes neuroblastoma in transgenic mice. *EMBO J,* 1997 16, 2985-2995.

[144] Griffin, CA; Baylin, SB. Expression of the c-myb oncogene in human small cell lung carcinoma. *Cancer Res,* 1985 45, 272-275.

[145] Raschella, G; Negroni, A; Skorski, T; Pucci, S; Nieborowska-Skorska, M; Romeo, A; Calabretta, B. Inhibition of proliferation by c-myb antisense RNA and oligodeoxynucleotides in transformed neuroectodermal cell lines. *Cancer Res,* 1992 52, 4221-4226.

[146] Brignole, C; Pastorino, F; Marimpietri, D; Pagnan, G; Pistorio, A; Allen, TM; Pistoia, V; Ponzoni, M. Immune cell-mediated antitumor activities of GD2-targeted liposomal c-myb antisense oligonucleotides containing CpG motifs. *J Natl Cancer Inst,* 2004 96, 1171-1180.

[147] Pagnan, G; Stuart, DD; Pastorino, F; Raffaghello, L; Montaldo, PG; Allen, TM; Calabretta, B; Ponzoni, M. Delivery of c-myb antisense oligodeoxynucleotides to

human neuroblastoma cells via disialoganglioside GD(2)-targeted immunoliposomes: antitumor effects. *J Natl Cancer Inst,* 2000 92, 253-261.

[148] Khan, J; Wei, JS; Ringner, M; Saal, LH; Ladanyi, M; Westermann, F; Berthold, F; Schwab, M; Antonescu, CR; Peterson, C; Meltzer, PS. Classification and diagnostic prediction of cancers using gene expression profiling and artificial neural networks. *Nat Med,* 2001 7, 673-679.

[149] Yamanaka, Y; Hamazaki, Y; Sato, Y; Ito, K; Watanabe, K; Heike, T; Nakahata, T; Nakamura, Y. Maturational sequence of neuroblastoma revealed by molecular analysis on cDNA microarrays. *Int J Oncol,* 2002 21, 803-807.

[150] Albino, D; Scaruffi, P; Moretti, S; Coco, S; Truini, M; Di Cristofano, C; Cavazzana, A; Stigliani, S; Bonassi, S; Tonini, GP. Identification of low intratumoral gene expression heterogeneity in neuroblastic tumors by genome-wide expression analysis and game theory. *Cancer,* 2008 113, 1412-1422.

[151] Berwanger, B; Hartmann, O; Bergmann, E; Bernard, S; Nielsen, D; Krause, M; Kartal, A; Flynn, D; Wiedemeyer, R; Schwab, M; Schafer, H; Christiansen, H; Eilers, M. Loss of a FYN-regulated differentiation and growth arrest pathway in advanced stage neuroblastoma. *Cancer Cell,* 2002 2, 377-386.

[152] Takita, J; Ishii, M; Tsutsumi, S; Tanaka, Y; Kato, K; Toyoda, Y; Hanada, R; Yamamoto, K; Hayashi, Y; Aburatani, H. Gene expression profiling and identification of novel prognostic marker genes in neuroblastoma. *Genes Chromosomes Cancer,* 2004 40, 120-132.

[153] Hiyama, E; Hiyama, K; Yamaoka, H; Sueda, T; Reynolds, CP;Yokoyama, T. Expression profiling of favorable and unfavorable neuroblastomas. *Pediatr Surg Int,* 2004 20, 33-38.

[154] McArdle, L; McDermott, M; Purcell, R; Grehan, D; O'Meara, A; Breatnach, F; Catchpoole, D; Culhane, AC; Jeffery, I; Gallagher, WM; Stallings, RL. Oligonucleotide microarray analysis of gene expression in neuroblastoma displaying loss of chromosome 11q. *Carcinogenesis,* 2004 25, 1599-1609.

[155] Janoueix-Lerosey, I; Novikov, E; Monteiro, M; Gruel, N; Schleiermacher, G; Loriod, B; Nguyen, C; Delattre, O. Gene expression profiling of 1p35-36 genes in neuroblastoma. *Oncogene,* 2004 23, 5912-5922.

[156] Alaminos, M; Mora, J; Cheung, NK; Smith, A; Qin, J; Chen, L;Gerald, WL. Genome-wide analysis of gene expression associated with MYCN in human neuroblastoma. *Cancer Res,* 2003 63, 4538-4546.

[157] Fischer, M; Oberthuer, A; Brors, B; Kahlert, Y; Skowron, M; Voth, H; Warnat, P; Ernestus, K; Hero, B; Berthold, F. Differential expression of neuronal genes defines subtypes of disseminated neuroblastoma with favorable and unfavorable outcome. *Clin Cancer Res,* 2006 12, 5118-5128.

[158] Wang, Q; Diskin, S; Rappaport, E; Attiyeh, E; Mosse, Y; Shue, D; Seiser, E; Jagannathan, J; Shusterman, S; Bansal, M; Khazi, D; Winter, C; Okawa, E; Grant, G; Cnaan, A; Zhao, H; Cheung, NK; Gerald, W; London, W; Matthay, KK; Brodeur, GM; Maris, JM. Integrative genomics identifies distinct molecular classes of neuroblastoma and shows that multiple genes are targeted by regional alterations in DNA copy number. *Cancer Res,* 2006 66, 6050-6062.

[159] Oberthuer, A; Berthold, F; Warnat, P; Hero, B; Kahlert, Y; Spitz, R; Ernestus, K; Konig, R; Haas, S; Eils, R; Schwab, M; Brors, B; Westermann, F;Fischer, M.

Customized oligonucleotide microarray gene expression-based classification of neuroblastoma patients outperforms current clinical risk stratification. *J Clin Oncol,* 2006 24, 5070-5078.

[160] Cheung, IY; Feng, Y; Gerald, W; Cheung, NK. Exploiting gene expression profiling to identify novel minimal residual disease markers of neuroblastoma. *Clin Cancer Res,* 2008 14, 7020-7027.

[161] Wei, JS; Greer, BT; Westermann, F; Steinberg, SM; Son, CG; Chen, QR; Whiteford, CC; Bilke, S; Krasnoselsky, AL; Cenacchi, N; Catchpoole, D; Berthold, F; Schwab, M; Khan, J. Prediction of clinical outcome using gene expression profiling and artificial neural networks for patients with neuroblastoma. *Cancer Res,* 2004 64, 6883-6891.

[162] Ohira, M; Oba, S; Nakamura, Y; Isogai, E; Kaneko, S; Nakagawa, A; Hirata, T; Kubo, H; Goto, T; Yamada, S; Yoshida, Y; Fuchioka, M; Ishii, S;Nakagawara, A. Expression profiling using a tumor-specific cDNA microarray predicts the prognosis of intermediate risk neuroblastomas. *Cancer Cell,* 2005 7, 337-350.

[163] Ohira, M; Oba, S; Nakamura, Y; Hirata, T; Ishii, S; Nakagawara, A. A review of DNA microarray analysis of human neuroblastomas. *Cancer Lett,* 2005 228, 5-11.

[164] Schramm, A; Vandesompele, J; Schulte, JH; Dreesmann, S; Kaderali, L; Brors, B; Eils, R; Speleman, F; Eggert, A. Translating expression profiling into a clinically feasible test to predict neuroblastoma outcome. *Clin Cancer Res,* 2007 13, 1459-1465.

[165] Yuza, Y; Agawa, M; Matsuzaki, M; Yamada, H; Urashima, M. Gene and protein expression profiling during differentiation of neuroblastoma cells triggered by 13-cis retinoic acid. *J Pediatr Hematol Oncol,* 2003 25, 715-720.

[166] Vitali, R; Mancini, C; Cesi, V; Tanno, B; Mancuso, M; Bossi, G; Zhang, Y; Martinez, RV; Calabretta, B; Dominici, C; Raschella, G. Slug (SNAI2) down-regulation by RNA interference facilitates apoptosis and inhibits invasive growth in neuroblastoma preclinical models. *Clin Cancer Res,* 2008 14, 4622-4630.

[167] Abe, M; Westermann, F; Nakagawara, A; Takato, T; Schwab, M; Ushijima, T. Marked and independent prognostic significance of the CpG island methylator phenotype in neuroblastomas. *Cancer Lett,* 2007 247, 253-258.

In: New Approaches in the Treatment of Cancer
Editors: Carmen Mejia Vazquez et al. pp.71-89
ISBN 978-1-62100-067-9

Chapter IV

THE ROLE OF PLANT LECTINS IN CANCER TREATMENT

Roberto A. Ferriz-Martinez[1], Iovanna C. Torres-Arteaga[1], Alejandro Blanco-Labra[2] and Teresa Garcia-Gasca[1,*]

[1]Universidad Autónoma de Querétaro, Querétaro, México
[2]Centro de Investigación y Estudios Avanzados del Instituto Politécnico Nacional, Unidad Irapuato, Gto., México

ABSTRACT

Social behavior of cells depends on membrane glycosylation, including cell communication, adhesion and migration. Malignant transformation is associated with alterations in cell surface carbohydrates expression, which suggests that such molecules play an important role in malignant transformation. Plant lectins are oligomeric proteins lacking enzymatic activity and are distinct from immunoglobulins. They can have several carbohydrate-binding sites per molecule that allow them to specifically interact with other carbohydrate moieties, hence the name lectin (from the Latin *legere*, to select or choose). Lectins are commonly used in biochemistry, cell biology and immunology, as well as for diagnostic and therapeutic purposes in cancer investigation. They are important tools for investigating structural and functional complex carbohydrates, for the evaluation of changes that occur in the cell surface during physiological and pathological processes and for the identification of cancer cells. Because of the ability of lectins to recognize cancer cells as well as for their cytotoxic activity against them, the role of plant lectins as anticancer agents is discussed.

* Correspondence concerning this article should be addressed to: Teresa Garcia-Gasca. Facultad de Ciencias Naturales. Universidad Autónoma de Querétaro. Av. de las Ciencias s/n. C.P. 76230, Querétaro, México. Tel. (+52442) 1921200 ext 5308; Fax (+52442) 2342958. E-mail: tggasca@gmail.com

INTRODUCTION

Lectins are proteins or glycoproteins from non-immune origin that specifically recognize cell surface molecules with at least two binding sites to carbohydrates (hence their ability to agglutinate cells), precipitating the corresponding glycoconjugates. They are found in all kinds of organisms, including animals, plants, fungi, bacteria and viruses [1, 2]. Lectins have no single action and a wide spectrum of functions has been related to them (Figure 1). Their relative abundance is not necessarily related to the importance of their function [3].

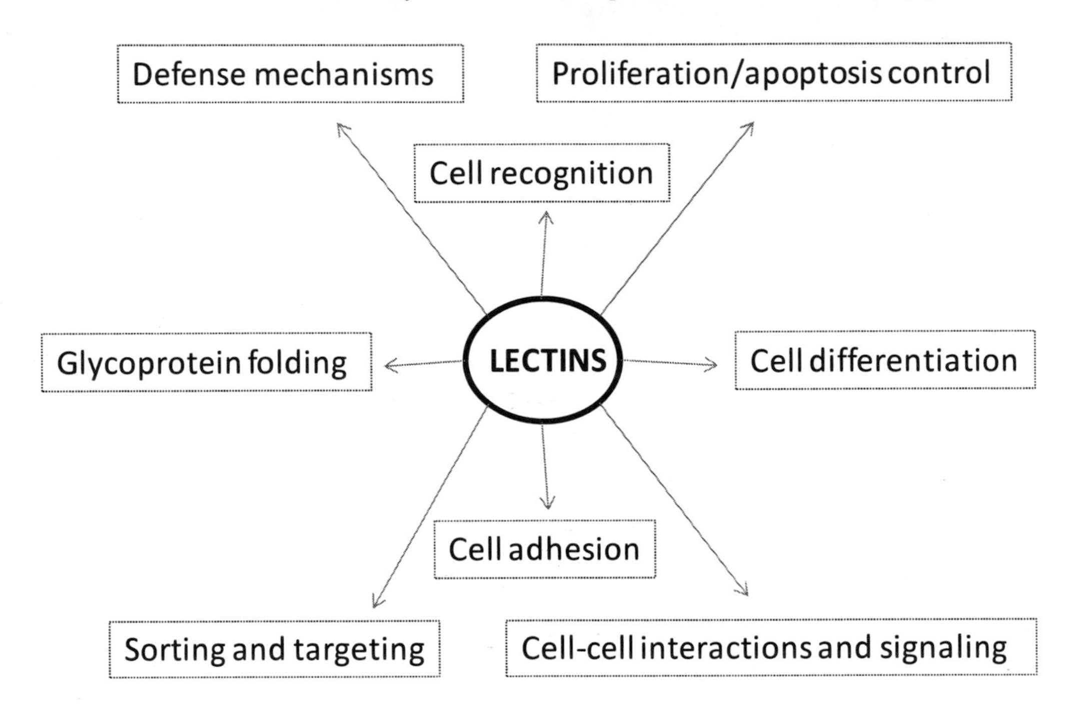

Figure 1. Some biological functions of lectins in live organisms [3,4].

Plant lectins can be defined as all plant proteins possessing at least one non-catalytic domain, which binds reversibly to a specific mono- or oligosaccharide [5]. Classification of plant lectins is based on different criteria. On the basis of the overall structure of the mature lectins they can be divided in four groups (Table 1) but analysis of the available sequences distinguishes seven families of evolutionary related proteins (Table 2). Some lectins, however, do not fit the classification system or cannot be classified because there is no sequence information available [6].

The main source of lectins in the human diet is found in plants. Lectins are mainly present in seeds cotyledons and kernels where they represent 2 to 10% of the total protein. It is suggested that, within the plant, these proteins may have different functions such as: physiological regulation, defense against microorganisms attack, storage protein, carbohydrate transport, mitogenic stimulation, recognition of the nitrogen-fixing bacteria of *Rhizobium* genus, and some more. Plant lectins represent a unique group of proteins with potent biological activity. They occur in foods like wheat, corn, tomato, peanut, kidney bean, banana, pea, lentil, soybean, mushroom, rice, and potato. Many lectins resist digestion, survive gut passage, and bind to gastrointestinal cells and/or enter the circulation intact, maintaining full biological activity including specific agglutination of lymphocytes, erythrocytes, spermatozoa, platelets, bacteria and tumor cells, induction of mitosis or cytotoxic effects on lymphocytes. Once they are consumed, different biological properties are observed at biochemical and molecular level. Binding between lectins and surface cell molecules or internalization into cells involve a wide variety of signals that are important for cell regulation, including [7, 8]:

1) Cell agglutination and/or aggregation.
2) Induction of apoptosis or cell cycle arrest.
3) Down regulation of telomerase activity and inhibition of angiogenesis.
4) Increase of drug sensitivity of tumor cells, hence their utility in the design of immunotoxins for cancer treatment.
5) Direct effects on the immune system by altering the production of various interleukins, or by activating certain protein kinases.
6) Ingestion of lectins also sequesters the available body pool of polyamines, thereby thwarting cancer cell growth.
7) Some lectins can bind to ribosomes, inhibiting protein synthesis.

Due to their ability to bind reversibly with specific carbohydrate structures, lectins have commonly been used as molecular tools in several disciplines of biology and medicine. Lectin affinity chromatography (LAC) and various histochemical methods, provide practical applications for the observation of changes occurring at the cell membrane in different stages of physiological and pathological development of human or animal organisms [9].

Table 1. Plant lectins classification based on mature lectin structure

Lectin type	Definition
Merolectins	Single carbohydrate-binding domain, they are monovalent and hence cannot precipitate in glycoconjugates or agglutinate cells.
Hololectins	Contain at least two carbohydrate-binding domains that are either identical or very homologous and bind either the same or structurally similar sugars. They are di- or multivalent and hence agglutinate cells and/or precipitate glyco-conjugates.
Chimerolectins	They are fusion proteins consisting of one or more carbohydrate-binding domains and a well-defined enzymatic domain or another biological activity that act independently from the carbohydrate-binding domain. Depending on the number of carbohydrate-binding sites, chimerolectins behave as merolectins or as hololectins.
Superlectins	Consist of at least two carbohydrate-binding domains that recognize structurally unrelated sugars. They can also be considered a special group of chimerolectins.

Adapted from [6].

Table 2. Plant lectins classification based on molecular structure

Lectin group	Definition
Legume lectins	Plant lectins that are found exclusively in the *Leguminoseae,* but not all lectins found in legume species belong to the legume lectins. All legume lectins are built up of protomers of approximately 30 kDa that give rise to the so-called 'one-chain' legume lectins. In some instances the protomers are cleaved into two smaller polypeptides. The legume lectins composed of such cleaved protomers are usually referred to as 'two chain' legume lectins. Legume lectins contain divalent cations (Mn^{2+} or Ca^{2+}) at specific metal-binding sites which are essential for the carbohydrate-binding activity. Many, but not all, legume lectins are glycosylated and possess one or two glycan chains of high-mannose or complex type that may be present on a single lectin protomer. Differences in glycosylation result in the formation of glycoforms, which can mistakenly be considered as isolectins. Native legume lectins are composed of two or four protomers held together by noncovalent interactions. The possible combinations imply that legume lectins can occur in eight different molecular forms.
Chitin-binding lectins	This family comprises all proteins containing at least one hevein domain (small 43 amino acid protein from the latex of the rubber tree, *Hevea brasiliensis*) but there are also chitin-binding lectins without hevein domains. The family of chitin-binding lectins comprises merolectins, hololectins, as well as different types of chimerolectins.
Type 2 RIP and related lectins	Ribosome-inactivating proteins (RIP) are commonly known as proteins that catalytically inactivate eukaryotic ribosomes, as a result, protein synthesis is arrested and the cell dies. All type 2 RIP are built up of similar protomers consisting of disulfide bridge linked A and B chains. The A chain (25 to 30 kDa) possesses *N*-glycosidase activity, whereas the B chain (30 to 35 kDa) has one or more carbohydrate-binding sites. Because the A chain of type 2 RIP shares a high sequence similarity with type 1 RIP, type 2 RIP are considered as chimerolectins composed of a RIP subunit and a lectin subunit. Native type 2 RIP consist of one or two, and, in a few exceptional cases, four identical [A-s-s-B]-pairs. Because the [A-s-s-B]-pair is a single structural unit, type 2 RIP consisting of one, two, and four [A-s-s-B]-pairs are considered as monomeric, dimeric, and tetrameric proteins, respectively.
Monocot mannose-binding lectins	Super families of strictly mannose-specific lectins, which have been found exclusively in a subgroup of the monocotyledonous plants, consist of subunits with a similar sequence and overall three-dimensional structure. According to the size of the protomers, these lectins can be divided into one-domain protomers of 11 to 14 kDa and two-domain protomers of about 30 kDa.
Jacalin-related lectins	Jacalin is the trivial name for the lectin from the seeds of jack fruit (*Artocarpus integrifolia*). All lectins that are structurally and evolutionary related to the jack fruit lectin belong to this group that comprises two subgroups of lectins. A first subgroup is the GalNAcspecific *Moraceae* seed lectins, which are very similar to the jack fruit lectin. The second subgroup is the *Convolvulaceae* lectins, which share sequence similarity with the *Moraceae* lectins but exhibit specificity toward mannose/maltose.
Amatanthin lectin family	The term amaranthin, from the seed lectin of *Amaranthus caudatus,* is now used as a collective name for the closely related GalNAc-specific seed lectins from various *Amaranthus* species. The amaranthins are not related to any other lectin family. Detailed specificity studies have been performed only with the *Amaranthus caudatus* lectin. The lectin is inhibited by GalNAc but has a much higher affinity for the disaccharide Galb(1,3)GalNAc.
***Cucurbitaceae* phloem lectins**	Small family of chitin-binding agglutinins found in the phloem exudates of *Cucurbitaceae* species. They are not related to other *Cucurbitaceae* lectins and do not contain the vein domains. The *Cucurbitaceae* phloem lectins exhibit specificity toward oligomers of GlcNAc.
No classified lectins	Plant families in which lectins occur that, in the absence of clear criteria, have not been classified: *Apiaceae, Araucariaceae, Celastraceae, Cucurbitaceae, Euphorbiaceae, Gramineae, Labiatae*

Adapted from [6].

Cell Membrane Glycosylation and Lectins: The Key of Selectivity

Tumor cells display aberrant patterns of glycosylation in carbohydrates linked to ceramides and cell surface proteins [10, 11, 12]. Alterations on membrane glycosylation are present in all cancer cells and some of them are well known as progression markers. Each type of cancer presents differential alteration patterns even during the different stages of the disease [13]. Two major glycosylation changes have been described in cancer cells: blockage of carbohydrate synthesis or neo synthesis [11]. Glycosylation alterations that occur in cancer cells may involve loss or changes in function of certain structures, presence of truncated structures or their precursors and, to a lesser extent, the appearance of new structures. Carbohydrates expressed in tumor cells are either adhesion molecules *per se* or modulate adhesion receptor functions. Among the more common changes are the increase of N-glycans and sialic acid content in the cell surface, the abnormal production of mucin, expression of Lewis X/A structures in glycosphingolipids (identified at first as a tumor antigen), and the increased expression of galectins (Figure 2). All these changes correlate with the ability of metastatic cancer cells and/or the increase in migration and their ability to evade the immune system [10,14]. In some cases membrane glycoproteins are also modified, so that they act as oncogenic antigens. Several lines of evidence accumulated in recent years implicate tumor cell lectins in cellular interactions such as adhesion, cell growth, tumor cell differentiation, and metastasis. The involvement of lectins in processes such as cell–cell and host–pathogen interactions, serum-glycoprotein turnover and innate immune responses are of particular relevance to tumor growth and metastatic spread [13].

Changes in glycosylation involve not only interactions with endogenous, but also with exogenous lectins, that can alter the response of cancer cells. The knowledge of the interaction of lectins with cancer cells and how they can affect the biology of the tumor will explain the role of carbohydrates in the acquisition of malignant status and therefore its inhibition [13]. The study of lectins as biological tools has led to the conclusion that their main significance lies in their properties in cell recognition (i.e. red blood cells, lymphocytes, platelets, sperm, bacteria, viruses and tumor cells) [7]. Several studies have focused on their ability to show preferential agglutination on cancer cells [16] therefore, one important area where lectins are used is in the detection of malignant changes in transformed cells due to the changes on cancer cells surface [7, 14, 17]. Higher affinity has been observed between human cancer cells and lectins, than between healthy cells and the same lectins [18]. Evidence of this is shown in the selective binding of plant lectins, such as Concanavalin A (ConA) and the wheat germ agglutinin (WGA) to tumor cells [13]. The link between membrane glycoproteins and lectins is weak, but a stronger one is formed by multiple binding sites of a lot weak joints. Through this mechanism, lectins can induce apoptosis, cytotoxicity, and inhibition of tumor growth [8, 17]. Selective binding of lectins to specific carbohydrates allows them to be used as diagnostic tools, some examples of differential recognition are:

- Mistletoe lectins, (MLs, ML-I, ML-II, and ML-III) in which the binding of the B-chain to carbohydrates inhibit their toxic activities. Digalactosides Gal-β-1,2Gal-β-allyl and Gal-β-1,3Gal-β-allyl were 60 and 30 times, respectively, more potent than D-galactose, protecting the cells from ML-I cytotoxicity. GalNAc and nitrophenyl galNAc protected mostly from the effects of ML-II and ML-III. The serum glycoproteins haptoglobin, 1-acid glycoprotein, and transferrin notably inhibited the toxicity of the lectins but deglycosylated haptoglobin had no protective activity on the Molt 4 cells [19].

- The potential and the applicability of different plant lectins using 5637 bladder cancer cells as a model for human urinary carcinoma were studied. As a result, wheat germ agglutinin (WGA) and *Ulex europaeus* agglutinin (UEA) revealed strongest interaction with single cells demonstrating a high presence of N-acetyl-d-glucosamine, sialic acid and α-l-fucose residues on the membrane surface [20].
- *Griffonia simplicifolia* lectin-I (GS-I) and *Vicia vilosa* agglutinin (VVA) showed significant associations with nuclear grade of ductal carcinoma in situ (DCIS). DCIS specimens with nuclear grades II and III showed significantly more intense reactivity than DCIS cases with nuclear grade I to GS-1 and VVA. Those results suggest that the expression of VVA- and GS-I-reactive carbohydrate antigens may contribute to forming higher grade DCIS and increase the recurrence risk [21].
- Different fluorescence labeled lectins: DBA (*Dolichos biflorus*) PNA, LCA (*Lens culinaris*), STL (*Solanum tuberosum*), UEA-I (*Ulex europaeus* I), and WGA showed binding specificity on three cell lines of human colorectal carcinoma (CaCo-2, HT-29 and HCT-8) [22].
- Bioadhesive properties of fluorescein-labeled plant lectins with different carbohydrate specificities, investigated by flow cytometry at 4 and 37°C using Du-145 prostate cancer cells. At both temperatures lectin association rate increased following the order: *Dolichos biflorus* agglutinin (DBA) peanut agglutinin, Ulex *europaeus* isoagglutinin I, *Lens culinaris* agglutinin, *Solanum tuberosum* lectin, wheat germ agglutinin (WGA), reflecting the glycosylation pattern of Du-145 cells [23]
- ABL (*Agaricus bisporus*) lectin specifically binds to a galactosilated disaccharide expressed in keratinocytes and this lectin reversibly inhibits proliferation of cancer cell lines without cytotoxicity [24].
- Comparative analysis of glycoproteins patterns from human melanoma cells using different lectins (SNA: *Sambucus nigra*, MAA: *Maackia amurensis* and PHA: *Phaseolus vulgaris*) suggest an increased expression of branching N-oligosaccharides in human melanoma from metastatic sites. It suggests that carbohydrates are associated with the acquisition of the metastatic potential of tumor cells [25].
- Peanut agglutinin lectin (PNA) binds the Thomsen–Friedenreich (TF) oncofetal carbohydrate antigen that is increased in colon cancer, adenomas, and inflammatory bowel disease. However, PNA has a mitogenic effect, both *in vitro* and *in vivo*, for colon epithelial cancer cells mediated by phosphorylation of c-Met and MAPK [26].
- Lymphatic invasion, lymph node metastasis, and peritoneal metastasis correlated with staining with lectins that bind galactose/N-acetylgalactosamine residues (Gal/GalNAc) such as Maclurapomifera (MPA), Arachishypogaea (PNA), Helixpomatia (HPA), and Viciavillosa (VVA). In contrast, hepatic metastasis correlated with staining with *Anguilla anguilla* lectin (AAA), anti-LewisX (LEX-2), anti-sialyl Lewisa (NS19-9), andanti-sialyl-dimeric LewisX (FH-6) MAbs, all of which bind preferentially to fucosylated carbohydrate chains. The five-year survival

rate of patients was related to the staining of cancers with MPA, HPA, FH-6 or NS19-9, and MPA and FH-6 staining were in dependent prognostic factors. Carbohydrate expression profiles of cancer cells are relevant to the route of tumor cell dissemination, metastatic pattern as well as prognosis of colorectal cancer [27].

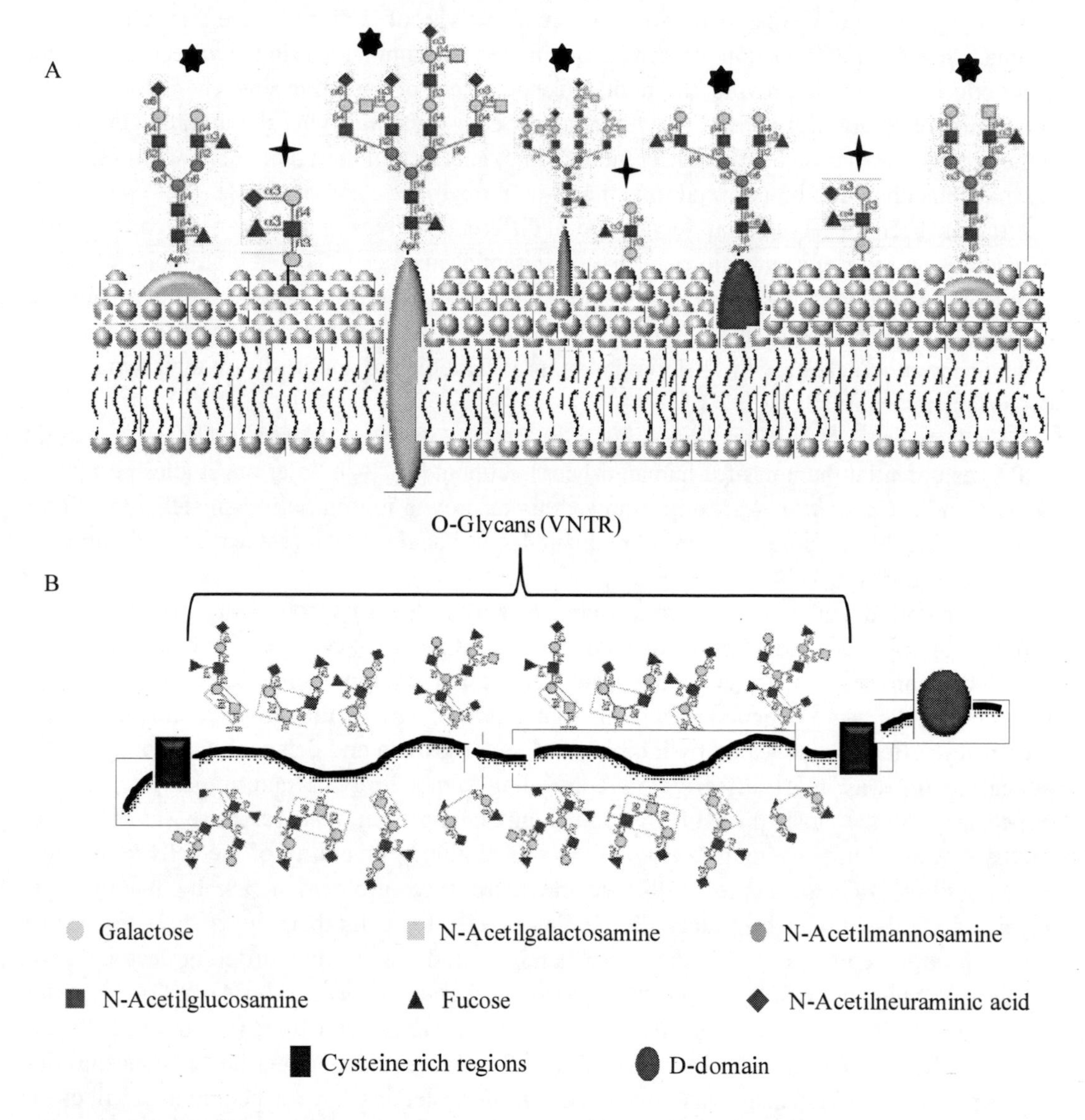

Figure 2. Simplified structure of cell oligosaccharides. (A) Glycoproteins and glycolipids of cell membrane with (✱)N-glycan structures and (✦)Type-1 and -2 Lewis determinants. (B) O-GalNAc glycans on a simplified model of mucin. The VNTR (variable number of tandem repeat) region rich in serine, threonine, and proline is highly O-glycosylated and the peptide assumes an extended "bottle brush" conformation. Hundreds of O-GalNAc glycans with many different structures may be attached to serine or threonine residues in the VNTR domains. The cysteine-rich regions at the ends of the molecules are involved in disulfide bond formation to form large polymers of several million daltons. D domains are also involved in polymerization [15].

LECTINS AS ANTICANCER AGENTS

Lectins have anticancer properties *in vitro* and *in vivo*, preferentially binding to cancer cell membranes or their receptors, causing cytotoxicity, apoptosis, and inhibition of tumor growth [8]. Antitumor effect and anticarcinogenic activity of lectins are due through different mechanisms as the induction of remission in certain tumors, having a direct anti-tumor cytotoxic effect, by improving the antineoplastic effect of radiation and chemotherapy, by promoting restoration of normal growth in cancer cells, by amplifying the immunogenicity of tumor cells and because of their differential cytotoxic effect on malignant cells with respect to normal cells, they exhibit minimal risk of anti-tumor cytotoxic activity [28].

It has been observed that lectins from different sources inhibit cancer cells growth depending on their concentration and in a differential manner [29]. They are able to induce apoptosis and activate the immune system by stimulating the proliferation of T lymphocytes [30] and also food lectins can stimulate differentiation of colon cancer cells [31]. The ability of lectins to modulate growth, differentiation, proliferation and apoptosis are mainly mediated by surface receptors [32].

First studies had focused on cytotoxic properties of lectins like ricin (RCA) and abrin (APA) as potential therapies for human cancer treatment [33, 34]. Later on, studies performed using Con A (*Canavalia ensiformis*) showed tumor growth inhibition in hamsters [35]. Some studies using either pure or semi-pure plant lectins against different cancer cell lines or tumors are shown in Table 3.

Comparative studies using several lectins as antitumoral or cytotoxic agents have shown differential effect depending on lectin source and cell line or cancer type. For example, lectins from common bean, soybean, and wheat were tested on lymphoma cells. After *in vitro* treatment, cells were inoculated into normal animals. All lectins were found to possess therapeutic effects, as revealed by inhibition of tumor growth and delayed tumor progression. Wheat lectin was most effective in controlling tumor growth and improving the life expectancy of the host, probably by activating the host immune response (macrophages increased three-fold). Although cell viability was retained, the ability of the cells to multiply was possibly affected. Tumor cells become more susceptible to attack by macrophage-mediated cytolysis, which induces the binding of effector cells that trigger the non-specific lysis of target cells [93]. On the other hand, a study with five different lectins: PHA (*Phaseolus vulgaris*) GSA (*Griffonia simplicifolia*) Con-A (*Concavalina A*), WGA (*Triticum vulgare*) and PNA (*Arachis hypogea*) on three colon cancer cell lines (Lovo, HCT-15 and SW837) showed that growth was affected in different ways depending on the concentration and type of lectin tested. It was concluded that these lectins have a potential to affect the growth of cancerous colonies *in vitro* [94]. Lectin from common bean (*Phaseolus vulgaris*) has mitogenic action on immune system cells and has the ability to specifically agglutinate malignant cells. This has developed a strong interest in research to use it as a treatment for tumor growth control [95].

Table 3. Cytotoxic and anticancer effects of some plant and mushroom lectins

Lectins or lectins extracts	Effects	Ref
AAL *Agrocybe aegerita*	Antitumoral effect via apoptosis with DNAase activity. Growth inhibition on HeLa, SW480, SCG-7901, MGC80-3, BGC-823, HL-60 cells and murine S-180 sarcoma.	[36]
ABL *Algaricus bisporus*	Cell proliferation inhibition on HT29 cells. Internalization and blockage NLS dependent nuclear channels.	[37, 38]
	Internalization, proliferation inhibition and blockage of nuclear proteins importation.	[39]
Abrin-a	Cytoagglutination against human cultured cell lines derived from acute lymphoblastic leukemia and adult T-cell leukemia, weak agglutination against normal lymphocytes.	[40]
Abrin	Antitumoral effects on transplanted mice.	[41]
AHL *Arisaema helleborifolium*	Inhibits proliferation of human cancer cell lines HOP-62 (95%), HCT-15 (92%), HEP-2 (66%), HT-29 (68%), PC-3 (39.4%), and A-549 (20.7%).	[42]
Alocasia cucullata	Inhibition of SiHa (human cervix) cancer cell line.	[43]
ATL (*Arisaema tortuosum*)	*In vitro* proliferation inhibition of human cancer cell lines HT29, SiHa and OVCAR-5.	[44]
DSA (*Datura stramonium*)	Irreversible differentiation induction on glioma C6 cells, dose-dependent proliferation inhibition and DNA synthesis suppression. Recognition between astrocitic and neuronal glycoreceptors.	[45]
GS-1 (*Griffonia simplicifolia*)	Tumoral growth inhibition in mice, cytotoxic effect.	[46, 47]
Iscador M (*Viscum album*)	Increase in life span, reduction in tumor growth, and hyperplasia of mice and rats with lymphoma and lung cancer.	[48]
Iscador M special, Iscador Qu special, and Iscador P. Aqueous mistletoe extracts (*Viscum album*)	Preparations containing high lectin concentration showed antitumor activity in the mammary cancer cell line MAXF 401NL. Apoptosis and cytotoxicity were positively correlated at low and intermediate concentrations, and the effects observed in long intervals and high concentrations of the lectin were mostly necrotic. Proliferation inhibition on 16 tumor cell lines.	[49]
Isorel Mistletoe extract (*Viscum album*)	Stimulation of immune system, protein synthesis inhibition in various malignant cell lines. Almost complete inhibition of tumor growth, increase of apoptosis and necrosis, and reduction in mitosis was apparent only for tumors in the vicinity of the tumor exposed to mistletoe. Reduction of lung metastases. Local and systemic effects.	[50]
	Prolonged survival time and a reduction in the number of tumor colonies. Histology revealed an increase of apoptosis and necrosis in the tumors, while a reduction in mitosis was noticed only for the tumors in the vicinity of the tumor exposed to Isorel. Immunomodulation combined with tumor growth inhibition and a reduction in metastasis was observed.	[51]
KM-110 Extract from korean mistletoe (*Viscum album* var. coloratum)	Inhibition of lung metastasis of melanoma and colon cells. Liver and spleen metastasis of lymphoma cells by various administration routes (subcutaneous, oral, intranasal and intravenous) was dose-dependent. Stimulation of host defense system and NK cell activation.	[52]
KML-C Korean mistletoe lectin (*Viscum album* var. coloratum)	Stimulation of immune system, NK cells and macrophages activation.	[53]
Kurokawa mushroom (*Boletopsis leucomelas*)	Inhibition of proliferation of human monoblastic leukemia U937 dose-dependently due to apoptosis induction.	[54]
Mesquite seed lectin (*Prosopis*)	Antiproliferative effect on cervical human tumor cells (HeLa) but no effect on normal cells.	[55]

Table 3. (Continued)

Lectins or lectins extracts	Effects	Ref
ML Mistletoe lectin (*Viscum album*)	Antitumor activity by cytotoxicity. Bladder carcinoma was reduced, and survival times were prolonged in mice as a function of concentration.	[56]
	Growth-inhibition on HeLa-S3, Molt-4, MFM-223, COR-L51, KPL-1 and VM-CUB1 tumor cell lines	[57]
	Blocks the growth of bladder carcinoma cells.	[58]
ML-I Mistletoe lectin (*Viscum album*)	Apoptosis induction on leukemic T and B cell lines. Ribosomal inactivation.	[59]
	Reduction of tumor growth of a murine non-Hodgkin lymphoma.	[60]
	Reduced mitotic activity of murine non-Hodgkin lymphoma tumors, lower degree of mitotic activity, CD3 cells infiltration in tumors, apoptotic bodies, poorly developed blood supply, and reduction in tumor weight.	[61]
ML II Mistletoe lectin (*Viscum album*)	Strong inducer of pro-oxidants that mediate the activation of caspase-9 and caspase 3-like proteases, apoptotic death of human myeloleukemic U937 cells.	[62]
ML-I and ML-III Mistletoe lectins (*Viscum album*)	Differential induction of apoptosis on leukemic B-cells from patients with B chronic lymphocytic leukemia and on the leukemic T-cell line Molt-4.	[63]
PCL *Polygonatum cyrtonema* Lectin	Induced HeLa cell apoptosis.	[64]
PHA Common bean agglutinin (*Phaseolus vulgaris*)	Reduction in number of Krebs II tumor cells in the ascitic fluid of mice and tumor-cell growth.	[65]
	Increase in the activity of polyamine oxidase.	[66]
	After including the lectin in the diet of mice, reduction of intraperitoneal tumors and subcutaneous no-Hodgkin lymphomas in mice.	[67, 68]
	Reduction of tumorogenesis in animals.	[69]
***Pleurotus ostreatus* lectin**	Differential effect on human hepatoma (H3B), human choriocarcinoma, mouse melanoma, and rat osteosarcoma cell lines. Lectin was more efficient on sarcoma S-180 than on hepatoma H-22 tumor inhibition, improvement of the host immune system.	[70]
Ricin	Protein synthesis inhibition by binding to ribosomes. Internalization and trigger cell proliferation.	[71]
rML Recombinant mistletoe lectin (*Viscum album*)	Immunomodulation can influence tumor growth in breast cancer patients	[72]
	The inhibitory effect not related with interferon gamma (IFN-γ) and/or interleukin-10-dependent mechanisms in rat urothelial carcinogenesis	[73]
	Antitumor activity if administered locally into the peritoneum of a human ovarian cancer harboring SCID mouse.	[74]
	Alone or in combination with ionizing radiation showed down regulation of the proliferative activity and cell killing of transformed murine tumor cells in a dose response manner.	[75]
SBA Soybean agglutinin	Inhibition of ascitic lymphoma cells and immune system stimulation.	[76]
	Inhibition of proliferation of breast cancer MCF7 cells and hepatoma HepG2 cells.	[77]
SVL (*Sauromatum venosum*)	Proliferation inhibition of murine cancer cell-lines (WEHI-279, J774, P388D1 and A-20). *In vitro* anti-proliferative activity on T-47D (breast), SiHa (cervix), SW-620 (colon), HT-29 (colon), HEP-2 (liver), OVCAR-5 (ovary) and PC-3 (prostate) cells except on SK-N-MC (CNS), SK-N-SH (CNS) cells.	[78]
Tepary bean lectin extracts (*Phaseolus acutifolius*)	Differential cytotoxic effect on breast, cervix and colon human cancer cell lines.	[79]
TMA I and TMA II (*Tricholoma mongolicum*)	Inhibition of sarcoma 180 cells and increment of life span.	[80]
VAA Mistletoe agglutinin (*Viscum album*)	VAA therapy alone stimulated tumor growth as well as lung metastasis.	[81]

Table 3. (Continued)

Lectins or lectins extracts	Effects	Ref
VAA-1 Mistletoe agglutinin-*1* (*Viscum album*)	Synergistic antineoplastic activity alone and in combination with other chemotherapeutic drugs on A549human lung carcinoma cell line. Induction of nonapoptotic G1-phase accumulation mechanisms.	[82]
VCA Korean mistletoe agglutinin (*Viscum album* var. corolatum)	Dose-dependent effect on promieloid leukemia HL-60 cells viability and apoptosis induction via caspase 3.	[83]
	Dose-dependent effect on melanoma B16-BL6 cells growth, apoptosis induction, antimetastasic effect, increased life span observed in inoculated mice, dose-dependent angiogenesis inhibition.	[84]
	Apoptosis induction on human hepatocarcinoma SK-Hep-1 and Hep3B cells via Bax activation and Bcl-2 inhibition, caspase 3 activation and telomerase inhibition.	[85]
VFA (*Vicia faba*)	Colorectal adenocarcinoma cell lines (LS174T, SW1222 and HT29) showed cell aggregation, morphologic differentiation and dose-dependent proliferation inhibition. Morphological differentiation and reduction of malignant phenotype of colon cancer cells. Aggregation of cancer cells binding directly to EpCAM.	[86, 87]
WGA	Inhibitory effect on the rat pancreatic tumor cell line AR42J, accompanied by a small decrease in α-amylase secretion.	[88]
	Highly toxic to human pancreatic carcinoma cells *in vitro*, with high membrane binding to sialic acid residues, with lectin internalization and apoptosis induction.	[89]
	Restriction of tumor growth of lymphoma cells.	[90]
	Isolectins showed differential interaction with leukemic cells and different cytoagglutinating and cytotoxic activities.	[91]
	Differential effects on cell growth of several human breast cancer cell lines *in vitro* (MCF-7, T47D, HBL 100, BT 20).	[92]

European mistletoe (*Viscum album*), used as complementary cancer therapies in Europe, has been used parenterally for more than 80 years as an anticancer agent with strong immunomodulating action. The quality of life of patients with pancreatic cancer stages III and IV improved as a result of exposure to Eurixor in a phase I and II study [96], on the opposite, patients with head and neck squamous cell carcinoma did not experience an improvement in their quality of life [97]. Mistletoe lectins or extracts from *Viscum album* (European variety, VAA) and *Viscum album* var. *coloratum* (Korean variety, VCA) have been widely studied against cancer. These varieties presented similar cytotoxic activity (IC50 of 1.2 ng/mL) against Molt-4 cells (T cell lymphoblasts, leukemia) [98]. Lectin from Chinese mistletoe showed important effects on human T cells cytotoxicity, apoptosis and cytokine production. ML increased tumor necrosis factor (TNF)-α release and inhibiting the release of anti-inflammatory interleukin (IL)-10 [99].

Specificity of lectins has triggered numerous applications in experimental medical sciences. Although the antitumor activity of lectins has been described, it is important to consider that their use may present, in some cases, adverse effects [7,16]. While not all lectins are toxic, many of them may cause different degrees of toxicity with severe negative effects, even death [100, 101]. Toxicity of lectins depends on the administration route and some of them had been reported to be highly allergenic under certain conditions [8, 16, 101, 102].

Due to the properties of some lectins as RIP, some studies have focused on using them for production of immunotoxins against cancer cells, where the lectin is attached to a monoclonal antibody, which has a specific receptor site for tumor cells. However, there have been reports after clinical trials that one of the major adverse effects, that limit the therapeutic dose in patients treated with immunotoxins formed by ricin A chain, is the vascular infiltration syndrome. This effect is even more frequent and severe in patients previously treated with radiotherapy [7]. Therefore, due to the toxicity of certain lectins, it is necessary to evaluate its systemic toxicity before testing their therapeutic effectiveness. On top of that, it will be recomended to take in consideration whether the patient has been receiving a special treatment which could pose an additional effect in the use of lectins.

Conclusion

Plant lectins have shown unique characteristics against different types of cancer cells and, in some cases, they present differences in the recognition between normal and transformed cells; their effects involve death and growth inhibition of cancer cells. The two main properties of lectins; selectivity and cytotoxicity, have become the focus of attention in research against cancer. Considering the extensive number of different lectins present in living organisms, and taking into account their different structures as well as differences in their mechanism of action, these compounds represent the opening of new avenues in the search for different cancer treatments. There is still the need to prove the inocuity of those lectins proposed for their possible use for the cancer treatment. Nonetheless, even those lectins that could be found to be toxic to humans or to animals, they still have the potential to be used as diagnostic tools, particularly oriented to the early recognition of different types of cancer cells.

Acknowledgments

The authors wish to thank the support from PROMEP (103.5/04/2830), FOMIX (QRO-2007-C01-78221) and CONACYT (Ciencia Básica 82349).

References

[1] Lotan, R; Raz, A. Lectins in cancer cells. *Ann. N. Y. Acad. Sci*. 1988. 551(1): 385–396.

[2] Wang, HX; Liu, WK; Ng, TB; Ooi, VEC; Chang, ST. The immunomodulatory and antitumor activities of lectins from the mushroom Tricholomamongolicum. *Immunopharmacology*. 1996. (31):205–211.

[3] Sharon, N; Lis, H. Lectins as Cell Recognition Molecules. *Science*. 1989. 246:227-234.

[4] Barondes, SH. Lectins: Their Multiple Endogenous Cellular Functions. *Annual Review of Biochemistry*. 1981. 50:207-231

[5] Peumans, WJ; Van Damme, EJM. Lectins as plant defense proteins. *Plant Physiol.* 1995. 109:347–352.

[6] Van Damme, EJM; Peumans, WJ; Barre, A; Rougé, P. Plant Lectins: A Composite of Several Distinct Families of Structurally and Evolutionary Related Proteins with Diverse Biological Roles. *Critical Reviews in Plant Sciences*. 1998. 17(6):575–692.

[7] Castillo-Villanueva, A; Abdullaev, F. Lectinas vegetales y sus efectos en el cáncer. *Revista de Investigación Clínica*. 2005. 57(1):55-64.

[8] González de Mejía, E; Prisecaru, VI. Lectins as bioactive plant proteins: a potential in cancer treatment. *Critical Reviews in Food Science and Nutrition*. 2005. 45:425-445

[9] Końska, G; Wójtowicz, U; Pituch-Noworolska, A. Possible application of lectins in diagnostics and therapy. Part I. Diagnostic application Przegl Lek. 2008. 65(4):189-94

[10] Hakomori, S. Tumor Malignancy Defined by Aberrant Glycosylation and Sphingo(glyco)lipid Metabolism. *Cancer Research*. 1996. 56:5309-5318

[11] Gorelik, E; Galili, U; Raz, A. On the role of cell surface carbohydrates and their binding proteins (lectins) in tumor metastasis. *Cancer and Metastasis Reviews*. 2001. 20:245–277

[12] Hakomori, S. Aberrant glycosylation in cancer cell membranes as focused on glycolipids: Overview and perspectives. *Cancer Res*. 1985. 45:2405–2414

[13] Nagata, Y. Function and structure of fungal lectins. *Chem. Biol*. 2000. 38:368–373

[14] Chrispeels, MJ. Glycobiology of Plan Cells. In: Varki A, Cummings R, Esko J, Freeze H, Hart G, Marth J editors. *Essentials of glycobiology*. Cold Spring Harbor Laboratory Press.2° Edition. Cold Spring Harbor, NY. USA. 1999. http://www.ncbi.nlm.nih.gov/books/bv.fcgi?rid=glyco.chapter.1520

[15] Marth, JD. O-Glycans. In: Varki A, Cummings R, Esko J, Freeze H, Hart G, Marth J editors. *Essentials of glycobiology*. Cold Spring Harbor Laboratory Press. 2° Edition. Cold Spring Harbor, NY. USA. 2009 http://www.ncbi.nlm.nih.gov /books/bv.fcgi?rid=glyco

[16] Hernández, P; Perez, E; Martínez, L; Ortiz, B; Martínez, G. Las Lectinas Vegetales como Modelo de Estudio de las Interacciones Proteína-Carbohidrato. *REB* 2005. 24(1):21-27.

[17] Nishimura, H; Nishimura, M; Oda, R; Yamanaka, K; Matsubara, T; Ozaki, Y; Sekiya, K; Hamada, T; Kato, Y. Lectins induce resistance to proteases and/or mechanical stimulus in all examided cells–including bone marrow mesenchymal stem cells–on various scaffolds. *Exp. Cell Res*. 2004. 295: 119-127.

[18] Kuwahara, I; Ikebuchi, K; Hamada, H; Niitsu, Y; Miyazawa, K; Furukawa, K. Changes in N-glycosilation of human stromal cells by telomerase expression. *Biochem Biophys Res Commun*. 2002. 301: 293–297.

[19] Frantz, M; Jung, ML; Ribereau-Gayon, G; Anton, R. Modulation of mistletoe (*Viscum album* L.) lectins cytotoxicity by carbohydrates and serum glycoproteins. *Arzneimittelforschung*. 2000. 50(5):471–478

[20] Verena, E; Plattner, M; Ratzinger, G; Gabor, F; Wirth, M. Targeted drug delivery: Binding and uptake of plant lectins using human 5637 bladder cancer cells. *Croat Med J*. 2008. 48(3):318-33

[21] Korourian, S; Siege, E; Kieber-Emmons, T; Monzavi-Karbassi. Expression analysis of carbohydrate antigens in ductal carcinoma in situ of the breast by lectin histochemistry. *BMC Cancer*. 2008. 8:138.

[22] Garbor F;Stangl M; Wirth M. Lectin-mediated bioadhesion: binding characteristics of plant lectins on the enterocyte-like cell lines Caco-2, HT-29 and HCT-8. *J Control Release* 1998; 55: 131-42

[23] Gabor, F; Klausegger, U; Wirth, M. The Interaction between wheat germ agglutinin and other plant lectins with prostate cancer cells Du-145. *Int J Pharm.* 2001. 221(1-2):35-47.

[24] Parslew, R; Jones, KT; Rhodes, JM; Sharpe, GR. The antiproliferative effect of lectin from the edible mushroom (*Agarics bisporus*) on human keratinocytes: preliminary studies on its use in psoriasis. *Br J Dermatol.* 1999. 140:56-60.

[25] Litynska, A; Przybylo, M; Pochec, E; Hoja-Lukowicz, D; Ciolczyk, D; Laidler, P; Gil, D. Comparison of the lectin-binding pattern in different human melanoma cell lines. *Melanoma Res.* 2001. 11:205-12.

[26] Ravinder, S; Subramanian, S; Rhodes, JM; Campbell, BJ. Peanut lectin stimulates proliferation of colon cancer cells by interaction with glycosylated CD44v6 isoforms and consequential activation of c-Met and MAPK: functional implications for disease-associated glycosylation changes. *Glycobiology*. 2006. 16(7): 594–601

[27] Konno, A; Hoshino, Y; Terashima, S; Motoki, R; Kawaguchi, T. Carbohydrate expression profile of colorectal cancer cells is relevant to metastatic pattern and prognosis. *Clin. Exp. Metastasis.* 2002. 19(1):61–70.

[28] Ruiz Álvarez V; Hernández-Triana M. 2002. Aspectos bioquímicos de la fitohemaglutinina. Aplicaciones en terapéutica médica. Instituto de Nutrición e Higiene de los Alimentos, Laboratorio de Bioquímica y Fisiología, Ciudad de La Habana, Cuba.http://www.monografias.com/trabajos20/fitohemaglutinina/fitohemaglutinina.shtml

[29] Pryme, IF; Bardocz, S. Anti-cancer therapy: Diversion of polyamines in the gut. *Eur. J. Gastroenterol. Hepatol.* 2001. 13(9):1041–1046.

[30] Lyu, SY; Choi, SH; Park, WB. Korean mistletoe lectin-induced apoptosis in hepatocarcinoma cells is associated with inhibition of telomerase via mitochondrial controlled pathway independent of p-53. *Arch. Pharm. Res*. 2002. 25(1): 93-101.

[31] Jordinson, M; El-Hariry, I; Calnan, D; Calam, J; Pignatelli, M. *Vicia faba* agglutinin, the lectin present in broad beans, stimulates differentiation of undifferentiated colon cancer cells. *Gut.* 1999. 44:709–714.

[32] Abdullaev, FI; Gonzalez de Mejia, E. Antitumor effect of plant lectins. *Natural toxins.* 1997. 5:157-63

[33] Lin, JK; Tserng, KY; Chen, CC; Lin, LT; Tung, TC. Abrin and ricin: new anti-tumor substances. *Nature.* 1970. 227:292-3.

[34] Dickers, KJ; Bradberry, SM; Rice, P; Griffiths, GD; Vale, JA. Abrin poisoning. *Toxicol Rev.* 2003. 22(3):137-42.

[35] Shoham, J; Inbar, M; Sachs, L. Differential toxicity on normal and transformed cells *in vitro* and inhibition of tumor development *in vivo* by Concanavalin A. *Nature.* 1970. 227:1244-6.

[36] Zhao, C; Sun, H; Tong, X; Qi, Y. An antitumor lectin from the edible mushroom *Agrocybe aegerita*. *Biochem J.* 2003. 374:321-7.

[37] Kent, D; Sheridan, CM; Tomkinson, HA; White, SJ; Hiscott, P; Yu, L; Grierson, I. Edible mushroom (*Agaricus bisporus*) lectin inhibits human retinal pigment epithelial cell proliferation *in vitro*. *Wound Repair Regen.* 2003. 11(4):285-91.

[38] Yu, LG; Fernig, DG; White, MRH; Spiller, DG; Appleton, P; Evans, RC; Grierson, I; Smith, JA; Davies, H; Gerasimenko, OV; Petersen, OH; Milton, JD; Rhodes, JM. Edible mushroom (*Agaricus bisporus*) lectin, which reversibly inhibits epithelial cell

proliferation, blocks nuclear localization sequence-dependent nuclear protein import. *J Biol Chem.* 1999. 274:4890-4899.

[39] Yu, LG; Andrews, N; Weldon, M; Gerasimenko, OV; Campbell, BJ; Singh, R; Grierson, I; Petersen, OH; Rhodes, JM. An N-terminal truncated form of Orp 150 is a cytoplasmic ligand for the anti-proliferative mushroom *Agaricus bisporus* lectin and is required for nuclear localization sequence-dependent nuclear protein import. *J Biol Chem.* 2002. 227:24538-24545

[40] Moriwaki, S; Ohba, H; Nakamura, O; Sallay, I; Suzuki, M; Tsubouchi, H; Yamasaki, N; Itoh, K. Biological activities of the lectin, abrin-a, against human lymphocytes, and cultured leukemic cell lines. *J Hematother Stem Cell Res.* 2000. 9(1):47–53.

[41] Ramnath, V; Kuttan, G; Kuttan, R. Antitumor effect of abrin on transplanted tumours in mice. *Indian J Physiol Pharmacol.* 2002. 46(1):69-77.

[42] Kaur, N; Singh, K; Rup, PJ; Saxena, AK; Khan, RH; Ashraf, MT; Kamboj SS; Singh, J. A tuber lectin from *Arisaema helleborifolium* Schott with anti-insect activity against melon fruit Xy, *Bactrocera cucurbitae* (Coquillett) and anti-cancer effect on human cancer cell lines. *Arch Biochem Biophys.* 2006. 445:156–165

[43] Kaur, A; Singh Kamboj, S; Singh, J; Saxena, AK; Dhuna, V. Isolation of a novel N-acetyl-D-lactosamine specific lectin from Alocasia cucullata (Schott.). *Biotech Letters.* 2005. 27:1815-1820

[44] Dhuna, V; Bains, JS; Kamboj, SS; Singh, J; Kamboj, S; Saxena, AK. Purification and characterization of a lectin from Arisaema tortuosum Schott having in-vitro anticancer activity against human cancer cell lines. *J Biochem Mol Biol.* 38(5):526-32

[45] Sasaki, T; Yamazaki, K; Yamori, T; Endo, T. Inhibition of proliferation and induction of differentiation of glioma cells with *Datura stramonium* agglutinin. *Br J Cancer.* 2002. 87:918-23.

[46] Chen, YF; Boland, CR; Kraus, ER; Goldstein, IJ. The lectin *Griffonia simplicifolia* I-A4 (GSI-A4) specifically recognizes terminal alpha-linked N-acetylgalactosaminyl groups and is cytotoxic to the human colon cancer cell lines LSII74 and SW1116. *Int J Cancer.* 1994. 57:561-7.

[47] Knibbs, RN; Mac-Callum, DK; Lillie, JH; Goldstein, IJ. Wild-type and cultured Ehrlich ascites tumor cells differ in tumorigenicity, lectin binding pattern and binding to basement membranes. *Glycobiology.* 1994. 4:419-28.

[48] Kuttan, G; Menon, LG; Antony, S; Kuttan, R. Anticarcinogenic and antimetastatic activity of Iscador. *Anticancer Drugs.* 1997. 8(Suppl 1):S15–S16.

[49] Maier, G; Fiebig, HH. Absence of tumor growth stimulation in a panel of 16 human tumor cell lines by mistletoe extracts *in vitro*. *Anti-Cancer Drugs.* 2002. 13:373-9

[50] Zarkovic, N; Vukovic, T; Loncaric, I; Miletic, M; Zarkovic, K; Borovic, S; Cipak, A; Sabolovic, S; Konitzer, M; Mang, S. An overview on anticancer activities of the *Viscum album* extract Isorel. *Cancer Biother Radiopharm.* 2001. 16(1):55–62.

[51] Schaffrath, B; Mengs, U; Schwarz, T; Hilgers, RD; Beuth, J; Mockel, B; Lentzen, H; Gerstmayer, B. Anticancer activity of rViscumin (recombinant mistletoe lectin) in tumor colonization models with immunocompetent mice. *Anticancer Res.* 2001. 21(6A):3981–3987.

[52] Yoon, TJ; Yoo, YC; Kang, TB; Baek, YJ; Huh, CS; Song, SK; Lee, KH; Azuma, I; Kim, JB. Prophylactic effect of Korean mistletoe (*Viscum album coloratum*) extract on

tumor metastasis is mediated by enhancement of NK cell activity. *Int. J. Immunopharmacol.* 1998. 20(4–5):163–172.

[53] Yoon, TJ; Yoo, YC; Kang, TB; Song, SK; Lee, KB; Her, E; Song, KS; Kim, JB. Antitumor activity of the Korean mistletoe lectin is attributed to activation of macrophages and NK cells. *Arch Pharm Res.* 2003. 26:861-7.

[54] Koyama, Y; Katsuno, Y; Miyoshi, N; Hayakawa, S; Mita, T; Muto, H; Isemura, S; Aoyagi, Y; Isemura, M. Apoptosis Induction by Lectin Isolated from Mushroom *Boletopsis leucomelas* in U937 Cells. *Biosci Biotechnol Biochem.* 2002. 66(4):784-9.

[55] González de Mejía, E; Rocha, N; Winter, HC; Goldstein, IJ.. Differential effect of a lectin from mesquite (*Prosopis juliflora*) on HeLa and normal human keratinocyte cells. *FASEB J.* 2002. 15(4):C 128.

[56] Mengs, U; Schwarz, T; Bulitta, M; Weber, K; Madaus, AG. Antitumoral effects of an intravesically applied aqueous mistletoe extract on urinary bladder carcinoma MB49 in mice. *Anticancer Res.* 2000, 20(5B):3565–3568.

[57] Knöpfl-Sidler F, Viviani A, Rist L, Hensel A. Human cancer cells exhibit in vitro individual receptiveness towards different mistletoe extracts. *Pharmazie.* 2005. 60(6):448-54.

[58] Urech, K; Buessing, A; Thalmann, G; Schaefermeyer, H; Heusser, P. Antiproliferative effects of mistletoe (Viscum album L.) extract in urinary bladder carcinoma cell lines. *Anticancer Res*. 2006. 26(4B):3049-55.

[59] Bantel, H; Engels, IH; Voelter, W; Schulze-Osthoff, K; Wesselborg, S. Mistletoes lectin activates caspase-8/FLICE independently of death receptor signaling and enhances anticancer drug-induced apoptosis. *Cancer Res.* 1999. 59:2083-90.

[60] Pryme, IF; Bardocz, S; Pusztai, A; Ewen, SW. Dietary mistletoe lectin supplementation and reduced growth of a murine non-Hodgkin lymphoma. *Histol Histopathol.* 2002. 17:261-71.

[61] Pryme, IF; Bardocz, S; Pusztai, A; Ewen, SW; Pfuller, U. A mistletoe lectin (ML-1)-containing diet reduces the viability of a murine non-Hodgkin lymphoma tumor. *Cancer Detect Prevent.* 2004. 28:52-6.

[62] Kim, MS; Lee, J; Lee, KM; Yang, SH; Choi, S; Chung, SY; Kim, TY; Jeong, WH; Park, R. Involvement of hydrogen peroxide in mistletoe lectin-II-induced apoptosis of myeloleukemic U937 cells. *Life Sci*. 2003. 73(10):1231–1243.

[63] Bussing, A; Stein, GM; Pfuller, U; Schietzel, M. Differential binding of toxic lectins from *Viscum album* L., ML I and ML III, to human lymphocytes. *Anticancer Res.* 1999. 19(6B):5095–5099.

[64] Liu,B; Xu, X; Cheng, Y; Huang, J; Liu, Y; Liu, Z; Min, M; Bian, H; Chen, J; Bao, J. Apoptosis-inducing effect and structural basis of Polygonatum cyrtonema lectin and chemical modification properties on its mannose-binding sites. *BMB Reports.* 2008. 369-65.

[65] Bardocz, S; Grant, G; Duguid, TJ; Brown, DS; Pusztai, A; Pryme, IF. Intracellular levels of polyamines in Krebs II lymphosarcoma cells in mice fed phytohaemagglutinin-containing diets are coupled with altered tumour growth. *Cancer Lett*. 1997. 121(1):25–29.

[66] Rabellotti, E; Sessa, A; Tunici, P; Bardocz, S; Grant, G; Pusztai, A; Perin, A. Oxidative degradation of polyamines in rat pancreatic hypertrophy. *Biochim. Biophys Acta*. 1998. 1406(3):321–326.

[67] Pryme, IF; Pustai; Bardocz, S; Ewen, SW. A combination of dietary protein depletion and PHA-induced growth gut reduce the mass of murine non-Hodgkin lymphoma. *Cancer Lett.* 1999a. 139:145-52.

[68] Pryme, IF; Bardocz, S; Pusztai, A; Ewen SW. The growth of an established murine non-Hodgkin lymphoma tumour is limited by switching to a phytohaemagglutinin-containing diet. *Cancer Lett.* 1999b. 146:87-91

[69] Pryme, IF; Pusztai, AJ; Bardocz, SA. Diet containing the lectin phytohaemagglutinin (PHA) slows the proliferation of Krebs II cell tumours in mice. *Cancer Lett.* 1994. 76:133-7.

[70] Wang, H; Ng, TB; Ooi, VE; Liu, WK. Effects of lectins with different carbohydrate-binding specificities on hepatoma, choriocarcinoma, melanoma and osteosarcoma cell lines. *Int. J. Biochem. Cell. Biol.* 2000. 32(3):365–372.

[71] Fang, K. A toxin conjugate containing transforming growth factor-alpha and ricin A specifically inhibits growth of A431 human epidermoid cancer cells. *Proc. Natl. Sci. Counc. Repub. China B.* 1998. 22(2):76–82.

[72] Stein, G; Henn, W; von Laue, H; Berg, P. Modulation of the cellular and humoral immune responses of tumor patients by mistletoe therapy. *Eur. J. Med. Res.* 1998. 3(4):194–202.

[73] Elsässer-Beile, U; Ruhnau, T; Freudenberg, N; Wetterauer, U; Mengs, U. Antitumoral effect of recombinant mistletoe lectin on chemically induced urinary bladder carcinogenesis in a rat model. *Cancer*. 2001. 91(5):998–1004.

[74] Schumacher, U; Feldhaus, S; Mengs, U. Recombinant mistletoe lectin (rML) is successful in treating human ovarian cancer cells transplanted into severe combined immunodeficient (SCID) mice. *Cancer Lett.* 2000. 150(2):171–175.

[75] Hostanska, K; Vuong, V; Rocha, S; Soengas, MS; Glanzmann, C; Saller, R; Bodis, S; Pruschy, M. Recombinant mistletoe lectin induces p53-independent apoptosis in tumour cells and cooperates with ionising radiation. *Br. J. Cancer*. 2003. 88(11):1785–1792.

[76] Mukhopadhyay, P; Gupta, JD; Sanyal, U; Das, S. Influence of dietary restriction and soybean supplementation on the growth of a murine lymphoma and host immune function. *Cancer Lett.* 1994. 78:151-7.

[77] Lin, P; Ye, X; Ng, T. Purification of melibiose-binding lectins from two cultivars of Chinese black soybeans. *Acta Biochim Biophys Sin.* 2008. 40(12):1029-1038.

[78] Singh Bains, J; Singh, J; Kamboj, SS; Nijjar, KK; Agrewala, JN; Kumar, V; Kumar, A; Saxena, AK. Mitogenic and anti-proliferative activity of a lectin from the tubers of Voodoo lily (Sauromatum venosum). *Biochim Biophys Acta*. 2005. 1723(1-3):163-74.

[79] Castañeda-Cuevas A, Yllescas-Gasca L, López-Martínez J, Mendiola-Olaya E, Blanco-Labra A, Garcia-Gasca T. 2007. Efecto Antiproliferativo *In Vitro* de una Lectina De Frijol Tépari sobre Diferentes Tipos de Cáncer Humano [online]. 2007. RESPYN Special edition No. 7. Available from: http://www.respyn.uanl.mx/especiales/2007/ee-07-2007/index.html.

[80] Wang, HX; Ng, TB; Ooi, VE; Liu, WK; Chang, ST. Actions of lectins from the mushroom *Tricholoma mongolicum* on macrophages, splenocytes and life-span in sarcoma-bearing mice. *Anticancer Res.* 1997.17:419-24

[81] Timoshenko, AV; Lan, Y; Gabius, HJ; Lala, PK. Immunotherapy of C3H/HeJ mammary adenocarcinoma with interleukin-2, mistletoe lectin or their combination.

effects on tumour growth, capillary leakage and nitric oxide (NO) production. *Eur J Cancer*. 2001. 37(15):1910–1920.

[82] Siegle, I; Fritz, P; McClellan, M; Gutzeit, S; Murdter, TE. Combined cytotoxic action of *Viscum album* agglutinin-1 and anticancer agents against human A549 lung cancer cells. *Anticancer Res.* 2001. 21(4A):2687–2691.

[83] Lyu, SY; Park, WB; Choi, KH; Kim, WH. Involvement of caspase-3 in apoptosis induced by *Viscum album* var. *coloratum* agglutinin in HL-60 cells. *Biosci Biotechnol Biochem.* 2001:65: 534-41.

[84] Park, WB; Lyu, SY; Kim, JH; Choi, SH; Chung, HK; Ann, SH; Hong, SY; Yoon, TJ; Choi, MJ. Inhibition of tumor growth and metastasis by Korean mistletoe lectin is associated with apoptosis and antiangiogenesis. *Cancer Biother Radiopharm.* 2001. 16:439-47.

[85] Lyu, SY; Choi, SH; Park, WB. Korean mistletoe lectin-induced apoptosis in hepatocarcinoma cells is associated with inhibition of telomerase via mitochondrial controlled pathway independent of p53. *Arch Pharm Res.* 2002. 25(1):1-8.

[86] Jordison, M; El-Hariry, I; Calnan, D; Calam, J; Pignatelli, M. *Vicia faba* agglutinin, the lectin present in broad beans, stimulates differentiation of undifferentiated colon cancer cells. *Gut.* 1999. 44:709-14.

[87] Litvinov, SV; Velders, MP; Bakker, HA; Fleuren, GJ; Warnaar, SO. Ep-CAM: A human epithelial is a homophilic cell-cell adhesion molecule. *J Cell Biol.* 1994. 125:437–446.

[88] Mikkat, U; Damm, I; Kirchhoff, F; Albrecht, E; Nebe, B; Jonas, L. Effects of lectins on CCK-8-stimulated enzyme secretion and differentiation of the rat pancreatic cell line AR42J. *Pancreas*. 2001. 23(4):368–374.

[89] Schwarz, RE; Wojciechowicz, DC; Picon, AI; Schwarz, MA; Paty, PB. Wheatgerm agglutinin-mediated toxicity in pancreatic cancer cells. *Br J Cancer.* 1999. 80(11):1754–1762.

[90] Ganguly, C; Das, S. Plant lectins as inhibitors of tumor growth and modulators of host immune response. *Chemotherapy.* 1994. 40:272-8.

[91] Ohba, H; Bakalova, R; Murakib, M. Cytoagglutination and cytotoxicity of Wheat Germ Agglutinin isolectins against normal lymphocytes and cultured leukemic cell lines—relationship between structure and biological activity. *Biochim Biophys Acta.* 2003. 1619:144–150.

[92] Valentiner, U; Fabian, S; Schumacher, U; Leathem, AJ. The influence of dietary lectins on the cell proliferation of human breast cancer cell lines *in vitro*. *Anticancer Res.* 2003. 23(2B):1197–206.

[93] Watzl, B; Neudecker, C; Hansch, GM; Rechkemmer, G; Pool-Zobel, BL. Dietary wheat germ agglutinin modulates ovalbumin-induced immune responses in Brown Norway rats. *Br J Nutr.* 2001. 85(4):483–490.

[94] Kiss, R; Camby, I; Duckworth, D; De-Decker, R; Salmon, I; Pasteels, JL; Danguy, A; Yeaton, P. *In vitro* influence of *Phaseolus vulgaris*, *Griffonia simplicifolia*, Concanavalin A, wheat germ and peanut agglutinins on HCT-15, LoVo and SW 837 human colorrectal cancer cell growth. *Gut.* 1997. 40:253-61.

[95] Riaño-Sánchez R. Importancia y aplicaciones de las lectinas [online]. 1997. Available from: http://www.monografias.com/trabajos11/lecti/lecti.shtml

[96] Friess, H; Beger, HG; Kunz, J; Funk, N; Schilling, M; Buchler, MW. Treatment of advanced pancreatic cancer with mistletoe: Results of a pilot trial. *Anticancer Res.* 1996. 16(2):915–920.

[97] Steuer-Vogt, MK; Bonkowsky, V; Ambrosch, P; Scholz, M; Neiss, A; Strutz, J; Hennig, M; Lenarz, T; Arnold, W. The effect of an adjuvant mistletoe treatment programme in resected head and neck cancer patients: A randomised controlled clinical trial. *Eur J Cancer*. 2001. 37(1):23–31.

[98] Lyu, SY; Park, SM; Choung, BY; Park, WB. Comparative study of Korean (*Viscum album* var. *coloratum*) and European mistletoes (*Viscum album*). *Arch Pharm Res.* 2000. 23:592-8.

[99] Gomg, F; Ma, Y; MA, A; Yu, Q; Zhang, J; Nie, H; Chen, X; Shen, B; Li, N; Zhang, D. A Lectin from Chinese Mistletoe Increases δγ T Cell-mediated Cytotoxicity through Induction of Caspase-dependent Apoptosis. *Acta Biochim Biophys Sinica.* 2007. 39(6):445–452.

[100] Rhodes, JM. Beans means lectins. *Gut.* 1999. 44:593-594.

[101] Tareq, al-Ati. Plant lectins. Poisonous Plants [online]. 2001. Available from: http://www.ansci.cornell.edu/plants/toxicagents/lectins.html

[102] Lajolo, F; Genovese, M. Nutricional significance of lectins and enzyme inhibitors from legumes. *J Agric Food Chem.* 2002. 50:6592-6598.

In: New Approaches in the Treatment of Cancer
Editors: Carmen Mejia Vazquez et al. pp.91-124
ISBN 978-1-62100-067-9

Chapter V

PROTEASE INHIBITORS AS ANTICANCER AGENTS

José Luis Castro-Guillén[1], Teresa García-Gasca[2] and Alejandro Blanco-Labra[1,*]

[1]Centro de Investigación y Estudios Avanzados del Instituto Politécnico Nacional Unidad Irapuato, Guanajuato, México

[2]Universidad Autónoma de Querétaro, Querétaro, México

ABSTRACT

Protease inhibitors (PIs) encompass a large group of proteins that regulate the hydrolytic activity of proteolytic enzymes and play important physiological roles in all the living organisms. The protease/PI balance is necessary for cellular homeostasis, though, when such balance is broken, pathological conditions like cancer development are induced. The study of PIs as anti-cancer agents has been an important subject of research since more than three decades ago. There are a variety of mechanisms by which PIs perform their effects which depend on two main aspects: the nature, structure and functions of PI and, the interaction with a complex microenvironment that differs, even between cancers originated on the same source. There are many promissory cases, as well as, failures and paradoxical examples of PIs in the treatment of cancer which must be taken into consideration to propouse PI as possible part of the pharmaceutilcal strategies against cancer. In the following chapter the recent knowledge regarding signaling pathways involved in the anti-cancer effect of different classes of PIs, as well as their main features and the current perspectives in regard with their application as anti-cancer drugs will be discussed.

* Correspondence concerning this article should be addressed to: Alejandro Blanco-Labra. Departamento de Biotecnología y Bioquímica. Centro de Investigación y Estudios Avanzados del Instituto Politécnico Nacional. Unidad Irapuato, Km. 9.6 Libramiento Norte carretera Irapuato-León. C. P. 36821 Irapuato, Guanajuato, México. Phone Number (+52 462) 62 39600; Fax: (+52 462) 6239611; e-mail: ablanco@ira.cinvestav.mx.

INTRODUCTION

PIs constitute a group of proteins widely distributed among all the organisms. Its main feature includes their ability to form strong protease-PI complex, inhibiting the protelytic activity [1]. Proteases play higly important roles in all physiological processes of living organisms; therefore, its regulation is a critical step in many physiological and pathological processes. Early reports indicate that proteolysis is an important factor in cancer development, since PIs were found to be highly effective suppressors of carcinogenesis both on *in vitro* and *in vivo* systems [2-5]. Initially, proteolysis was related with the invasive process of tumors, where destruction of adjacent blood vessels and cellular tissues was necessary for migration of tumor cells. Presently, it is known that proteolysis participate in the whole process of cancer development, progresion and metastasis, making the regulation of proteases by PIs become more important as anti-tumor agents. On top of that, the complex molecular network of proteins that communicate with other proteins which play different functions, explain the importance that a molecule such as the PIs could play, some times favoring and some others impairing physiologycal processess. These molecules also have a great potential for their use as prognostic as well as for terapeutical agents against cancer.

SERINE PROTEASE INHIBITORS

The first proteinaceous PIs used against cancer and so far the once that have been more extensively studied, were serine proteases inhibitors, specifically the potato, Kunitz and Bowman-Birk families, which presented anti-carcinogenesis and anti-metastatic properties [6-10]. The importance of this class of inhibitors was based on their diversity of *in vitro* and *in vivo* effects in a variety of cancers. Several examples of plant- and animal-origin inhibitors have been studied and they will be dicussed in relation to their anti-tumor effects.

Bowman-Birk Protease Inhibitors

This family of protease inhibitors was one of the first PIs reported with anticarcinogenic properties. The soybean Bowman-Birk protease inhibitor (BBI), isolated from soybean, has the ability to inhibit trypsin and chymotrypsin activities [11,12]. BBI can suppress carcinogenesis both *in vitro* transformation systems and *in vivo* carcinogenesis assay systems [10,4,13,14,15]. The effect of BBI has beeen succesfully tested in mice, rats, hamsters and humans; in several tissues, organs and cells and with different types of cancers, including lung tumors, esophageal neoplasms and pancreatic neoplasms [5,16,17,18].

BBI is a metalloprotein containing magnesium, calcium and zinc. Interestingly, the demineralized state of BBI can inhibit even better the matrix metallo proteinase-1 [19]. The chymotrypsin inhibitory domain plays a main role in the suppressive effects on carcinogenesis [13,14,20], and it has been demonstrated that the photo- and radio-protective effect of this inhibitor is independent of its three-dimensional conformation [20,21]. BBI has an irreversible effect on transformation process, and it also been shown an extended effect against radiation-induced transformation after carcinogen exposure [13]. Even directly, soybean crude extract (BBIC) was able to exert the same effect *in vitro* that BBI alone. Both tested samples presented the same effectiveness on inhibition of growth, invasion and survival of human and mouse prostate and colon cancer cells, without affecting normal cells [22,23,24]. Also, BBI in both forms could act as normal tissue radio-protector on *in vitro* and *in vivo* assays in mice [24,25]. Since 1992, BBIC was approved by the FDA as "investigational new drug" status. A phase I human chemoprevention trial in patients with oral leukoplakia demonstrated that BBIC had no acute toxicity [26], and it was also demonstrated its clinical activity after oral administration in a dose dependent manner in oral leukoplakia lesion. BBI also lacks of clinical toxicity or drug allergy [27].

However, the mechanism of action for this inhibitor remains elusive. The first proposed mechanism was based on the hypothesis of the inhibition of intra cellular proteases involved in the induction and/or expression of transformed phenotype [28]. The radioprotective effect of BBI involves a DNA repairing mechanism dependent of the protein TP53 and, of the induction of DNA-dependent protein kinase, which in turn is activated through the internalization of epidermal growth factor receptor (EGFR) into cytoplasm and it is further transport into the nucleus. BBI also promotes a reduced formation of dicentric chromosomes and this effect is correlated with an increased in cell survival [29,30]. BBI is also a potent inhibition of the chymotrypsin-like activity present in the proteasome 26S of MCF7 cells [31], provoking growth arrests at G_1/S phases by decreasing the activity of extracellular-signal-regulated kinase (ERK1/2) caused for the up-regulation of mitogen activated protein kinase phosphatase-1 (MAP kinase phosphatase-1), as well as by the accumulation of the proteins $p21^{Cip1/WAF1}$ and $p27^{Kip1}$, and the down-regulation of cyclin D1 and E [31]. On the other hand, the inhibitory activity of BBI on proteasome prevents the degradation of the protein Connexin-43 (Cx43) which is a tumor suppresor gen. Out of that effect and without a clear mechanism, BBI is able to increase the expression of *Cx43* gen, resulting in a negative growth control in human osteosarcoma cells [32]. The effect of BBI on oncogenes has been also tested. This inhibitor can inhibit the over-exppression of two oncogenes, c-*myc* and c-*fos* in unirradiated rat mucosa cells [33] and BBI is also able to diminish proteolytic activity correlated with the *neu* oncogen [34].

Other members of this family have proved their effectiveness regarding their anti-cancer effect. For example, the field bean protease inhibitor (FBPI) is able to supress skin tumorogenesis in mice and it could act as anti-metastatic agent, inhibiting pulmonary metastasis of B16F10 melanoma cells through its anti-plasmin inhibitory activity [35,36]. Another member is found in the protein fraction of tepary bean seeds with protease inhibitory activity, which can potentially affect proliferation and metastasis of 3T3/*v-mos* transformed fibroblast, affecting cell survival and proliferation and partially restoring the adhesion patterns of transformed fibroblast [37,38].

Kunitz Trypsin Inhibitors

Many inhibitors of the Kunitz family have been reported to be active against cancer. It is interesting how Kunitz PIs can act with different signaling molecules, including key proteases in cancer invasion and other signaling-related proteins. This inhibitors act principally as anti-angiogenesis and anti-metastatic agents. Some examples of this type of inhibitors will be discused.

Bikunin

One of most studied Kunitz inhibitors is bikunin, known also as urinary trypsin inhibitor. Bikunin is produced by the liver and it is prevailing on human amniotic fluid and to a lesser extent, in urine and serum, usually as covalently linked to the light chain of the inter-α-inhibitor [39]. Bikunin is a multifunctional glycoprotein with two Kunitz-type protease inhibitor domains, and two glycosilations [40]. It is able to inhibit trypsin, chymotrypsin, human leukocyte elastase, plasmin, tissue kallikreins, plasma kallikreins, factor XIa, and granzyme K [41,42,43] and it has a variety of biological functions which depends on its broad spectrum of molecular targets that participate on different signaling cascades [44].

The anti-cancer activity of bikunin resides on the ability to inhibit both *in vitro* cell invasion, and *in vivo* metastasis in animal and human cancers [45,46,47]. Bikunin can suppress directly the cell surface-associated plasmin activity and reduce cell invasion by modulating urokinase-type plasminogen activator (uPA) expression at gene and protein levels, as well as uPAR (uPA receptor); both of them, through suppression of the MAP kinase-dependent signaling cascade, probably with events such as phosphorylation of MEK (mitogen-activated protein kinase) and ERK. [40,46,48]. The suppression of MAPK-dependent uPA up-regulation could suppress angiogenesis due to altered tube-like formation of endothelial cells [49]. In addition, bikunin is able to reduce cell invasion, but not proliferation, adhesion or migration, by means of suppression of ERK1/2 activation and the consequent inhibition of uPA exppression [44,48]. Another report suggest that the inhibitory response by bikunin, on the expression of (transforming growth factor β1) TGF-β1 and TGF-β1 mediated, Src- and ERK-dependent uPA signaling cascades, is due to the inhibition of a Ca^{2+} channel [50].

On the other hand, glycosilations of bikunin play an important role on its signaling transduction properties. The bikunin-mediated suppression of cell invasiveness is given for the interaction of bikunin with specific receptors at the cell membrane, including the one that initiate the modulation of *uPA* mRNA expression. Two receptors expressed by cancer cells have been studied, one of them of 45 kDa was called bikunin receptor and the other one, a 40 kDa protein was called link protein (LP) [51]. Bikunin reduces cell invasion through reduction of cell interactions with hyaluronan (HA) by suppression of dimerization of CD44 [51], which is related to the promotion of tumor cell adhesion, migration, invasion and angiogenesis [52]. Other receptors are also affected by bikunin: TGF-β receptor type I and type II (TβRI and TβRII, respectively). The oligomerization of TGF-β receptors is disrupted only by glycosilated bikunin, suppressing the expression of uPA, PAI-1 (plasminogen activator inhibitor type 1) and collagen [53]. Target genes have been identifying by cDNA microarray hybridization, finding 11 bikunin-stimulated genes and 29 bikunin-repressed genes such as CDC-like kinase, Ets domain transcription factor, Rho GTPase-activating protein, tyrosine phosphorilation-regulated kinase, HA-binding protein, matriptase, and pregnancy-associated plasma protein-A (PAPP-A) which are implicated in tumor promotion. Therefore, all down-regulated genes by bikunin were shown to promote invasion and tumor metastasis and, up-regulated genes promote apoptosis and tumor suppression. The effect of bikunin could be related mainly with the suppression of matriptase, PAPP-A, and of other genes, as a consequence of the down-regulation of uPA signaling; probably reestablishing the proteolytic imbalance of transformed cells [54].

Bikunin is considering as a favorable prognostic factor in ovarian cancer and its measurement has been introduced as a new diagnostic tool for the evaluation of prognosis [55]. As therapeutic agent, bikunin was tested on its efficacy of once-daily oral administration firstly on ovarian HRA cancer cells growing in the peritonea of nude mice, and afterwards, on human phase I trial. In both cases there were no dose-limiting toxicities, suggesting that this inhibitor could suppress both invasion and angiogenesis in a safety way [56].

Hepatocyte Growth Factor Inhibitor Type-1 (HAI-1)

Hepatocyte growth factor activator inhibitor type 1 (HAI-1) is a multidomain Kunitz protease inhibitor. Like bikunin, HAI-1 has two Kunitz domains; however, it lacks glycosilations and it belongs to a unique class of PIs with a type-1 transmembrane domain and can act at the cell surface [57,58]. Due to its location, HAI-1 has a critical role regulating proteolytic activities on pericellular microenvironment in both normal and malignant conditions. HAI-1 was first identified as a potent inhibitor of hepatocyte growth factor activator (HGFA), a 53-kDa serine protease [59] that is able to activate the hepatocyte growth factor (HGF) zimogen. The cytokine HGF is involved in the regeneration of the injured tissue and it can influence cancer metastasis [60]. Besides HAI-1, another HAI is reported: HAI-2 [61] characterized for its lack of the ability to bind HGFA, though, both inhibitors possesses an anti-invasive activity on transformed cells [62].

The anti-proteolytic activity, specifically, the N-terminal Kunitz domain (KD-1) of HAI-1 inhibits HGFA and its other cognates, matriptase and prostatin [63,64,65]; as well as other serine proteases implicated in cancer metastasis, including hepsin, plasma kallikrein and trypsin [58,63]. It has been demonstrated that KD-1 is directly responsible for the anti-migration/invasion effects of HAI-1 *in vitro* [66]. A recent report, demonstrated the interactions between HAI-1 and its membrane serine protease target, using a stable knockout of HAI-1 gene (*SPINT1*) [67]. In that study, HAI-1/*SPINT1* was involved in transcriptional and functional changes in a carcinoma phenomenon known as EMT (the epithelial to mesenchymal transition) [68]. HAI-1/*SPINT1* knockout induced an elongated spindle-like morphology associated with accelerated invasion, mimicking the EMT process; presenting also a decreased expression of E-cadherin and up-regulation of its transcriptional repressor, Smad-interacting protein 1 (SIP-1) and matrix metalloproteinase 9 (MMP-9) [67]. The key role of HAI-1 on activation of pro-matriptase [64] suggests that HAI-1 might be not only a negative regulator but also a cofactor for optimal activities of such proteases [69]. However, it is important to mention that the complete molecule of HAI-1 promoted glioblastoma cell malignity *in vivo* and this effect was dependent of its localization at cellular surface. Nonetheless, the secreted form of HAI-1 show no pro-malignant activity but rather a suppressive effects both *in vitro* and *in vivo* [69].

Other Kunitz Inhibitors

One of most studied plant PIs is the Kunitz tripsin inhibitor from soybean (KTI). This inhibitor has anti-invasiveness properties since it is able to block the ERK-dependent uPA signaling cascades through the reduction of TGF-β1-mediated activation of ERK1/2 and by suppression of TGF-β1-induced phosphorilation of Src, and Akt [70,71]. Otherwise, KTI is able to affect cell migration and tubulogenesis without toxic effects on epithelial cells [72]. Another member of Kunitz family that is the one present in *Peltophorum dubium* seeds, called *Peltophorum dubium* trypsin inhibitor (PDTI) with a N-terminal sequence with homology with the N-terminal sequence of KTI. This protein inhibits both bovine trypsin and chymotrypsin [73]. Comparing PDTI with KTI, an interesting feature is that both inhibitors are capable of inducing apoptosis of Nb2 rat lymphoma and human leukemia Jurkat cells with recruitment of Fas-associated death domain (FADD) to the cell membrane [73,74]. Nevertheless, each inhibitor had different specificity, for example: KTI had more potency than PDTI on Jurkat cell apoptosis, contrary to Nb2 rat lymphoma cells, where PDTI was more potent. Otherwise KTI is more specific for human cells than PDTI [73,74].

Serpins

Serpins are a superfamily of proteins vastly distributed among higher eukaryotes and viruses. Members of this family share a common structural arrangement [75,76]. Their mechanism of action, represent a common characteristic of these inhibitors, which consist in two pathways: the non-inhibitory or substrate pathway and the inhibitory pathway [76,77]. In the non-ihibitory pathway, the reactive site loop is hydrolized as substrate; otherwise, in the inhibitory pathway, the reactive site loop when it is cutted, suffer a conformational change, in which serpin kinetically "trap" the enzyme, forming a covalent and irreversible bond with the protease, locking the inhibitor-protease complex [77]. Many members of this family of proteins possess anti-cancer effects, acting as tumor suppressors but with some paradoxical effects in some cases. Most of reviewed serpins are highlighted for its anti-antiangiogenic effect.

Maspin

This inhibitor represents an outstanding member of the serpin family related to anticancer features. It is a 42 kDa protein that was found to be down-regulated in mammary carcinoma cells [78]; since its promoter is silenced during cancer progression, it is consider therefore, a tumor suppressor gene [78,79]. Maspin is a protein epigenetically regulated and with its tissue-specific expression related with DNA methylation [80]. Its promoter region is especially important since it has a hormone-responsive element and a p53 binding site. Also maspin expression is regulated by both p53 and TGF-β tumor suppressive pathways [81,82,83]. Maspin has been widely studied due to its inhibition of tumor growth, angiogenesis, invasion, motility, and metastasis; as well as for its apoptosis promotion [82,84,85,86]. There are divergent effects related to maspin activities, since in some cases it has been correlated with better prognosis in breast, prostatic, oral, colorectal, bladder, and lung cancers [84,87-92], but in other cases, contradictory results are found, indicating that high maspin expression could enhance invasion and metastasis on breast, gastric, ovarian, and non–small cell lung carcinomas [93-97]. Nevertheless, Kashima *et al.* [98] found that maspin may be involved in the occurrence and progression of intraductal papillary mucinous neoplasm, but the pro-apoptotoc effect of this inhibitor can suppress further invasion and progression. These differences in their behaviour could be explained probably by the differences between tumors that have lost p53 or $p16^{ink4A}$ tumor suppressor genes [99,100], as well as by the surrounding microenvironment.

Maspin is a no inhibitory serpin [101] that affects the pro-uPA/uPA/plasmin cascade directly related to metastasis promotion [102], and its anti-metastatic feature is ascribed to its reactive site loop [103]. Maspin can bind both uPA and tissue-type PA (tPA), at "*an exosite on maspin close to, but outside of, the reactive center loop*", having no effect in plasminogen activators (PAs) activity themselves [104]. This inhibitor can bind the complex between PA and PAI, the PA single chain and the complex uPA/uPAR [102,104,105]. The latter union may contribute to block the pericellular proteolysis which is dependent on the interaction between uPA and uPAR [102,105]. Maspin may also internalize uPA/uPAR complex even when uPA remains inactive as zymogen, implicating the down-regulation of the expression of both uPA and uPAR and, consequently, counteracting the uPA-mediated cell detachment [105,106]. The ability of maspin to inhibit cell motility is related with the Rho GTPase pathway and its ability to promote cell adhesion via phosphatidylinositol 3-kinase (PI3K)/ERK pathway [107]. The latter plays an important role in regulating cell migration [108]. It can also stimulate cell adhesion through its direct interaction with β1 integrin [109], through its interaction with matrix proteins such as type I and III collagen [110], and by changing the expression profiles of integrins and through up-regulation of several matrix proteins as focal adhesion contacts [102,103,111]. Anti-metastatic and anti-angiogenesis abitily of maspin have been confirmed on *in vivo* models [85]. Inhibitory activity of maspin against angiogenesis was first shown when maspin inhibited migration of endothelial cells through the inhibition of basic fibroblast growth factor (FGF) and vascular endothelial growth factor (VEGF) *in vitro,* and when it blocked neovascularization *in vivo* [112]. Further works correlated maspin expression with decreased tumor-induced angiogenesis in breast, colon, ovarian and skin cancer [113,114,115]. The anti-angiogenic activity of maspin is not ascribed to its reactive site loop [112], whereas the N-terminal region of maspin where collagen-binding site is located was necessary for such activity [110].

Expression of maspin varies between cells and conditions; maspin as protein is found on cytoplasm, nucleus, on cellular vesicles, on cell surface and parcially as secreted protein [116]. Evidence suggest that intracellular maspin play an important role in the maintenance of cellular homeostasis and response to cellular stress induced by immflamation, tissue injury and remodeling, through regulation of the glutathione S-transferase (GST) redox system in cytoplasm and through regulation of gene transcription of stress-related genes in nucleus [117,118]. Also, maspin is linked with receptor activator of nuclear factor-κB (RANK) ligand/IκB kinase α pathway that causes metastatic progression by repressing expression of maspin in prostate tumors [119]. In ovarian, pancreatic and lung cancinoma, cytoplasmatic maspin has been related with poor prognosis. In contrast when maspin is located at nucleus a favourable prognosis exist in breast, lung ovarian cancer, and laryngeal squamous cell carcinoma [95,120,91,114,121].

Jiang *et al.* [86] demonstrated that maspin enhances apoptosis in breast cancer cells through over-expression of Bcl-2 family of proteins via the mitochondrial apoptosis pathway [122,123,124]. Also, the nuclear expression of maspin may restore sensitivity towards many apoptosis-inducing chemotherapeutic agents [121,125]. Furthermore, ectopic maspin may improve the efficacy of proteasome inhibitors which in turn, induce endogen maspin expression through p38 MAPK pathway [126]. It has been demonstrated that maspin itself may reduce the chymotrypsin-like activity of the proteasome 26S similarly to BBI [31,127]. Nuclear maspin act as transcriptional regulator directly interacting with transcription factors and proteins that participate in chromatin remodeling through the inhibition of histone deacetylase 1 (HDAC1) activity [128]. Proteomic studies showed that maspin can up-regulate proteins that promote apoptosis and down-regulate the anti-apoptotic proteins. In the same way maspin produce changes in the pattern of cytoskeletal proteins, up-regulating proteins known to restrict cell migration and down-regulating those proteins that promote the same process [127]. Interestingly, maspin could produce in breast cancer cells an effect characterized by regression from a fibroblast-like phenotype back to epithelial-like phenotype, phenomenon known as EMT [68]. This phenomenon involve changes in cytoskeletal proteins [107,127], which is probably regulated by TGF-β pathway, since maspin is regulated directly for this pathway [83]; in a similar way to the effect of HAI-1 Kunitz inhibitor have on human pancreatic cancer [67].

Pigment Epithelium-Derived Factor (PEDF)

PEDF is a 50 kDa glycosilated non-inhibitory serpin, isolated from conditioned medium of cultured primary human fetal retinal pigment epithelial cells [129,130]. This inhibitor is largely distributed among several tissues including liver, testis, ovaries, placenta and pancreas [131]. An outstanding feature of PEDF is its potent anti-angiogenic effect [132,133,134] and its multipotent neurotrophic effect [134]; aditionally, PEDF possess pro-apoptotic anti-tumorogenic effect and induces neuronal differentiation [133,135,136]. The multiple functions of PEDF in normal cells have been related with different segments of its structure [137]; recently, it has been found a peculiar region located near of the anti-angiogenesis segment, which binds specifically to endothelial cell membranes, inhibits FGF-induced angiogenesis by pro-apoptotic and anti-migration effect, and interacts with a novel non-integrin 37/67-kDa laminin receptor of PEDF [138].

A poor prognosis has been found when the expression of PEDF is low, and it has been linked with poor prognosis and high levels of metastasis in prostate and pancreatic cancers and in neuroblastomas and gliomas [139-142], whereas its overexpression produces a decrease of angiogenesis and cell growth of melanoma, neuroblastoma, osteosarcoma, and pancreatic cancer cells [142,144,145]. PEDF was found to reduce glioma angiogenesis by the down-regulation of angiogenesis inducers VEGF and FGF and by the up-regulation of angiogenesis inhibitor thrombospondin-2; and it also reduces invasiveness, migration and metastasis, probably through the down-regulation of MMP-9 in melanoma and osteosarcoma, with the increased cell adhesion to collagen type-1 in the latter case [146,147,144]. Early studies established that PEDF can promote apoptosis in tumor cells and normal stress-induced epithelial cells [146], probably do to death receptor Fas (Fas)/membrane-bound Fas ligand (FasL) death pathway [143,148]. Apoptosis due to PEDF could depend also of the VEGF/VEGF receptor-1–induced angiogenesis [149], and through the induction of p53, Bax and the repression of Bcl-2 [150]. The dual effects of PEDF on apoptosis between different kinds of cells could be explained by the union of PEDF with more than one cell surface receptor which could activate different cell signal cascades [146]. Recent works revealed the intracellular mechanism of PEDF, consisting in the sequential activation/induction of p38 MAPK, cytosolic calcium-dependent phospholipase A_2-α (cPLA$_2$-α), peroxisome proliferator-activated receptor gamma (PPAR-γ) and p53 [151,152].

Other Serpins

Antithrombin (AT) is a heparin-binding protein known as the major plasma inhibitor of coagulation proteases, including thrombin and factor Xa [154]. Its reactive site loop can be cleaved by other type of proteases, inactivating this serpin [155]. However, this inactive-cleaved form of AT (C-AT) and another inactive form produced by heat treatment known as latent form (L-AT) have been related with anti-angiogenic activity [156]. The mechanism of the anti-angiogenic effect of L-AT and C-AT, basically consist on the disruption of cell-matrix interactions, the increasing of apoptosis and cell cycle arrest, and the inhibition of tumor growth and metastasis, via changes on the focal adhesion kinase and endothelial cell ligand-receptor signalling pathways [157,158,159]. Several important genes are affected by L-AT and C-AT in endothelial cells, acting on the down-regulation of pro-angiogenic genes, including cell-surface and matrix proteoglycans (perlecan, biglycan, and syndecans 1 and 3) and mitogenesis-related and signal transducers and transcription activators (STAT) of signaling proteins (MAPK-3, STAT 2, 3, and 6 and early growth response factor 1); as well as the up-regulation of anti-angiogenic genes such as p21, caspase 3 and tissue inhibitor of metalloprotease 1, 2, 3 [158].

Angiotensinogen (AGT) is the precursor of angiotensin I in the renin-angiotensin system (RAS) and as maspin and PEDF AGT is a non-inhibitory serpin with anti-angiogenic activity [159,160]. Interestingly, AGT is able to inhibit angiogenesis through the induction of apoptosis and suppression of endothelial cell proliferation, but unlike other serpins, without altering the exppression of vascular growth factors [161]. It has been demonstrated that AGT exert its anti-angiogenic and anti-metastatic effect in different mice models probably through the modulation of intramembrane proteolysis made patent by Noch activation [162,163].

Headpin (SERPINB13, Hurpin, PI13) is a serpin that is normally expressed in squemous epithelium of the oral mucosa, skin and cervix [164]. This serpin specifically inhibits lisosomal cysteine proteases as cathepsins K and L [165], and it is able to block *in vivo* angiogenesis by reducing the IL-8 and VEGF expression at transcriptional and protein level. Also, extracellular presence of headpin reduce invasion, migration, and tube formation of endothelial cells, and when headpin is located at nucleus, it is able to regulate the transcription of mediators of cell proliferation [166]. The down-regulation of *headpin* gene by means of hypermethylation is linked with the development, aggressiveness and poor clinical outcome of oral, head and neck squamous cell carcinomas [167,168].

Kallistatin or kallikrein-binding protein (KBP) is a serpin firstly discovered as an inhibitor of the kininogenase and amidolytic activities of tissue kallikrein *in vitro* with [169]. KBP can suppress VEGF- and FGF-induced proliferation, migration, and adhesion to endothelial cells and inhibit angiogenesis through its heparin-binding domain [170,171]. In addition, the anti-angiogenic effect of KBP requires the down-regulation of VEGF expression through the inhibition of hypoxia-inducible factor 1α (HIF-1α) [172].

Squamous cell carcinoma antigen (SCCA) is an inhibitory serpin that was found originally from squamous cell carcinoma of the uterine cervix [173,174]. SCCA comprises two distinct isoforms named SCCA1 and SCCA2, which differ in properties [175]. The main feature is that both isoforms are able to protect tumor cells from apoptosis [176]. The mechanism through SCCA isoforms act is due, in part, to their effect in the stimulation on the production of pro-metaloproteinase 9 (pro-MMP-9) independent to their protease inhibitory activity [177]. Also, caspase-3 was suggested the as upstream target of SCCA1 and cathepsin

G as target of SCCA2 [176,178]. In addition, SCCA1 can inhibit the UV-induced apoptosis via its translocation into the nucleus by the direct or indirect interaction with the c-Jun NH_2-terminal kinase-1 (JNK1) after UV radiation [179]. Both SCCA isoforms have been proposed as serological biomarkers in the detection of early steps of tumor development, especially on smaller hepatocellular carcinoma (HCC) [180].

The protease inhibitor 9 (PI-9) is the unique serpin that inhibits granzyme B, caspase-1 and, to a lesser extent, caspase-4 and -8 [181,182]. It is expressed by tumor derived from both T and B cells [183]. PI-9 is associated with poor prognosis and poor clinical outcome since it may protect tumor cell from immune response. The mechanism by which PI-9 is able to protect the tumor cell is based on its ability to inhibit death receptor-mediated apoptosis, specifically inhibiting TNF, TNF-related apoptosis-inducing ligand (TRAIL) and FasL in some sarcoma cells, and subsequently, by binding to the intermediate active forms of caspase-8 and caspase-10, preventing the caspase-3 activation, which in turn inhibits the whole process of apoptosis [184].

Neuroserpin is a serpin expressed only in nervious system, specifically in neurons [185,186]. *Neuroserpin* gene is highly expressed in prostate cancer and it may be associated to progression and agresiveness of this kind of cancer [187].

MATRIX METALLOPROTEINASE INHIBITORS

Matrix metalloproteinases (MMPs) is a group of zinc-dependent proteases which are consider as one of the most important factors in cancer metastasis, since they participate in extracellular matrix (ECM) degradation and subsequent cancer cell invasion [188-193]. Novel biological functions in early stages of cancer development have been attributed to MMPs in as much as they promote malignant transformation through the formation of a complex microenvironment by the activation of growth factors, suppression of tumor cell apoptosis or release of angiogenic factors [194-197]. Thus, it is evident that the control of MMP activity could be important in the whole process of cancer development. Physiologically, the proteolytic activity of MMPs is inhibited by non-specific PIs, such as α2-macroglobulin and α1-antiprotease and, by specific PIs, called tissue inhibitors of MMPs (TIMPs) [198]; in addition, the latter ones are able to inhibit also, the catalytic activation process of MMPs [198,199]. TIMPs are variably glycosylated secreted proteins with molecular mass between 21 and 28 kDa that occasionally are found in association with membrane-bound proteins [200,201]. TIMPs are involved in the homeostasis of ECM due to their biological activity determined by the complex interactions with ECM- and non-ECM-proteins into the extracellular milieu and with receptors in other cells [201]. The application of TIMPs in cancer was demonstrated by their ability to inhibit tumor growth in transgenic mouse models [202,203], and the ability to decrease tumor metastasis and growth in cancer cells as well as protecting normal tissue, with favourable prognosis in cancer patients [204-207]. However, by the nature of MMPs' roles, TIMPs also present promotion of cancer development [201,208,209]. Considering the complex biological activities of TIMPs, the technical difficulties and the lack of effective methods of systemic gene delivery, their application into useful drugs was hindered [196]. On the other hand, small-molecule synthetic inhibitors of MMPs (MMPIs) have been rapidly developed and evaluated into human clinical trials as anticancer agents and, unfortunately, those trials have been largely disappointing and fail so far to produce statistically significant results, due mainly to the non-selective broad spectrum of MMPIs which in turn cause adverse side-effects [196,210-214]. According to pharmacologic approaches directed to extracellular MMPs the synthetic inhibitors have been divided in four categories: peptidomimetics, non-peptidomimetics, tetracycline derivatives and bisphophonates [211,212]. Peptidomimetic inhibitors mimic the cleavage site of collagen acting as competitive inhibitors and chelating the zinc atom of MMP active site. [215]. Non-peptidomimetics inhibitors are designed according the active site of MMPs [216]. Tetracycline derivates are able to bind metal ions and to downregulate MMP gene transcription [217], whereas biphosphonates binds to hydroxyapatite crystal and, they are able to inhibit 2 key enzymes in the mevalonate pathway [218].

The inhibition of many MMP subtypes by a single MMPI is the main reason for the adverse results, since some MMPs have tumor-suppressive effects or even both, anti-cancer and cancer-promoting effects depending on the kind of tissue and/or stage of cancer development [214,219]. In addition, the interconnection between proteolyitc pathways in which MMPs are implicated and the balance between MMPs and PIs, needs to be consider for further strategies with MMPs as drug targets. Several factors must be taken into consideration when studying the clinical performance of MMPIs; the difference between proteolytic systems of animal models and humans, the physiological state of groups of patients regarding to cancer development, the adequate doses and correct standard criteria of evaluation, and the correct identification of MMP expression profiles at different physiological stages of tumor [214]. Therefore, it becomes urgent to study the drug side effects which produced unexpected perturbations in the protease web resulting from therapeutic inhibition of key nodal MMPs that could control the activity of other proteases in the degradome [220]. The therapeutic potential in controlling MMP signaling cascades that promote tumorogenesis is a great and necessary challenge and that emphasize the need to continue in the search of a better understanding of the chemical mechanisms that control those process, to be able to propose new more selective alternatives for the specific control of MMP in the process of cancer.

CISTEINE PROTEASE INHIBITORS

Cysteine proteases as other proteases, belong to a tangled signaling system of cellular regulation, though, is not surprising that misregulation of this kind of proteases led to pathological conditions. Lysosomal cysteine proteases can participate both negatively or positively in different stages of tumor progression, including immortalization, transformation, tumor invasion, angiogenesis, apoptosis and drug resistance; attributed greatly to the lost of balance cystein protease/PI [221-226]. Generally, mammalian cysteine proteases belong to the cathepsin superfamily and their activity is tightly regulated by cysteine protease inhibitors (CPIs) that are members of cystatin superfamily [227-229]. By virtue of their targets, CPIs are implicated in cell survival, proliferation, differentiation, immunomodulation and disorders such as cancer, since CPIs have both tumor promoting as well as tumor suppressing activities [222,230].

Some examples of important CPIs in cancer development will be discussed. Stefin A and B, also called Cystatin A and B, are able to regulate initiation or propagation of the lysosomal cell death pathway [225,231]. In various cancer cell lines stefin A strongly reduces their susceptibility to cell death-inducing agents, however, few cancers can use stefin A as protective agent and it is related with malignant transformation [225,232]. Stefin A has been shown to reduce tumor cell invasion and metastasis, and it could play a role in the prevention [233,234]. Otherwise, stefin B and cystatin C are correlated with survival, whereas stefin A is not. Similar to stefin A, exogenous stefin B also inhibit motility of melanoma cells [235]. Cystatin C is the most potent inhibitor of cysteine proteases and it is ubiquitously expressed in all tissues and cell types. This protein, unlike most cystatins, is considered a housekeeping type protein [236]. Cystatin C has recently been described as a tumor growth factor-b (TGF-β) receptor antagonist [237], whose expression is regulated by TGF-β in mouse cells. By binding to TGF-β, cystatin C could inhibit TGF- β signaling [237], a multifunctional cytokine endowed with both tumor-promoting and tumor-suppressing function, which could explain the dual action of cystatin C. The effect of cystatin C illustrates the dual nature of the cystatins: in general they are potent protease inhibitors but, in addition, they also show cytokine-like activities. Another example is Cystatin E/M which is not expressed in breast and in brain tumors, and in melanoma cells, but is highly expressed in prostate cancer cells and in oropharyngeal squamous cell carcinoma [230,238,239,240]. Cystatin E/M is able to supress breast tumor growth and to diminish metastatic burden at secondary sites [241]. Though, cystatin E/M is considered as tumor suppressor in breast cancer, since the expression of this gene is considerably decreased [230,238,241]. Cystatin F that is also referred as a cystatin-like metastasis-associated protein (CMAP) [242], unlike cystatin E/M, it is identified as the most important factor of liver metastasis and it has been proposed to be use as diagnosis tool [242].

OTHER PIs

Secretory Leukocyte Protease Inhibitor (SLPI)

Secretory leukocyte protease inhibitor (SLPI) is an 11.7 kDa protein of the Kazal family that is produced at mucosal surfaces, principally at the upper respiratory tract [243,244]. SLPI inhibits granulocyte and elastases, cathepsin B and G, trypsin, chymotrypsin, mast cell chymase, and tryptase [243-247]. Devoogdt *et al.* [248], demonstrated that although SLPI protects broad tissue functions, counteracting inflammatory process and invading pathogens, and participating in the process of tissue repairing, SLPI also increased malignancy of cancer cells and it is therefore correlated, principally through its protease inhibitor activity, with tumor progression [248-250]. In addition, evidence demonstrated that SLPI is up-regulated in non-small cell lung cancer, gastric cancer, and in ovarian, cervix and pancreas cancinomas, confirming those results with the fact that lung carcinogenesis is suppressed if SLPI is absent [251-253]. As a consequence SLPI has the potential to become a prognostic marker in those types of cancer.

Devoogdt *et al.* [254] demonstrated that high levels of *SLPI* gene expression increased both the tumorigenicity and lung-colonizing potential of low-malignant Lewis Lung Carcinoma cells (3LL-S) and this function was dependent on its protease inhibitor activity, but not on its proliferation stimulating properties [254,255]. Otherwise, the promotion of malignant potential of cancer cells that is correlated with the increasing expression of SLPI is also influenced by the local tumor microenvironment in which cytokines and steroid hormones are responsible for SLPI expression [248,256]. King *et al.* [257] reported that progesterone is able to increase SLPI in both ways, directly by increasing SLPI levels, and indirectly by acting in synergy with the pro-inflammatory cytokines, IL-1β and TNF-α. The latter cytokine is able to act as an endogenous tumor promoter by means of the promotion of SLPI [258]. Devoogdt *et al.* [259] found that SLPI stimulated significant proliferation and survival of Hey-A8 ovarian cancer cells *in vitro*, and that SLPI protected HEY-A8 cells from degradation and apoptosis due to neutrophil elastase. They concluded the existence of a PI independent function for SLPI in ovarian cancer growth and dissemination. Luo *et al.* [260] found the expression of SLPI in the bronchi and lung tissues of chronic obstructive pulmonary disease (COPD) models, finding that the increased expression of SLPI is linked to the increased expression of TGF-β1, and this process is probably related to the activation of Smads signal pathway. On the other hand, SLPI can act as protective gene against liver metastasis, since it can decrease the liver-metastasizing potential of carcinoma cells through decreasing in TNF-α and E-selectin production due to the attenuation of host proinflammatory response [261]. Consequently, SLPI expression can differently affect tumor behavior in different anatomic sites [261]. An interesting feature of SLPI is that even when it can act as anti-angiogenesis factor by suppressing the migration of newly formed blood vessels and it is able to inhibit the migration activity of vascular endothelial cells, both *in vitro* and *in vivo* assays; SLPI can induce a sinusoidal vasculature in primary tumors which is the first step of an invasion-independent pathway of cancer metastasis [262].

A NEW APPROACH TO OBTAIN PI BASED CANCER TREATMENTS

An interesting alternative that has been proved to reduce the cost of testing new drugs consists of testing on a particular type cancer, a drug that has already been successfully used on a different disease. Such is the case of different PIs that have been used to treat Human Immunodeficiency virus (HIV). The strategy consist in the use of small molecules, referred as HIV-1 protease inhibitors (HIV-PIs), that target the viral aspartyl protease which cleaves precursor proteins into components of viral core in the HIV-replication process [263]. Considering that the basis to the activity in both diseases is the control of specific target enzymes which are required for the cell to develop the malignancy or in the case of virus, the patogenicity. The main benefit will be that those drugs have already been tested to be safe, and in general, the way they act is known, since there are already studies on their absorption, the way they are excreted, and their undesired effects they present [264]. HIV-PIs have been used for HIV treatments since 1993, and their safety, toxicity and the different effects they caused in human, are well established. The development of new treatments according to an analysis of 68 approved drugs estimated that it takes an average of 15 years and US$802 million to successfully develop a new drug, and nearly $900 million when including postmarketing safety costs [264]. In addition, HIV-PIs are the foundation of multidrug HIV treatment regimens, called ''highly active antiretroviral therapy'' (HAART) that combines different strategies against HIV, and is characterized by an increase of survival, restoration of immunity and decrease of viral resistance [265,266]. The interest showed on HIV-PIs in regard with their anti-tumor effects was discovered from the unexpected observation in which patients on HAART reduced the risk to develop HIV-associated malignancies such as Kaposi's sarcoma and non–Hodgkin's lymphoma [267]. Later on, it was demonstrated that the HIV-PIs, saquinavir, indinavir, and ritonavir decreased proliferation and increased differentiation of all-*trans*-retinoic acid for myelocytic leukemia cells [268]. Moreover, HIV-PIs proved to be potent anti-angiogenic, pro-apoptotic agents who also could inhibit the cell growth and induce regression in Kaposi's sarcoma as well as prostate cancer cells [269,270]. The different mechanisms proposed to explain these effects comprise the inhibition of NF-κB activity, the suppression of production of pro-angiogenic cytokines (TNFα, interleukin 6, and VEGF), the partial inhibition of the chaperone function of heat shock protein 90 (Hsp90), the suppression of proteasomal chymotrypsin-like activities with its subsequent accumulation of missfolded proteins, the blockage of (PI3K)–Akt, STAT3 and androgen receptor signal pathways [270-275]. A recent report links the pro-apoptotic effect of nelfinavir and atazanavir with a proteasome inhibition-derivate stress pathway: the endoplasmic reticulum stress response (ESR), which is also responsible for insulin resistance, a common HIV-PI–side effect [276].

The anti-tumor effect of HIV-PIs varies between each kind of inhibitor. Comparing some of most potent HIV-PIs, the most efficient inhibitor was nelfinavir [277]. This inhibitor proved to have interesting results regarding to its mechanism; it was able to inhibit the activation of Akt signaling pathway in human non–small cell lung cancer cell lines and in human umbilical vein endothelial cells, but not in human melanoma cells, where nelfinavir activate the Akt pathway [277,278,279]. This result indicated that this process is cell-dependent and it probably could not be a direct result of anti-tumor effect but rather reflects cellular responses to stress condition provoked by nelfinavir [279]. In addition, nelfinavir was able to inhibit angiogenesis, tumor cell migration and it could contribute to the increase of radiation sensitivity [278]. Nelfinavir by itself promotes cell death in two different ways: with caspase-dependent apoptosis and caspase-independent apoptosis accompanied with autophagy and induction of ESR [277]. The inhibition of cell growth by nelfinavir is given for a G_0-G_1 cycle arrest that is related to nelfinavir-mediated proteasome-degradation of Cdc25A phosphatase, without inhibition of chymotrypsin-like activity of the proteasome; the degradation of Cdc25A triggers the inhibition of cyclin dependent kinase 2 (CDK2) and concomitant dephosphorylation of retinoblastoma tumor suppressor [279]. Finally, the toxicity of nelfinavir in pancreatic ductal adenocarcinoma (PDAC) was determined in a phase I clinical trial, in combination with chemoradiotherapy, giving as a result the assurance that nelfinavir is safe in locally advanced PDAC, consolidating this combination for next phase II trial [280].

Conclusion

PIs have shown to be an interesting group of molecules from the viewpoint of the modulation of physiological and pathological functions. Since PIs showed a great potential against cancer, the elucidation of their mechanisms of action has demostrated the extraordinarily intrincate processess implicated in cancer development. The differences in the way different PIs work make difficult to stablish exactly the main pathway responsible for their anti-tumor effect, and in most cases it is still unknown the target enzyme or enzymes that interacts with a particular inhibitor. However, recent studies have set the basis for elucidation of the mechanisms by which PIs exert their anti-tumor effect and their effect on the signaling pathways involved. The anti-cancer effect of PIs can affect the genetic expression level, as well as at the protein level, different signaling molecules. In some cases, the mechanisms by which PIs exert their anti-cancer effect involved the inhibition of chymotrypsin-like activity of the proteasome 26 S, giving us an idea of the key role that this activity fulfill in cancer progression and the complex network of metabolic pathways affected by it. We could conclude by stating that some PIs have demostrated their importance in the regulation of different events that interfere with the development and/or metastasis of cancer. However, there is not a general mechanism for these kinds of molecules, which can interact at different levels, including the possibility that they can in some instances favor the cancer process. Therefore, while encouraging the continuation of studies directed to the understanding the molecular bases for each particular PI, it is relevant to point out that caution must be taken to ensure no negative effects would be present. Altogether, PI constitude a promissory type of molecules with potential for their possible application in prognosis, diagnosis and therapy in cancer.

REFERENCES

[1] Laskowsky Jr., M; Kato, I. Protein inhibitors of proteinases. *Ann Rev Biochem,* 1980 49, 593–626.

[2] Kennedy, AR; Liltle, JB. Protease inhibitors suppress radiation induced malignant transformation *in vitro*. *Nature,* 1978 276, 825–826.

[3] Troll, W; Frenkel, K; Wiesner, R. Protease inhibitors as anticarcinogens. *J. Natl Cancer Inst,* 1984 73, 1245–1250.

[4] Messadi, DV; Billings, P; Shklar, G; Kennedy, AR. Inhibition of oral carcinogenesis by a protease inhibitor. *J. Natl Cancer Inst.* 1986 76, 447–452.

[5] Kennedy, AR. Chemopreventive agents: protease inhibitors. *Pharmacol Ther*, 1998 78, 167–209.

[6] Yagi, T; Ishizaki, K; Takebe, H. Cytotoxic effects of protease inhibitors on human cells. 2. Effect of elastatinal. *Cancer Lett,* 1980 10, 301–307.

[7] Billings, PC; Morrow, AR; Ryan, CA; Kennedy, AR. Inhibition of radiation-induced transformation of C3H/10T1/2 cells by carboxypeptidase inhibitor I and inhibitor II from potatoes. *Carcinogenesis,* 1989 10, 687–691.

[8] Billings, PC; Jin, T; Ohnishi, N; Liao, DC; Habre, JM. The interaction of the potato-derived chymotrypsin inhibitor with C3H/101/2 cells. *Carcinogenesis*, 1991 12, 653–657.

[9] Prange, E; Schroyens, W; Pralle, H. The influence of the protease inhibitor aprotinin on tumor invasion of three cell lines *in vitro*. *Clin Expl Metastasis*, 1988 6, 107–113.

[10] Weed, H; McGandy, RB; Kennedy, AR. Protection against dimethylhydrazine induced adenomatous tumors of the mouse colon by the dietary addition of an extract of

soybeans containing the Bowman-Birk protease inhibitor. *Carcinogenesis,* 1985 6, 1239–1241.

[11] Birk, Y. Purification and some properties of a highly active inhibitor of trypsin and chymotrypsin from soybeans. *Biochim Biophys Acta*, 1961 54, 378–438.

[12] Birk, Y. The Bowman-Birk inhibitor. *Int J Peptide Protein Res,* 1985 25, 113–131.

[13] Yavelow, J; Collins, M; Birk, Y; Troll, W; Kennedy, AR. Nanomolar concentrations of Bowman-Birk soybean protease inhibitor suppress x-ray-induced transformation *in vitro*. *Proc Natl Acad Sci USA.* 1985 82, 5395–5399.

[14] Kennedy, AR. The Bowman-Birk inhibitor from soybeans as an anticarcinogenic agent, *Am J Clin Nutr*, 1998 68, 1406s–1412s.

[15] St. Clair, WH. Suppresion of 3-methylcholanthrene-induced cellular transformation by timed administration of the Bowman-Birk protease inhibitor. *Carcinogenesis,* 1991 12, 935–937.

[16] Witschi, H; Kennedy, AR. Modulation of lung tumor development in mice with the soybean-derived Bowman- Birk protease inhibitor. *Carcinogenesis,* 1989 10, 2275–2277.

[17] von Hofe, E; Newberne, PM; Kennedy, AR. Inhibition of N-nitrosomethylbenzylamine-induced esophageal neoplasms by the Bowman- Birk protease inhibitor. *Carcinogenesis,* 1991 12, 2147–2150.

[18] Furukawa, F; Imaida, K; Okamiya, H; Shinoda, K; Sato, M; Imazawa, T; Hayashi, Y; Takahashi, M. Inhibitory effects of soybean trypsin inhibitor on induction of pancreatic neoplastic lesions in hamsters by N-nitrosobis(2-oxopropyl)amine. *Carcinogenesis,* 1991 12, 2123–2125.

[19] Losso, JN; Munene, CN; Bansode, RR; Bawadi, HA. Inhibition of matrix metalloproteinase-1 activity by the soybean Bowman–Birk inhibitor. *Biotechnol Lett,* 2004 26, 901–905.

[20] Gueven, N; Dittmann, K; Mayer, C; Rodemann HP. The radioprotective potential of the Bowman-Birk protease inhibitor is independent of its secondary structure. *Cancer Lett,* 1998 125, 77–82.

[21] Dittmann, KH; Gueven, N; Mayer, C; Rodemann, HS. Characterization of the amino acids essential for the photo- and radioprotective effects of Bowman-Birk protease inhibitor-derived nonapeptidde. *Protein Eng Des Sel,* 2001 14, 157–160.

[22] Wan, XS; Ware, JH; Zhang, L; Newberne, PM; Evans, SM; Clark, LC; Kennedy, AR. Treatment With Soybean-Derived Bowman Birk Inhibitor Increases Serum Prostate-Specific Antigen Concentration While Suppressing Growth of Human Prostate Cancer Xenografts in Nude Mice. *Prostate,* 1999 41, 243–252.

[23] Kennedy, AR; Wan, XS. Effects of the Bowman-Birk inhibitor on growth, invasion, and clonogenic survival of human prostate epithelial cells and prostate cancer cells. *Prostate,* 2002 50, 125–133.

[24] Kennedy, AR; Billings, PC; Wan, XS; Newberne, PM. Effects of Bowman-Birk Inhibitor on Rat Colon Carcinogenesis. *Nutr and Cancer,* 2002 43, 174–186.

[25] Dittmann, KH; Toulany, M; Classen, J; Heinrich, V; Milas, L; Rodemann, HP. Selective Radioprotection of Normal Tissues by Bowman-Birk Proteinase Inhibitor (BBI) in Mice. *Strahlenther Onkol,* 2005 181, 191–196.

[26] Armstrong, WB; Kennedy, AR; Wan, XS; Atiba, J; Mc-Claren, CE; Meyskens, FL Jr. Single-dose administration of Bowman-Birk inhibitor concentrate in patients with oral leukoplakia. *Cancer Epidemiol Biomark Prev,* 2000 9, 43–47.

[27] Armstrong, WB; Kennedy, AR; Wan, XS; Taylor, TH; Nguyen, QA; Jensen, J; Thompson, W; Lagerberg, W; Meyskens, FL Jr. Clinical Modulation of Oral Leukoplakia and Protease Activity by Bowman-Birk Inhibitor Concentrate in a Phase IIa Chemoprevention Trial. *Clin cancer res,* 2000 6, 4684–4691.

[28] Billings, PC; St Clair, W; Owen, AJ; Kennedy, AR. Potential intracellular target proteins of the anticarcinogenic Bowman-Birk protease inhibitors identified by affinity chromatography. *Cancer Res,* 1988 48, 1798–1802.

[29] Dittmann, K; Virsik-Köpp, P; Mayer, C; Rave-Fränk, M; Rodemann, HP. Bowman–Birk protease inhibitor activates DNA-dependent protein kinase and reduces formation of radiation-induced dicentric chromosomes. *Int J Radiat Biol,* 2003 79, 801–808.

[30] Dittmann, KH; Mayer, C; Kehlbach, R; Rodemann, HP. The radioprotector Bowman–Birk proteinase inhibitor stimulates DNA repair via epidermal growth factor receptor phosphorylation and nuclear transport. *Radiother Oncol,* 2008 86, 375–382.

[31] Chen, YW; Huang, SC; Lin-Shiau, SY; Lin, JK. Bowman-Birk inhibitor abates proteasome function and suppresses the proliferation of MCF7 breast cancer cells through accumulation of MAP kinase phosphatase-1. *Carcinogenesis,* 2005 26, 1296–1306.

[32] Saito, T; Sato, H; Virgona, N; Hagiwara, H; Kashiwagi, K; Suzuki, K; Asano, R; Yano, T. Negative growth control of osteosarcoma cell by Bowman–Birk protease inhibitor from soybean; involvement of connexin 43. *Cancer Lett,* 2007 253, 249–257.

[33] St. Clair, WH; St. Clair, DK. Effect of the Bowman-Birk Protease Inhibitor on the Expression of Oncogenes in the Irradiated Rat Colon. *Cancer Res,* 1991 51, 4539–4543.

[34] Wan, XS; Meyskens, Jr. FL; Armstrong, WB; Taylor, TH; Kennedy, AR. Relationship between Protease Activity and neu Oncogene Expression in Patients with Oral Leukoplakia Treated with the Bowman Birk Inhibitor. *Cancer Epidemiol Biomark Prev,* 1999 8, 601–608.

[35] Fernandes, AO; Banerji, AP. The field bean protease inhibitor can effectively suppress 7,12-dimethylbenz(a)anthracene-induced skin tumorigenesis in mice. *Cancer Lett,* 1996 104, 219–224.

[36] Banerji, A; Fernandes, A; Bane, S; Ahire, S. The field bean protease inhibitor has the potential to suppress B16F10 melanoma cell lung metastasis in mice. *Cancer Lett*, 1998 129, 25–20.

[37] Campos, J; Martinez-Gallardo, N; Mendiola-Olaya, E; Blanco-Labra, A. Purification and partial characterization of a proteinase inhibitor from tepary bean (*Phaseolus acutifolius*) seeds. *J Food Biochem*, 1997 21, 203–218.

[38] García-Gasca, T; Salazar-Olivo, LA; Mendiola-Olaya, E; Blanco-Labra, A. The effects of a protease inhibitor fraction from tepary bean (*Phaseolus acutifolius*) on *in vitro* cell proliferation and cell adhesion of transformed cells. *Toxicol In Vitro*, 2002 16, 229–233.

[39] Yoshida, E; Maruyama, M; Sugiki, M; Mihara, H. Immunohistochemical demonstration of bikunin, a light chain of inter-α-trypsin inhibitor, in human brain tumors. *Inflammation,* 1994 18, 589–596.

[40] Suzuki, M; Kobayashi, H; Tanaka, Y; Hirashima, Y; Terao, T. Structure and function analysis of urinary trypsin inhibitor (UTI): identification of binding domains and signaling property of UTI by analysis of truncated proteins. *Biochim. Biophys. Acta,* 2001 1547, 26–36.

[41] Bromke, BJ; Kueppers, F. The major urinary protease inhibitor: simplified purification and characterization. *Biochem Med,* 1982 27, 56–67.

[42] Balduyck, M; Davril, M; Mizon, C; Smyrlaki, M; Hayem, A; Mizon, J. Human urinary proteinase inhibitor: inhibitory properties and interaction with bovine trypsin. *Biol Chem Hoppe-Seyler,* 1985 366, 9–14.

[43] Delaria, KA; Muller, DK; Marlor, CW; Brown, JE; Das, RC; Roczniak, SO; Tamburini, PP. Characterization of placental bikunin, a novel human serine protease inhibitor. *J Biol Chem,* 1997 272, 12209–12214.

[44] Suzuki, M; Kobayashi, H; Tanaka, Y; Hirashima, Y; Kanayama, N; Takei, Y; Saga, Y; Suzuki, M; Itoh, H; Terao, T. Suppression of invasion and peritoneal carcinomatosis of ovarian cancer cell line by overexpression of bikunin. *Int J Cancer*, 2003 104, 289–302.

[45] Kobayashi, H; Shinohara, H; Fujie, M; Gotoh, J; Itoh, M; Takeuchi, K; Terao, T. Inhibition of metastasis of Lewis lung carcinoma by urinary trypsin inhibitor in experimental and spontaneous metastasis models. *Int J Cancer*, 1995 63, 455–462.

[46] Kobayashi, H; Suzuki, M; Hirashima, Y; Terao, T. The Protease Inhibitor Bikunin, a Novel Anti-Metastatic Agent. *Biol Chem*, 2003 384, 749–754.

[47] Yagyu, T; Kobayashi, H; Matsuzaki, H; Wakahara, K; Kondo, T; Kurita, N; Sekino, H; Inagaki, K. Enhanced spontaneous metastasis in bikunin-deficient mice. *Int J Cancer,* 2006 118, 2322–2328.

[48] Kobayashi, H; Suzuki, M; Tanaka, Y; Hiroshima, Y; Terao, T. Suppression of urokinase expression and invasiveness by urinary trypsin inhibitor is mediated through inhibition of protein kinase C- and MEK/ERK/c-Jun-dependent signaling pathways. *J Biol Chem*, 2001 276, 2015–22.

[49] Giuliani, R; Bastaki, M; Coltrini, D; Presta, M. Role of endothelial cell extracellular signal-regulated kinase1/2 in urokinase-type plasminogen activator upregulation and *in vitro* angiogenesis by fibroblast growth factor-2. *J. Cell Sci,* 1999 112, 2597–2606.

[50] Kobayashi, H; Suzuki, M; Tanaka, Y; Kanayama, N; Terao, T. A Kunitz-type Protease Inhibitor, Bikunin, Inhibits Ovarian Cancer Cell Invasion by Blocking the Calcium-dependent Transforming Growth Factor-β1 Signaling Cascade. *J Biol Chem*, 2003 278, 7790–7799.

[51] Suzuki, M; Kobayashi, H; Fujie, M; Nishida, T; Takigawa, M; Kanayama, N; Terao, T. Kunitz-type protease inhibitor bikunin disrupts phorbol ester-induced oligomerization of CD44 variant isoforms containing epitope v9 and subsequently suppresses expression of urokinase-type plasminogen activator in human chondrosarcoma cells. *J Biol Chem,* 2002 277, 8022–8032.

[52] Herrera-Gayol, A; Jothy, S. Adhesion proteins in the biology of breast cancer: contribution of CD44. *Exp Mol Pathol*, 1999 66, 149–156.

[53] Yagyu, T; Kobayashi, H; Wakahara, K; Matsuzaki, H; Kondo, T; Kurita, N; Sekino, H; Inagaki, K; Suzuki, M; Kanayama, N; Terao, T. A Kunitz-type protease inhibitor bikunin disrupts ligand-induced oligomerization of receptors for transforming growth

factor (TGF)-β and subsequently suppresses TGF-β signalings. *FEBS Lett,* 2004 576, 408–416.

[54] Suzuki, M; Kobayashi, H; Tanaka, Y; Hirashima, Y; Kanayama, N; Takei, Y; Saga, Y; Suzuki, M; Itoh, H; Terao, T. Bikunin Target Genes in Ovarian Cancer Cells Identified by Microarray Analysis. *J Biol Chem*, 2003 278, 14640–14646.

[55] Matsuzaki, H; Kobayashi, H; Yagyu, T; Wakahara, K; Kondo, T; Kurita, N; Sekino, H; Inagaki, K; Suzuki, M; Kanayama, N; Terao, T. Plasma Bikunin As a Favorable Prognostic Factor in Ovarian Cancer. *J Clin Oncol*, 2005 23, 1463–1472.

[56] Kobayashi, H; Yagyu, T; Inagaki, K; Kondo, T; Suzuki, M; Kanayama, N; Terao, T. Therapeutic Efficacy of Once-Daily Oral Administration of a Kunitz-Type Protease Inhibitor, Bikunin, in a Mouse Model and in Human Cancer. *Cancer,* 2004 100, 869–877.

[57] Shimomura, T; Denda, K; Kitamura, A; Kawaguchi, T; Kito, M; Kondo, J; Kagaya, S; Qin, L; Takata, H; Miyazawa, K; Kitamura, N. Hepatocyte growth factor activator inhibitor, a novel Kunitz-type serine protease inhibitor. *J Biol Chem,* 1997 272, 6370–6376.

[58] Kataoka, H; Miyata, S; Uchinokura, S; Itoh, H. Roles of hepatocyte growh factor (HGF) activator and HGF activator inhibitor in the pericellular activation of HGF/scatter factor. *Cancer Metastasis Rev,* 2003 22, 223–236.

[59] Kataoka, H; Itoh, H; Hamasuna, R; Meng, JY; Koono, M. Pericellular activation of hepatocyte growth factor/scatter factor (HGF/SF) in colorectal carcinomas. roles of HGF activator (HGFA) and HGFA inhibitor type 1 (HAI-1). *Hum. Cell,* 2001 14, 83–93.

[60] Miyazawa, K; Shimomura, T; Naka, D; Kitamura, N. Proteolytic activation of hepatocyte growth factor in response to tissue injury. *J Biol Chem,* 1994 269, 8966–8970.

[61] Kawaguchi, T; Qin, L; Shimomura, T; Kondo, J; Matsumoto, K; Denda, K; Kitamura, N. Purification and cloning of Hepatocyte growth factor activator inhibitor type 2, a Kunitz-type serine protease inihibitor. *J Biol Chem*, 1997 272, 27558–27564.

[62] Parr, C; Jiang, WG. Hepatocyte growth factor activation inhibitors (HAI-1 and HAI-2) regulate HGF-induced invasion of human breast cancer cells. *Int J Cancer*, 2006 119, 1176–1183.

[63] Kirchhofer, D; Peek, M; Li, W; Stamos, J; Eigenbrot, C; Kadkhodayan, S; Elliot, JM; Corpuz, RT; Lazarus, RA; Moran, P. Tissue expression, protease specificity, and Kunitz domain functions of hepatocyte growth factor activator inhibitor-1B (HAI-1B), a new splice variant of HAI-1. *J Biol Chem,* 2003 278, 36341–36349.

[64] Oberst, MD; Williams, CA; Dickson, RB; Johnson, MD; Lin, CY. The activation of matriptase requires its noncatalytic domains, serine protease domain, and its cognate inhibitor, *J Biol Chem*, 2003 278, 26773–26779.

[65] Fan, B; Wu, TD; Li, W; Kirchhofer, D. Identification of hepatocyte growth factor activator inhibitor-1B as a potential physiological inhibitor of prostasin. *J Biol Chem*, 2005 280, 34513–34520.

[66] Miyata, S; Fukushima, T; Kohama, K; Tanaka, H; Takeshima, H; Kataoka, H. Roles of Kunitz domains in the anti-invasive effect of hepatocyte growth factor activator inhibitor type 1 in human glioblastoma cells. *Hum Cell*, 2007 20, 100–106.

[67] Cheng, H; Fukushima, T; Takahashi, N; Tanaka, H; Kataoka, H. Hepatocyte Growth Factor Activator Inhibitor Type 1 Regulates Epithelial to Mesenchymal Transition through Membrane-Bound Serine Proteinases. *Cancer Res*, 2009 69, 1828–1835.

[68] Christiansen, JJ; Rajasekaran, AK. Reassessing epithelial to mesenchymal transition as a prerequisite for carcinoma invasion and metastasis. *Cancer Res*, 2006 66, 8319–8326.

[69] Miyata, S; Uchinokura, S; Fukushima, T; Hamasuna, R; Itoh, H; Akiyama, Y; Nakano, S; Wakisaka, S; Kataoka, H. Diverse roles of hepatocyte growth factor activator inhibitor type 1 (HAI-1) in the growth of glioblastoma cells *in vivo*. *Cancer Lett*, 2005 227, 83–93.

[70] Kobayashi, H; Suzuki, M; Kanayama, N; Terao, T. A soybean Kunitz trypsin inhibitor suppresses ovarian cancer cell invasion by blocking urokinase upregulation. *Clin Exp Metastasis*, 2004 21, 159–166.

[71] Inagaki, K; Kobayashi, H; Yoshida, R; Kanada, Y; Fukuda, Y; Yagyu, T; Kondo, T; Kurita, N; Kitanaka, T; Yamada, Y; Sakamoto, Y; Suzuki, M; Kanayama, N; Terao, T. Suppression of Urokinase Expression and Invasion by a Soybean Kunitz Trypsin Inhibitor Are Mediated through Inhibition of Src-dependent Signaling Pathways. *J Biol Chem*, 2005 280, 31428–31437.

[72] Shakiba, Y; Mansouri, K; Mostafaie, A. Anti-angiogenic effect of soybean Kunitz trypsin inhibitor on human umbilical vein endothelial cells. *Fitoterapia*, 2007 78, 587–589.

[73] Troncoso, MF; Zolezzi, PC; Hellman, U; Wolfenstein-Todela, C. A novel trypsin inhibitor from *Peltophorum dubium* seeds, with lectin-like properties, triggers rat lymphoma cell apoptosis. *Arch Biochem Biophys*, 2003 411, 93–104.

[74] Troncoso, MF; Biron, VA; Longhi, SA; Retegui, LA; Wolfenstein-Todel, C. *Peltophorum dubium* and soybean Kunitz-type trypsin inhibitors induce human Jurkat cell apoptosis. *Int Immunopharmacol*, 2007 7, 625–636.

[75] Huber, R; Carrell, RW. Implications of the three-dimensional structure of α1-antitrypsin for structure and function of serpins. *Biochem*, 1989 28, 8951–8966.

[76] Gettins, PG. Serpin structure, mechanism, and function. *Chem Rev*, 2002 102, 4751–4804.

[77] Wilczynska, M; Fa, M; Ohlsson, PI; Ny, T. The Inhibition Mechanism of Serpins. Evidence that the mobile reactive center loop is cleaved in the native protease-inhibitor complex. *J Biol Chem*, 1995 270, 29652–29655.

[78] Zou, Z; Anisowicz, A; Hendrix, MJ; Thor, A; Neveu, M; Sheng, S; Rafidi, K; Seftor, E; Sager, R. Maspin, a serpin with tumor-suppressing activity in human mammary epithelial cells. *Science,* 1994 263, 526–529.

[79] Maass, N; Biallek, M; Rosel, F; Schem, C; Ohike, N; Zhang, M; Jonat, W; Nagasaki, K. Hypermethylation and histone deacetylation lead to silencing of the *maspin* gene in human breast cancer. *Biochem Biophys Res Comm*, 2002 297, 125– 128.

[80] Domann, FE; Rice, JC; Hendrix, MJC; Futscher, BW. Epigenetic silencing of maspin gene expression in human breast cancers. *Int J Cancer*, 2000 85, 805–810.

[81] Zhang, M; Magit, D; Sager, R. Expression of maspin in prostate cells is regulated by a positive ets element and a negative hormonal response element site recognized by androgen receptor. *Proc Nat Acad Sci USA*, 1997 94, 5673–5678.

[82] Zou, Z; Gao, C; Nagaich, AK; Connell, T; Saito, S; Moul, JW; Seth, P; Appella, E; Srivastava, S. p53 regulates the expression of the tumor suppressor gene *maspin*. *J Biol Chem*, 2000 275, 6051–6054.

[83] Wang, SE; Narasanna, A; Whitell, CW; Wu, FY; Friedman, DB; Arteaga, CL. Convergence of p53 and transforming growth factor β (TGFβ) signaling on activating expression of the tumor suppressor gene *maspin* in mammary epithelial cells. *J Biol Chem*, 2007 282, 5661–5669.

[84] Sheng, S; Carey, J; Seftor, EA; Dias, L; Hendrix, MJ; Sager, R. Maspin acts at the cell membrane to inhibit invasion and motility of mammary and prostatic cancer cells. *Proc Natl Acad Sci USA*, 1996 93, 11669–11674.

[85] Zhang, M; Shi, Y; Magit, D; Furth, PA; Sager, R. Reduced mammary tumor progression in WAP-TAg/WAP-maspin bitransgenic mice. *Oncogene*, 2000 19, 6053–6058.

[86] Jiang, N; Meng, Y; Zhang, S; Mensah-Osman, E; Sheng, S. Maspin sensitizes breast carcinoma cells to induced apoptosis. *Oncogene*, 2002 21, 4089–4098.

[87] Maass, N; Hojo, T; Rosel, F; Ikeda, T; Jonat, W; Nagasaki, K. Down regulation of the tumor suppressor gene *maspin* in breast carcinoma is associated with a higher risk of distant metastasis. *Clin Biochem*, 2001 34, 303–307.

[88] Machtens, S; Serth, J; Bokemeyer, C; Bathke, W; Minssen, A; Kollmannsberger, C; Hartmann, J; Knüchel, R; Kondo, M; Jonas, U; Kuczyk, M. Expression of the p53 and Maspin protein in primary prostate cancer: correlation with clinical features. *Int J Cancer*, 2001 95, 337–342.

[89] Xia, W; Lau, YK; Hu, MC; Li, L; Johnston, DA; Sheng, S; El-Naggar, A; Hung, MC. High tumoral maspin expression is associated with improved survival of patients with oral squamous cell carcinoma. *Oncogene*, 2000 19, 2398–2403.

[90] Beecken, WD; Engl, T; Engels, K; Blumenberg, C; Oppermann, E; Camphausen, K; Shing, Y; Reinecke, G; Jonas, D; Blaheta, R. Clinical relevance of maspin expression in bladder cancer. *World J Urol*, 2006 24: 338–44.

[91] Lonardo, F; Li, X; Siddiq, F; Singh, R; Al-Abbadi, M; Pass, HI; Sheng, S. Maspin nuclear localization is linked to favorable morphological features in pulmonary adenocarcinoma. *Lung Cancer*, 2006 51, 31–39.

[92] Katakura, H; Takenaka, K; Nakagawa, M; Sonobe, M; Adachi, M; Ito, S; Wada, H; Tanaka, F. Maspin gene expression is a significant prognostic factor in resected non-small cell lung cancer (NSCLC). Maspin in NSCLC. *Lung Cancer,* 2006 51, 323–328.

[93] Umekita, Y; Ohi, Y; Sagara, Y; Yoshida H. Expression of maspin predicts poor prognosis in breast-cancer patients. *Int J Cancer*, 2002 100, 452–455.

[94] Yu, M; Zheng, H; Tsuneyama, K; Takahashi, H; Nomoto, K; Xu, H; Takano, Y. Paradoxical expression of maspin in gastric carcinomas: correlation with carcinogenesis and progression. *Hum Pathol*, 2007 38, 1248–1255.

[95] Sood, AK; Fletcher, MS; Gruman, LM; Coffin, JE; Jabbari, S; Khalkhali-Ellis, Z; Arbour, N; Seftor, EA; Hendrix, MJ. The paradoxical expression of maspin in ovarian carcinoma. *Clin Cancer Res*, 2002 8, 2924–2932.

[96] Bolat, F; Gumurdulu, D; Erkanli, S; Kayaselcuk, F; Zeren, H; Vardar, MA; Kuscu, E. Maspin overexpression correlates with increased expression of vascular endothelial growth factors A, C, and D in human ovarian carcinoma. *Pathol Res Pract*, 2008 204, 379–387.

[97] Hirai, K; Koizumi, K; Haraguchi, S; Hirata, T; Mikami, I; Fukushima, M; Yamagishi, S; Kawashima, T; Okada, D; Shimizu, K; Kawamoto, M. Prognostic significance of the tumor suppressor gene *maspin* in non–small cell lung cancer. *Ann Thorac Surg*, 2005 79, 248–253.

[98] Kashima, K; Ohike, N; Mukai, S; Sato, M; Takahashi, M; Morohoshi, T. Expression of the tumor suppressor gene *maspin* and its significance in intraductal papillary mucinous neoplasms of the pancreas. *Hepatobiliary Pancreat Dis Int*, 2008 7, 86—90.

[99] Arbiser, JL. Molecular regulation of angiogenesis and tumorigenesis by signal transduction pathways: evidence of predictable and reproducible patterns of synergy in diverse neoplasms. *Semin Cancer Biol*, 2004 14, 81–91.

[100] Denk, AE; Bettstetter, M; Wild, PJ; Hoek, K; Bataille, F; Dietmaier, W; Bosserhoff, AK. Loss of maspin expression contributes to a more invasive potential in malignant melanoma. *Pigment Cell Res*, 2007 20, 112–119.

[101] Bass, R; Fernandez, AM; Ellis, V. Maspin inhibits cell migration in the absence of protease inhibitory activity. *J Biol Chem*, 2002 277, 46845–46848.

[102] Yin, S; Lockett, J; Meng, Y; Biliran, H Jr; Blouse, GE; Li, X; Reddy, N; Zhao, Z; Lin, X; Anagli, J; Cher, ML; Sheng, S. Maspin retards cell detachment via a novel interaction with the urokinase-type plasminogen activator/urokinase-type plasminogen activator receptor system. *Cancer Res*, 2006 66, 4173–4181.

[103] Ngamkitidechakul, C; Warejcka, DJ; Burke, JM; O'Brien, WJ; Twining, SS. Sufficiency of the reactive site loop of maspin for induction of cell-matrix adhesion and inhibition of cell invasion. Conversion of ovalbumin to a maspin-like molecule. *J Biol Chem*, 2003 278, 31796–31806.

[104] Al-Ayyoubi, M; Schwartz, BS; Gettins, PG. Maspin binds to urokinase-type and tissue-type plasminogen activator through exosite-exosite interactions. *J Biol Chem*, 2007 282, 19502–19509.

[105] McGowen, R; Biliran, H Jr; Sager, R; Sheng, S. The surface of prostate carcinoma DU145 cells mediates the inhibition of urokinase-type plasminogen activator by maspin. *Cancer Res*, 2000 60, 4771–4778.

[106] Lockett, J; Yin, S; Li, X; Meng, Y; Sheng, S. Tumor suppressive maspin and epithelial homeostasis. *J Cell Biochem*, 2006 97, 651–660.

[107] Odero-Marah, VA; Khalkhali-Ellis, Z; Chunthapong, J; Amir, S; Seftor, RE; Seftor, EA; Hendrix, MJ. Maspin regulates different signaling pathways for motility and adhesion in aggressive breast cancer cells. *Cancer Biol Ther*, 2003 2, 398–403.

[108] Evers, EE; Zondag, GCM; Malliri, A; Price, LS; ten Klooster, JP; van der Kammen, RA; Collard, JG. Rho family proteins in cell adhesion and cell migration. *Eur J Cancer*, 2000 36, 1269–74.

[109] Cella, N; Contreras, A; Latha, K; Rosen, JM; Zhang, M. Maspin is physically associated with β1 integrin regulating cell adhesion in mammary epithelial cells. *FASEB J*, 2006 20, 1510–1512.

[110] Blacque, OE; Worrall, DM. Evidence for a direct interaction between the tumor suppressor serpin, maspin, and types I and III collagen. *J Biol Chem*, 2002 277, 10783–10788.

[111] Seftor, RE; Seftor, EA; Sheng, S; Pemberton, PA; Sager, R; Hendrix, MJ. Maspin suppresses the invasive phenotype of human breast carcinoma. *Cancer Res*, 1998 58, 5681–5685.

[112] Zhang, M; Volpert, O; Shi, YH; Bouck, N. Maspin is an angiogenesis inhibitor. *Nat Med*, 2000 6, 196–199.

[113] Hojo, T; Akiyama, Y; Nagasaki, K; Maruyama, K; Kikuchi, K; Ikeda, T; Kitajima, M; Yamaguchi, K. Association of maspin expression with the malignancy grade and tumor vascularization in breast cancer tissues. *Cancer Lett*, 2000 171, 103–110.

[114] Solomon, LA; Munkarah, AR; Schimp, VL; Arabi, MH; Morris, RT; Nassar, H; Ali-Fehmi, R. Maspin expression and localization impact on angiogenesis and prognosis in ovarian cancer. *Gynecol Oncol*, 2006 101, 385–389.

[115] Chua, R; Setzer, S; Govindarajan, B; Sexton, D; Cohen, C; Arbiser, JL. Maspin expression, angiogenesis, prognostic parameters, and outcome in malignant melanoma. *J Am Acad Dermatol*, 2009 60, 758–66.

[116] Pemberton, PA; Tipton, AR; Pavloff, N; Smith, J; Erickson, JR; Mouchabeck, ZM; Kiefer, MC. Maspin is an intracellular serpin that partitions into secretory vesicles and is present at the cell surface. *J Histochem Cytochem*, 1997 45, 1697–1706.

[117] Yin, S; Li, X; Meng, Y; Finley, RL Jr; Sakr, W; Yang, H; Reddy, N; Sheng, S. Tumor-suppressive maspin regulates cell response to oxidative stress by direct interaction with glutathione S-transferase. *J Biol Chem*, 2005 280, 34985–34996.

[118] Bailey, CM; Khalkhali-Ellis, Z; Seftor, EA; Hendrix, MJC. Biological functions of maspin. *J Cell Physiol*, 2006 209, 617–624.

[119] Luo, JL; Tan, W; Ricono, JM; Korchynskyi, O; Zhang, M; Gonias, SL; Cheresh, DA; Karin, M. Nuclear cytokine-activated IKKα controls prostate cancer metastasis by repressing Maspin. *Nature,* 2007 446, 690–694.

[120] Nicolai Maass, LR; Martin, Z; Koichi, N; Pierre, R. Maspin locates to the nucleus in certain cell types. *J Pathol*, 2002 197, 274–275.

[121] Marioni, G; Giacomelli, L; D'Alessandro, E; Marchese-Ragona, R; Staffieri, C; Ferraro, SM; Staffieri, A; Blandamura, S. Nuclear localization of mammary serine protease inhibitor (MASPIN): is its impact on the prognosis in laryngeal carcinoma due to a proapoptotic effect? *Am J Otolaryngol*, 2008 29, 156–162.

[122] Liu, J; Yin, S; Reddy, N; Spencer, C; Sheng, S. Bax Mediates the Apoptosis-Sensitizing Effect of Maspin. *Cancer Res*, 2004 64, 1703-1711.

[123] Zhang, W; Shi, HY; Zhang, M. Maspin overexpression modulates tumor cell apoptosis through the regulation of Bcl-2 family proteins. *BMC Cancer,* 2005 5, 50. doi:10.1186/1471-2407-5-50.

[124] Latha, K; Zhang, W; Cella, N; Shi, HY; Zhang, M. Maspin mediates increased tumor cell apoptosis upon induction of the mitochondrial permeability transition. *Mol Cell Biol*, 2005 25, 1737–1748.

[125] Klasa-Mazurkiewicz, D; Narkiewicz, J; Milczek, T; Lipińska, B; Emerich, J. Maspin overexpression correlates with positive response to primary chemotherapy in ovarian cancer patients. *Gynecol Oncol*, 2009 113, 91–98.

[126] Li, X; Chen, D; Yin, S; Meng, Y; Yang, H; Landis-Piwowar, KR; Li, Y; Sarkar, FH; Reddy, GPV; Dou, QP; Sheng, S. Maspin Augments Proteasome Inhibitor-Induced Apoptosis in Prostate Cancer Cells. *J Cell Physiol*, 2007 212, 298–306.

[127] Chen, EI; Florens, L; Axelrod, FT; Monosov, E; Barbas III, CF; Yates III, JR; Felding-Habermann, B; Smith, JW. Maspin alters the carcinoma proteome. *FASEB J*, 2005, Express Article. doi:10.1096/fj.04-2970fje.

[128] Li, X; Yin, S; Meng, Y; Sakr, W; Sheng, S. Endogenous inhibition of histone deacetylase 1 by tumor suppressive maspin. *Cancer Res*, 2005 66, 9323–9329.

[129] Tombran-Tink, J; Johnson, LV. Neuronal differentiation of retinoblastoma cells induced by medium conditioned by human RPE cells. *Invest Ophthalmol Vis Sci*, 1980 30, 1700–1707.

[130] Steele, FR; Chader, GJ; Johnson, LV; Tombran-Tink, J. Pigment epithelium-derived factor: neurotrophic activity and identification as a member of the serine protease inhibitor gene family. *Proc Natl Acad Sci USA*, 1992 90, 1526–1530.

[131] Tombran-Tink, J; Mazuruk, K; Rodriguez, IR; Chung, D; Linker, T; Englander, E; Chader, GJ. Organization, evolutionary conservation, expression, and unusual Alu density of the human gene for pigment epithelium-derived factor, a unique neurotrophic serpin. *Mol Vision*, 1996 2, 1–5.

[132] Dawson, DW; Volpert, OV; Gillis, P; Crawford, SE; Xu, HJ; Benedict, W; Bouck, NP. Pigment epithelium-derived factor: a potent inhibitor of angiogenesis. *Science*, 1999 285, 245–248.

[133] Bouck, N. PEDF: anti-angiogenic guardian of ocular function. *Trends Mol Med*, 2002 8, 330–334.

[134] Amaral, J; Becerra, SP. Pigment epithelium-derived factor and angiogenesis. Therapeutic Implications. In: Penn, JS. *Retinal and Choroidal Angiogenesis*. Dordrecht, The Netherlands: Springer; 2008; 311–337.

[135] Steele, FR; Chader, GJ; Johnson, LV; Tombran-Tink, J. Pigment epitheliumderived factor: neurotrophic activity and identification as a member of the serine protease inhibitor gene family. *Proc Natl Acad Sci USA*, 1993 90, 1526–1530.

[136] Tombran-Tink, J; Chader, GG; Johnson, LV. PEDF: a pigment epithelium-derived factor with potent neuronal differentiative activity. *Exp Eye Res*, 1991 53, 411–414.

[137] Ek, ETH; Dass, CR; Choong, PFM. PEDF: a potential molecular therapeutic target with multiple anti-cancer activities. *TRENDS in Mol Med*, 2006 12, 497–502.

[138] Bernard, A; Gao-Li, J; Franco, CA; Bouceba, T; Huet, A; Li, Z. Laminin Receptor Involvement in the Anti-angiogenic Activity of Pigment Epithelium-derived Factor. *J Biol Chem*, 2009 284, 10480–10490.

[139] Halin, S; Wikstrom, P; Rudolfsson, SH; Stattin, P; Doll, JA; Crawford, SE; Bergh, A. Decreased pigment epithelium-derived factor is associated with metastatic phenotype in human and rat prostate tumors. *Cancer Res*, 2004 64, 5664–5671.

[140] Uehara, H; Miyamoto, M; Kato, K; Ebihara, Y; Kaneko, H; Hashimoto, H; Murakami, Y; Hase, R; Takahashi, R; Mega, S; Shichinohe, T; Kawarada, Y; Itoh, T; Okushiba, S; Kondo, S; Katoh, H. Expression of pigment epithelium-derived factor decreases liver metastasis and correlates with favorable prognosis for patients with ductal pancreatic adenocarcinoma. *Cancer Res*, 2004 64, 3533–3537.

[141] Crawford, SE; Stellmach, V; Ranalli, M; Huang, X; Huang, L; Volpert, O; De Vries, GH; Abramson, LP; Bouck, N. Pigment epitheliumderived factor (PEDF) in neuroblastoma: a multifunctional mediator of Schwann cell antitumor activity. *J Cell Sci*, 2001 114, 4421–4428.

[142] Guan, M; Yam, HF; Su, B; Chan, KP; Pang, CP; Liu, WW; Zhang, WZ; Lu, Y. Loss of pigment epithelium derived factor expression in glioma progression. *J Clin Pathol*, 2003 56, 277–282.

[143] Abe, R; Shimizu, T; Yamagishi, SI; Shibaki, A; Amano, S; Inagaki, Y; Watanabe, H; Sugawara, H; Nakamura, H; Takeuchi, M; Imaizumi, T; Shimizu, H. Overexpression of Pigment Epithelium-Derived Factor Decreases Angiogenesis and Inhibits the Growth of Human Malignant Melanoma Cells *in Vivo*. *Am J Pathol*, 2004 164, 1225–1232.

[144] Ek, ETH; Dass, CR; Contreras, KG; Choong, PFM. Pigment epithelium-derived factor overexpression inhibits orthopic osteosarcoma growth, angiogenesis and metastasis. *Cancer Gene Ther*,2007 14, 616–626.

[145] Hase, R; Miyamoto, M; Uehara, H; Kadoya, M; Ebihara, Y; Murakami, Y; Takahashi, R; Mega, S; Li, L; Shichinohe, T; Kawarada, Y; Kondo, S. Pigment epithelium-derived factor gene therapy inhibits human pancreatic cancer in mice. *Clin Cancer Res*, 2005 11, 8737–8744.

[146] Guan, M; Pang, CP; Yam, HF; Cheung, KF; Liu, WW; Lu, Y. Inhibition of glioma invasion by overexpression of pigment epithelium-derived factor. *Cancer Gene Ther*, 2004 11, 325–332.

[147] Zhang, SM; Wang, JJ; Gao, G; Parke, K; Ma, JX. Pigment epithelium-derived factor downregulates vascular endothelial growth factor (VEGF) expression and inhibits VEGF–VEGF receptor 2 binding in diabetic retinopathy. *J Mol Endocrinol*, 2006 37, 1–12.

[148] Volpert, OV; Zaichuk, T; Zhou, W; Reiher, F; Ferguson, TA; Stuart, PM; Amin, M; Bouck, NP. Inducer-stimulated Fas targets activated endothelium for destruction by anti-angiogenic thrombospondin-1 and pigment epithelium-derived factor. *Nat Med*, 2002 8, 349–357.

[149] Cai, J; Jiang, WG; Grant, MB; Boulton, M. Pigment Epithelium-derived Factor Inhibits Angiogenesis via Regulated Intracellular Proteolysis of Vascular Endothelial Growth Factor Receptor 1. *J Biol Chem*, 2006 281, 3604–3613.

[150] Zhang, T; Guan, M; Xu, C; Chen, Y; Lu, Y. Pigment epithelium-derived factor inhibits glioma cell growth *in vitro* and *in vivo*. *Life Sci*, 2007 81, 1256–1263.

[151] Chen, L; Zhang, SSM; Barnstable, CJ; Tombran-Tink, J. PEDF induces apoptosis in human endothelial cells by activating p38 MAP kinase dependent cleavage of multiple caspases. *Biochem Biophys Res Commun*, 2006 348, 1288–1295.

[152] Ho, TC; Chen, SL; Yang, YC; Lo, TH; Hsieh, JW; Cheng, HC; Tsao, YP. Cytosolic phospholipase A_2-α is an early apoptotic activator in PEDF-induced endothelial cell apoptosis. *Am J Physiol Cell Physiol*, 2009 296, C273–C284.

[153] Mirochnik, Y; Aurora, A; Schulze-Hoepfner, FT; Deabes, A; Shifrin, V; Beckmann, R; Polsky, C; Volpert, OV. Short Pigment Epithelial-Derived Factor-Derived Peptide Inhibits Angiogenesis and Tumor Growth. *Clin Cancer Res*, 2009 15, 1655–1663.

[154] Björk, I; Olson, ST. Antithrombin. A bloody important serpin. *Adv Exp Med Biol*, 1997 425, 17–33.

[155] Björk, I; Fish, WW. Production in vitro and properties of a modified form of bovine antithrombin, cleaved at the active site by thrombin. *J Biol Chem*, 1982 257, 9487–9493.

[156] O'Reilly, MS; Pirie-Shepherd, S; Lane, WS; Folkman, J. Antiangiogenic activity of the cleaved conformation of the serpin antithrombin. *Science*, 1999 285, 1926–1928.

[157] Larsson, H; Sjöblom, T; Dixelius, J; Östman, A; Ylinenjärvi, K; Björk, I; Claesson-Welsh, L. Antiangiogenic Effects of Latent Antithrombin through Perturbed Cell-

Matrix Interactions and Apoptosis of Endothelial Cells. *Cancer Res*, 2000 60, 6723–6729.

[158] Zhang, W; Chuang, YJ; Jin, T; Swanson, R; Xiong, Y; Leung, L; Olson, ST. Antiangiogenic Antithrombin Induces Global Changes in the Gene Expression Profile of Endothelial Cells. *Cancer Res*, 2006 66, 5047–5055.

[159] Doolittle, RF. Angiotensinogen Is Related to the Antitrypsin-Antithrombin-Ovalbumin Family. *Science*, 1983 222, 417–419.

[160] Célérier, J; Cruz, A; Lamandé, N; Gasc, JM; Corvol, P. Angiotensinogen and Its Cleaved Derivatives Inhibit Angiogenesis. *Hypertension*. 2002 39, 224–228.

[161] Brand, M; Lamande, N; Larger, E; Corvol, P; Gasc, JM. Angiotensinogen impairs angiogenesis in the chick chorioallantoic membrane. *J Mol Med*, 2007 85, 451–460.

[162] Bouquet, C; Lamandé, N; Brand, M; Gasc, JM; Jullienne, B; Faure, G; Griscelli, F; Opolon, P; Connault, E; Perricaudet, M; Corvol, P. Suppression of angiogenesis, tumor growth, and metastasis by adenovirus-mediated gene transfer of human angiotensinogen. *Mol Ther*, 2006 14, 175–182.

[163] Vincent, F; Bonnin, P; Clemessy, M; Contrerès, JO; Lamandé, M; Gasc, JM; Vilar, J; Hainaud, P; Tobelem, G; Corvol, P; Dupuy, E. Angiotensinogen Delays Angiogenesis and Tumor Growth of Hepatocarcinoma in Transgenic Mice. *Cancer Res*, 2009 69, 2853–2860.

[164] Spring, P; Nakashima, T; Frederick, M; Henderson, Y; Clayman, G. Identification and cDNA cloning of headpin, a novel differentially expressed serpin that maps to chromosome 18q. *Biochem Biophys Res Commun*, 1999 264, 299–304.

[165] Jayakumar, A; Kang, Y; Frederick, MJ; Pak, SC; Henderson, Y; Holton, PR; Mitsudo, K; Silverman, GA; EL-Naggar, AK; Brömme, D; Clayman, GL. Inhibition of the cysteine proteinases cathepsins K and L by the serpin headpin (SERPINB13): a kinetic analysis. *Arch Biochem Biophys*, 2003 409, 367–374.

[166] Shellenberger, TD; Mazumdar, A; Henderson, Y; Briggs, K; Wang, M; Chattopadhyay, C; Jayakumar, A; Frederick, M; Clayman, GL. Headpin: A Serpin with Endogenous and Exogenous Suppression of Angiogenesis. *Cancer Res*, 2005 65, 11501–11509.

[167] Kawasaki, K; Uzawa, K; Kurasawa, Y; Yoshida, N; Shimada, K; Uesugi, H; Murano, A; Hayashi, Y; Yamaki, M; Moriya, T; Shiiba, M; Tanzawa, H. Reduced expression and hypermethylation of headpin, a serine proteinase inhibitor (serpin), in human oral squamous cell carcinoma. *千葉医学 [Chiba Medical Journal]*, 2008 84, 179–185.

[168] de Koning, PJA; Bovenschen, N; Leusink, FKJ; Broekhuizen, R; Quadir, R; van Gemert, JTM; Hordijk, GJ; Chang, WSW; van der Tweel, I; Tilanus, MGJ; Kummer, JA. Downregulation of SERPINB13 expression in head and neck squamous cell carcinomas associates with poor clinical outcome. *Int J Cancer*, 2009, DOI 10.1002/ijc.24507.

[169] Zhou, GX; Chao, L; Chao, J. Kallistatin: a novel human tissue kallikrein inhibitor. Purification, characterization, and reactive center sequence. *J Biol Chem*, 1992 267, 25873–25880.

[170] Miao, RQ; Agata, J; Chao, L; Chao, J. Kallistatin is new inhibitor of angiogenesis and tumor growth. *Blood,* 2002 100, 3245–3252.

[171] Miao, RQ; Chen, V; Chao, L; Chao, J. Structural elements of kallistatin required for inhibition of angiogenesis. *Am J Physiol Cell Physiol*, 2003 284, C1604–C1613.

[172] Zhu, B; Lu, L; Cai, W; Yang, X; Li, C; Yang, Z; Zhan, W; Ma, JX; Gao, G. Kallikrein-binding protein inhibits growth of gastric carcinoma by reducing vascular endothelial growth factor production and angiogenesis. *Mol Cancer Ther*, 2007 6, 3297–3306.

[173] Kato, H; Torigoe, T. Radioimmunoassay for tumor antigen of human cervical squamous cell carcinoma. *Cancer*, 1977 40, 1621–1628.

[174] Kato, H. Expression and function of squamous cell carcinoma antigen. *Anticancer Res*, 1996 16, 2149–2154.

[175] Schneider, SS; Schick, C; Fish, KE; Miller, JC; Pena, SD; Treter, SM; Hui, GA; Silverman, A. A serine proteinase inhibitor locus at 18q21.3 contains a tandem duplication of the human squamous cell carcinoma antigen gene. *PNAS*, 1995 92, 3147–3151.

[176] Suminami, Y; Nagashima, S; Vujanovic, NL; Hirabayashi, K; Kato, H; Whiteside, TL. Inhibition of apoptosis in human tumour cells by the tumour-associated serpin, SCC antigen. *Br J Cancer*, 2000 82, 981–989.

[177] Sueoka, K; Nawata, S; Nakagawa, T; Murakami, A; Takeda, O; Suminami, Y; Kato, H; Sugino, N. Tumor-associated serpin, squamous cell carcinoma antigen stimulates matrix metalloproteinase-9 production in cervical squamous cell carcinoma cell lines. *Int J Oncol*, 2005 27, 1345–1353.

[178] McGettrick, AF; Barnes, RC; Worrall, DM. SCCA2 inhibits TNF-mediated apoptosis in transfected HeLa cells: The reactive centre loop sequence is essential for this function and TNF-induced cathepsin G is a candidate target. *Eur J Biochem*, 2001 268, 5868–5875.

[179] Katagiri, C; Nakanishi, J; Kadoya, K; Hibino, T. Serpin squamous cell carcinoma antigen inhibits UV-induced apoptosis via suppression of c-JUN NH2-terminal kinase. *J Cell Biol*, 2006 172, 983–90.

[180] Trerotoli, P; Fransvea, E; Angelotti, U; Antonaci, G; Lupo, L; Mazzocca, A; Mangia, A; Antonaci, S; Giannelli, G. Tissue expression of Squamous Cellular Carcinoma Antigen (SCCA) is inversely correlated to tumor size in HCC. *Mol Cancer*,2009 8, 29. doi:10.1186/1476-4598-8-29.

[181] Bird, CH; Sutton, VR; Sun, J; Hirst, CE; Novak, A; Kumar, S; Trapani, JA; Bird, PI. Selective regulation of apoptosis: the cytotoxic lymphocyte serpin proteinase inhibitor 9 protects against granzyme B-mediated apoptosis without perturbing the Fas cell death pathway. *Mol Cell Biol*, 1998 18, 6387–6398.

[182] Annand, RR; Dahlen, JR; Sprecher, CA; De Dreu, P; Foster, DC; Mankovich, JA; Talanian, RV; Kisiel, W; Giegel, DA. Caspase-1 (interleukin-1beta-converting enzyme) is inhibited by the human serpin analogue proteinase inhibitor 9. *Biochem J*, 1999 342, 655–665.

[183] Bladergroen, BA; Meijer, CJLM; ten Berge, RL; Hack, CE; Muris, JJF; Dukers, DF; Chott, A; Kazama, Y; Oudejans, JJ; van Berkum, O; Kummer, JA. Expression of the granzyme B inhibitor, protease inhibitor 9, by tumor cells in patients with non-Hodgkin and Hodgkin lymphoma: a novel protective mechanism for tumor cells to circumvent the immune system? *Blood*, 2002 99, 232–237.

[184] Kummer, JA; Micheau, O; Schneider, P; Bovenschen, N; Broekhuizen, R; Quadir, R; Strik, MCM; Hack, CE; Tschopp, J. Ectopic expression of the serine protease inhibitor PI9 modulates death receptor-mediated apoptosis. *Cell Death Differ*, 2007 14, 1486–1496.

[185] Stoeckli, ET; Lemkin, PF; Kuhn, TB; Ruegg, MA; Heller, M; Sonderegger, P. Identification of proteins secreted from axons of embryonic dorsal-root-ganglia neurons. *Eur J Biochem*, 1989 180, 249–258.

[186] Osterwalder, T; Contartese, J; Stoeckli, ET; Kuhn, TB; Sonderegger, P. Neuroserpin, an axonally secreted serine protease inhibitor. *EMBO J*, 1996 15, 2944–2953.

[187] Hasumi, H; Ishiguro, H; Nakamura, M; Sugiura, S; Osada, Y; Miyoshi, Y; Fujinami, K; Yao, M; Hamada, K; Yamada-Okabe, H; Kubota, Y; Uemura, H. Neuroserpin (PI-12) is upregulated in high-grade prostate cancer and is associated with survival. *Int J Cancer*, 2005 115, 911–916.

[188] Liotta, LA; Tryggvason, K; Garbisa, S; Hart, I.; Foltz, CM; Shafie, S. Metastatic potential correlates with enzymatic degradation of basement-membrane collagen. *Nature*, 1980 284, 67–68.

[189] Woessner, JF Jr. The family of matrix metalloproteinases. *Ann. N.Y. Acad. Sci.* 1994 732, 11–21.

[190] Nagase, H; Woessner, JF Jr. Matrix metalloproteinases. *J. Biol. Chem.* 1999 274, 21491–21494.

[191] Chambers AF; Matrisian L. Changing views of the role of matrix metalloproteinases in metastasis. J Natl Cancer Inst, 1997 89, 1260–70.

[192] Wilson, CL; Heppner, KJ; Labosky, PA; Hogan, BL; Matrisian, LM. Intestinal tumorigenesis is suppressed in mice lacking the metalloproteinase matrilysin. *Proc Natl Acad Sci USA*, 1997 94, 1402–1407.

[193] Deryugina, EI; Quigley, JP. Matrix metalloproteinases and tumor metastasis. *Cancer Metastasis Rev.*, 2006 25, 9–34.

[194] Egeblad, M; Werb, Z. New functions for the matrix metalloproteinases in cancer progression. *Nat Rev Cancer*, 2002 2, 161–174.

[195] Hojilla, CV; Mohammed, FF; Khokha, R. Matrix metalloproteinases and their tissue inhibitors direct cell fate during cancer development. *Br J Cancer*, 2003 89, 1817–21.

[196] Coussens, LM; Fingleton, B; Matrisian, LM. Matrix Metalloproteinase Inhibitors and Cancer: Trials and Tribulations. *Science*, 2002 295, 2387–2392.

[197] Overall, CM; Kleifeld, O. Tumour microenvironment-opinion: Validating matrix metalloproteinases as drug targets and anti-targets for cancer therapy. Nat Rev Cancer, 2006 6, 227–239.

[198] Kahari, VM; Saarialho-Kere, U. Matrix metalloproteinases and their inhibitors in tumour growth and invasion. *Ann. Med*, 1999 31, 34–45.

[199] Gomez, DE; Alonso DF; Yoshiji H; Thorgeirsson UP. Tissue inhibitors of metalloproteinases: structure, regulation and biological functions. *Eur J Cell Biol*, 1997 74, 111–22.

[200] Brew, K; Dinakarpandian, D; Nagase, H. Tissue inhibitors of metalloproteinases: evolution, structure and function. *Biochim Biophys Acta*, 2000 1477, 267-283.

[201] DeClerck, YA. Chapter 9: Tissue Inhibitors of Metalloproteinases in Cancer. In: Foidart, JM, Muschel, RJ editors. *Proteases and Their Inhibitors in Cancer Metastasis*. New York, Boston, Dordrecht, London, Moscow: Kluwer Academic Publishers; 2004; 169-194.

[202] Kruger, A; Fata, JE; Khokha, R. Altered tumor growth and metastasis of a T-cell lymphoma in Timp-1 transgenic mice. *Blood,* 1997 90, 1993–2000.

[203] Martin, DC; Sanchez-Sweatman, OH; Ho, AT; Inderdeo, DS; Tsao, MS; Khokha, R. Transgenic TIMP-1 inhibits simian virus 40 T antigen-induced hepatocarcinogenesis by impairment of hepatocellular proliferation and tumor angiogenesis. *Lab Invest*, 1999 79, 225–34.

[204] Montgomery, AM; Mueller, BM; Reisfeld, RA; Taylor, SM; DeClerck, YA. Effect of tissue inhibitor of the matrix metalloproteinases-2 expression on the growth and spontaneous metastasis of a human melanoma cell line. Cancer Res, 1994 54,5467–5473.

[205] Khokha, R. Suppression of the tumorigenic and metastatic abilities of murine B16-F10 melanoma cells in vivo by the overexpression of the tissue inhibitor of the metalloproteinases-1. J Natl Cancer Inst, 1994 86, 299–304.

[206] Henriet, P; Blavier, L; Declerck, YA. Tissue inhibitors of metalloproteinases (TIMP) in invasion and proliferation. Apmis, 1999 107, 111–119.

[207] Brand, K; Baker, A; Perez-Canto, A; Possling, A; Sacharjat, M; Geheeb, M. Arnold, W. Treatment of colorectal liver metastases by adenoviral transfer of tissue inhibitor of metalloproteinases-2 into the liver tissue. Cancer Res, 2000 60, 5723–5730.

[208] Soloway PD; Alexander CM; Werb Z; Jaenisch R. Targeted mutagenesis of Timp-1 reveals that lung tumor invasion is influenced by Timp-1 genotype of the tumor but not by that of the host. *Oncogene*, 1996 13, 2307–2314.

[209] Kopitz, C; Gerg, M; Bandapalli, OR; Ister, D; Pennington, CJ; Hauser, S; Flechsig, C; Krell, HW; Antolovic, D; Brew, K; Nagase, H; Stangl, M; von Weyhern, CWH; Brücher, BLDM; Brand, K; Coussens, LM; Edwards, DR; Krüger, A. Tissue Inhibitor of Metalloproteinases-1 Promotes Liver Metastasis by Induction of Hepatocyte Growth Factor Signaling. *Cancer Res*, 2007 67, 8615–8623.

[210] Brown PD. Clinical studies with matrix metalloproteinase inhibitors. *APMIS*, 1999 107, 174–80.

[211] Hidalgo, M; Eckhardt, SG. Development of matrix metalloproteinase inhibitors in cancer therapy. *J Natl Cancer Inst*, 2001 93, 178–193.

[212] Nelson, AR; Fingleton, B; Rothenberg, ML; Matrisian, LM. Matrix metalloproteinases: Biologic activity and clinical implications. *J Clin Oncol*, 2000 18, 1135–1149.

[213] Zucker S; Cao J; Chen WT. Critical appraisal of the use of matrix metalloproteinase inhibitors in cancer treatment. *Oncogene*, 2000 19, 6642–6650.

[214] Konstantinopoulos, PA; Karamouzis, MV; Papatsoris, AG; Papavassiliou, AG. Matrix metalloproteinase inhibitors as anticancer agents. *Int J Biochem Cell Biol*, 2008 40, 1156–1168.

[215] Betz, M; Huxley, P; Davies, SJ; Mushtaq, Y; Pieper, M; Tschesche, H; Bode, W; Gomis-Rüth, FX. 1,8-A crystal structure of the catalytic domain of human neutrophil collagenase (matrix metalloproteinase-8) complexed with a peptidomimetic hydroxamate primed-side inhibitor with a distinct selectivity profile. *Eur J Biochem*, 1997 247, 356–363.

[216] Hu, J; Van den Steen, PE; Sang, QX; Opdenakker, G. Matrix metalloproteinase inhibitors as therapy for inflammatory and vascular diseases. *Nat Rev Drug Discov*, 2007 6, 480–498.

[217] Sapadin, AN; Fleischmajer, R. Tetracyclines: Nonantibiotic properties and their clinical implications. *J Am Acad Dermatol*, 2006 54, 258–265.

[218] Coxon, FP; Thompson, K; Rogers, MJ. Recent advances n understanding the mechanism of action of bisphosphonates. *Curr Opin Pharmacol*, 2006 6, 307–312.
[219] López-Otín, C; Matrisian, LM. Emerging roles of proteases in tumour suppression. *Nature*, 2007 7, 800–808.
[220] Overall, CM; Kleifeld, O. Towards third generation matrix metalloproteinase inhibitors for cancer therapy. *Brit J Cancer*, 2006 94, 941–946.
[221] Bervar, A; Zajc, I; Sever, N; Katunuma, N; Sloane, BF; Lah, TT. Invasiveness of Transformed Human Breast Epithelial Cell Lines Is Related to Cathepsin B and Inhibited by Cysteine Proteinase Inhibitors. *Biol Chem*, 2003 384, 447–455.
[222] Vasiljeva, O; Turk, B. Dual contrasting roles of cysteine cathepsins in cancer progression: Apoptosis versus tumour invasion. *Biochimie*, 2008 90, 380–386.
[223] Kim, K; Cai, J; Shuja, S; Kuo, T; Murnane, MJ. Presence of activated ras correlates with increased cysteine proteinase activities in human colorectal carcinomas. *Int J Cancer*, 1998 79, 324–333.
[224] Ravanko, K; Jarvinen, K; Helin, J; Kalkkinen, N; Holtta, E. Cysteine cathepsins are central contributors of invasion by cultured adenosylmethionine decarboxylasetransformed rodent fibroblasts. *Cancer Res*, 2004 64, 8831–8838.
[225] Joyce, JA; Baruch, A; Chehade, K; Meyer-Morse, N; Giraudo, E; Tsai, FY; Greenbaum, DC; Hager, JH; Bogyo, M; Hanahan, D. Cathepsin cysteine proteases are effectors of invasive growth and angiogenesis during multistage tumorigenesis. *Cancer Cell*, 2004 5, 443–453.
[226] Zheng, X; Chou, PM; Mirkin, BL; Rebbaa, A. Senescenceinitiated reversal of drug resistance: specific role of cathepsin L. *Cancer Res*, 2004 64, 1773–1780.
[227] Barrett, AJ. The cystatins: a diverse superfamily of cysteine peptidase inhibitors. *Biomed Biochim Acta*, 1986 45, 1363–1374.
[228] Turk, V; Bode, W. The cystatins: protein inhibitors of cysteine proteinases. *Fed Eur Biochem Soc Lett*, 1991 285, 213–219.
[229] Kos, J; Lah, TT. Cysteine proteinases and their endogenous inhibitors: Target proteins for prognosis, diagnosis and therapy in cancer (review). *Oncol Rep*, 1998 5, 1349–1361.
[230] Keppler, D. Towards novel anti-cancer strategies based on cystatin function. *Cancer Lett*, 2006 235, 159–176.
[231] Jones, B; Roberts, PJ; Faubion, WA; Kominami, E; Gores, GJ. Cystatin A expression reduces bile salt-induced apoptosis in a rat hepatoma cell line. *Am J Physiol*, 1998 275, G723–G730.
[232] Leinonen, T; Pirinen, R; Böhm, J; Johansson, R; Rinne, A; Weber, E; Kosma, VM. Biological and prognostic role of acid cysteine proteinase inhibitor (ACPI, cystatin A) in non-small-cell lung cancer. *J Clin Pathol*, 2007 60, 515–519.
[233] van Eijk, M; de Groot, C. Germinal center B cell apoptosis requires both caspase and cathepsin activity. *J Immunol*, 1999 163, 2478–2482.
[234] Parker, BS; Ciocca, DR; Bidwell, BN; Gago, FE; Fanelli, MA; George, J; Slavin, JL; Möller, A; Steel, R; Pouliot, N; Eckhardt, BL; Henderson, MA; Anderson, RL. Primary tumour expression of the cysteine cathepsin inhibitor Stefin A inhibits distant metastasis in breast cancer. *J Pathol*, 2008 214, 337-46.
[235] Boike, G; Lah, T; Sloane, BF; Rozhin, J; Honn, K; Guirguis, R; Stracke, ML; Liotta, LA; Schiffmann, E. A possible role for cysteine proteinase and its inhibitors in motility of malignant melanoma and other tumour cells, *Melanoma Res*, 1992 1, 333–340.

[236] Abrahamson, M; Barrett, AJ; Salvesen, G; Grubb, A. Isolation of six cysteine proteinase inhibitors from human urine. Their physicochemical and enzyme kinetic properties and concentrations in biological fluids. *J Biol Chem*, 1986 261, 11282–11289.

[237] Sokol, JP; Schiemann, WP. Cystatin C antagonizes transforming growth factor beta signaling in normal and cancer cells. *Mol Cancer Res*, 2004 2, 183–195.

[238] Sotiropoulou, G; Anisowicz, A; Sager, R. Identification, cloning, and characterization of cystatin M, a novel cysteine proteinase inhibitor, down-regulated in breast cancer. *J Biol Chem*, 1997 272, 903–910.

[239] Qiu, J; Ai, L; Ramachandran, C; Yao, B; Gopalakrishnan, S; Fields, CR; Delmas, AL; Dyer, LM; Melnick, SJ; Yachnis, AT; Schwartz, PH; Fine, HA; Brown, KD; Robertson, KD. Invasion suppressor cystatin E/M (CST6): High-level cell typespecific expression in normal brain and epigenetic silencing in gliomas. *Lab Invest*, 2008 88, 910–925.

[240] Vigneswaran, N; Wu, J; Zacharias, W. Upregulation of cystatin M during the progression of oropharyngeal squamous cell carcinoma from primary tumor to metastasis. Oral Oncol, 2003 39, 559–568.

[241] Zhang, J; Shridhar, R; Dai, Q; Song, J; Barlow, SC; Yin, L; Sloane, BF; Miller, FR; Meschonat, C; Li, BDL; Abreo, F; Keppler, D. Cystatin M: A Novel Candidate Tumor Suppressor Gene for Breast Cancer. *Cancer Res*, 2004 64, 6957–6964.

[242] Morita, M; Yoshiuchi, N; Arakawa, H; Nishimura, S. CMAP: a novel cystatin-like gene involved in liver metastasis. *Cancer Res*, 1999 59, 151–158.

[243] Zhang, Z; Li, Y; Li, C; Yuan, J; Wang, Z. Expression of a Buckwheat Trypsin Inhibitor Gene in Escherichia coli and its Effect on Multiple Myeloma IM-9 Cell Proliferation. *Acta Biochim Biophys Sin*, 2007 39, 701–707.

[244] Gauthier, F; Fryksmark, U; Ohlsson, K; Bieth, JG. Kinetics of the inhibition of leukocyte elastase by the bronchial inhibitor. *Biochim Biophys Acta*, 1982 700, 178–183.

[245] Abe, T; Kobayashi, N; Yoshimura, K; Trapnell, BC; Kim, H; Hubbard, RC; Brewer, MT; Thompson, RC; Crystal, RG. Expression of the secretory leukoprotease inhibitor gene in epithelial cells. *J Clin Inves*, 1991 87, 2207–2215.

[246] Thompson, RC; Ohlsson, K. Isolation, properties, and complete amino acid sequence of human secretory leukocyte protease inhibitor, a potent inhibitor of leukocyte elastase. *Proc Natl Acad Sci USA*, 1986 83, 6692–6696.

[247] Cox, SW; Rodríguez-Gonzalez, EM; Booth, V; Eley, BM; Secretory leukocyte protease inhibitor and its potential interactions with elastase and cathepsin B in gingival crevicular fluid and saliva from patients with chronic periodontitis. *J Periodont Res*, 2006 41, 477–485.

[248] Devoogdt, N; Revets, H; Ghassabeh, GH; De Baetselie, P. Secretory leukocyte protease inhibitor in cancer development. *Ann NY Acad Sci*, 2004 1028, 380–389.

[249] Morita, M; Arakawa, H; Nishimura, S. Identification and cloning of a novel isoform of mouse secretory leukocyte protease inhibitor, mSLPI-β, overexpressed in murine leukemias and a highly liver metastatic tumor, IMC-HA1 cells. *Adv Enzyme Regul*, 1999 39, 341-355.

[250] Hough, CD; Sherman-Baust, CA; Pizer, ES; Montz, FJ; Im, DD; Rosenshein, NB; Cho, KR; Riggins, GJ; Morin, PJ. Large-Scale Serial Analysis of Gene Expression Reveals Genes Differentially Expressed in Ovarian Cancer. *Cancer Res*, 2000 60, 6281–6287.

[251] Bouchard, D; Morisset, D; Bourbonnais, Y; Tremblay, GM. Proteins with whey-acidic-protein motifs and cancer. *Lancet Oncol*, 2006 7, 167–74.

[252] Cheng, WL; Wang, CS; Huang, YH; Liang, Y; Lin, PY; Hsueh, C; Wu, YC; Chen, WJ; Yu, CJ; Lin, SR; Lin, KH. Overexpression of a secretory leukocyte protease inhibitor in human gastric cancer. *Int J Cancer*, 2008 123, 1787–1796.

[253] Nukiwa, T; Suzuki, T; Fukuhara, T; Kikuchi, T. Secretory leukocyte peptidase inhibitor and lung cancer. *Cancer Sci*, 2008 99, 849–855.

[254] Devoogdt, N; Ghassabeh, GH; Zhang, J; Brys, L; De Baetselier, P; Revets, H. Secretory leukocyte protease inhibitor promotes the tumorigenic and metastatic potential of cancer cells. *PNAS*, 2003 100, 5778–5782.

[255] Zhang, D; Simmen, RCM; Michel, FJ; Zhao, G; Vale-Cruz, D; Simmen, FA. Secretory Leukocyte Protease Inhibitor Mediates Proliferation of Human Endometrial Epithelial Cells by Positive and Negative Regulation of Growth-associated Genes. *J Biol Chem*, 2002 277, 29999–30009.

[256] Auersperg, N; Wong, AST; Choi, KC; Kang, SK; Leung, PCK. Ovarian surface epithelium: biology, endocrinology, and pathology. *Endocr Rev*, 2001 22, 255–288.

[257] King, AE; Morgan, K; Sallenave, JM; Kelly, RW. Differential regulation of secretory leukocyte protease inhibitor and elafin by progesterone. *Biochem Biophys Res Commun*, 2003 310, 594–599.

[258] Devoogdt, N; Revets, H; Kindt, A; Liu, YQ; De Baetselier, P; Ghassabeh, GH. The Tumor-Promoting Effect of TNF-α Involves the Induction of Secretory Leukocyte Protease Inhibitor. *J Immunol*, 2006 177, 8046–8052.

[259] Devoogdt, N; Rasool, N; Hoskins, E; Simpkins, F; Tchabo, N; Kohn, EC. Overexpression of protease inhibitor-dead secretory leukocyte protease inhibitor causes more aggressive ovarian cancer *in vitro* and *in vivo*. *Cancer Sci*, 2009 100, 434–440.

[260] Luo, BL; Niu, RC; Feng, JT; Hu, CP; Xie, XY; Ma, LJ. Downregulation of Secretory Leukocyte Proteinase Inhibitor in Chronic Obstructive Lung Disease: The Role of TGF-β/Smads Signaling Pathways. *Arch Med Res*, 2008 39, 388–396.

[261] Wang, N; Thuraisingam, T; Fallavollita, L; Ding, A; Radzioch, D; Brodt, P. The Secretory Leukocyte Protease Inhibitor Is a Type 1 Insulin-Like Growth Factor Receptor–Regulated Protein that Protects against Liver Metastasis by Attenuating the Host Proinflammatory Response. *Cancer Res*, 2006 66, 3962-3070.

[262] Sugino, T; Yamaguchi, T; Ogura, G; Kusakabe, T; Goodison, S; Homma, Y; Suzuki, T. The secretory leukocyte protease inhibitor (SLPI) suppresses cancer cell invasion but promotes blood-borne metastasis via an invasion-independent pathway. *J Pathol*, 2007 212, 152–160.

[263] Flexner, C. HIV-protease inhibitors. *N Engl J Med*, 1998 338, 1281–1292.

[264] Chow, WA; Jiang, C; Guan, M. Anti-HIV drugs for cancer therapeutics: back to the future? *Oncology*, 2009 10, 61–71.

[265] Palella, FJ; Delaney, KM; Moorman, AC; Loveless, MO; Fuhrer, J; Satten, GA; Aschman, DJ; Holmberg, SD. Declining morbidity and mortality among patients with advanced human immunodefi ciency virus infection. *N Engl J Med*, 1998 338, 853–860.

[266] Perrin, L; Telenti, A. HIV treatment failure: testing for HIV resistance in clinical practice. *Science*, 1998 280, 1871–1873.

[267] Monini, P; Sgadari, C; Toschi, E; Barillari, G; Ensoli, B. Antitumour effects of antiretroviral therapy. *Nat Rev Cancer*, 2004 4, 861–875.

[268] Ikezoe, T; Daar, ES; Hisatake, J; Taguchi, H; Koeffler, HP. HIV-1 protease inhibitors decrease proliferation and induce differentiation of human myelocytic leukemia cells. *Blood*, 2000 96, 3553–3559.

[269] Sgadari, C; Barillari, G; Toschi, E; Carlei, D; Bacigalupo, I; Baccarini, S; Palladino, C; Leone, P; Bugarini, R; Malavasi, L; Cafaro, A; Falchi, M; Valdembri, D; Rezza, G; Bussolino, F; Monini, P; Ensoli, B. HIV protease inhibitors are potent anti-angiogenic molecules and promote regression of Kaposi sarcoma. *Nat Med*, 2002 8, 225–232.

[270] Pati, S; Pelser, CB; Dufraine, J; Bryant, JL; Reitz, MS Jr.; Weichold, FF. Antitumorigenic effects of HIV protease inhibitor ritonavir: inhibition of Kaposi sarcoma. *Blood*, 2002 99, 3771–3779.

[271] Pajonk, F; Himmelsbach, J; Riess, K; Sommer, A; McBride, WH. The human immunodeficiency virus (HIV)-1 protease inhibitor saquinavir inhibits proteasome function and causes apoptosis and radiosensitization in non-HIVassociated human cancer cells. *Cancer Res*, 2002 62, 5230–5235.

[272] Gaedicke, S; Firat-Geier, E; Constantiniu, O; Lucchiari-Hartz, M; Freudenberg, M; Galanos, C; Niedermann, G. Antitumor effect of the human immunodeficiency virus protease inhibitor ritonavir: induction of tumor-cell apoptosis associated with perturbation of proteasomal proteolysis. *Cancer Res*, 2002 62, 6901–6908.

[273] Gupta, AK; Cerniglia, GJ; Mick, R; McKenna, WG; Muschel, RJ. HIV protease inhibitors block Akt signaling nd radiosensitize tumor cells both *in vitro* and *in vivo*. *Cancer Res*, 2005 65, 8256–8265.

[274] Yang, Y; Ikezoe, T; Takeuchi, T; Adachi, Y; Ohtsuki, Y; Takeuchi, S; Koeffler, HP; Taguchi, H. HIV-1 protease inhibitor induces growth arrest and apoptosis of human prostate cancer LNCaP cells *in vitro* and *in vivo* in conjunction with blockade of androgen receptor STAT3 and AKT signaling. *Cancer Sci*, 2005 96, 425–433.

[275] Srirangam, A; Mitra, R; Wang, M; Gorski, JC; Badve, S; Baldridge, LA; Hamilton, J; Kishimoto, H; Hawes, J; Li, L; Orschell, CM; Srour, EF; Blum, JS; Donner, D; Sledge, GW; Nakshatri, H; Potter, DA. Effects of HIV protease inhibitor ritonavir on Akt-regulated cell proliferation in breast cancer. *Clin Cancer Res*, 2006 12, 1883–1896.

[276] Pyrko, P; Kardosh, A; Wang, W; Xiong, W; Schönthal, AH; Chen, TC. HIV-1 Protease Inhibitors Nelfinavir and Atazanavir Induce Malignant Glioma Death by Triggering Endoplasmic Reticulum Stress. *Cancer Res*, 2007 67, 10920–10928.

[277] Gills, JJ; LoPiccolo, J; Tsurutani, J; Shoemaker, RH; Best, CJM; Abu-Asab, MS; Borojerdi, J; Warfel, NA; Gardner, ER; Danish, M; Hollander, MC; Kawabata, S; Tsokos, M; Figg, WD; Steeg, PS; Dennis, PA. Nelfi navir, a lead HIV protease inhibitor, is a broad-spectrum, anticancer agent that induces endoplasmic reticulum stress, autophagy, and apoptosis *in vitro* and *in vivo*. *Clin Cancer Res*, 2007 13, 5183–5194.

[278] Cuneo, KC; Tu, T; Geng, L; Fu, A; Hallahan, DE; Willey, CD. HIV Protease Inhibitors Enhance the Efficacy of Irradiation. *Cancer Res*, 2007 67, 4886–4893.

[279] Jiang, W; Mikochik, PJ; Ra, JH; Lei, H; Flaherty, KT; Winkler, JD; Spitz, FR. HIV Protease Inhibitor Nelfinavir Inhibits Growth of Human Melanoma Cells by Induction of Cell Cycle Arrest. *Cancer Res*, 2007 67, 1221–1227.

[280] Brunner, TB; Geiger, M; Grabenbauer, GG; Lang-Welzenbach, M; Mantoni, TS; Cavallaro, A; Sauer, R; Hohenberger, W; McKenna, WG. Phase I trial of the human immunodefi ciency virus protease inhibitor nelfinavir and chemoradiation for locally advanced pancreatic cancer. *J Clin Oncol*, 2008 26, 2699–2706.

In: New Approaches in the Treatment of Cancer
Editors: Carmen Mejia Vazquez et al. pp.125-138

ISBN 978-1-62100-067-9

Chapter VI

PHOTOTHERMAL TECHNIQUE APPLIED TO THE CHARACTERIZATION OF NANOPARTICLES INCORPORATED INTO PPIX FOR APPLICATION IN THE CANCEROUS CELLS THERAPY

José Luis Jiménez Pérez[1,*], Alfredo Cruz Orea[2] and Eva Ramón Gallegos[3]

[1]UPIITA, Instituto Politecnico Nacional (IPN), México
[2]Centro de Investigación y de Estudios Avanzados del IPN, México
[3]ENCB, Instituto Politecnico Nacional (IPN), México

ABSTRACT

In this chapter are shown some applications of two photothermal techniques (Photoacoustic Spectroscopy, PAS, and Thermal Lens Spectrometry, TLS) to determine the characteristic non-radiative relaxation time (NRRT) and the thermal diffusivity. In addition, complementary techniques as Fluorescence Spectroscopy, Optical Absorption Spectrometry and TEM were used to determine the florescence intensity, the optical absorption and the particle sizes, respectively, of metallic solutions with gold nanoparticles (Au-np) and protoporphyrin IX (PpIX) for its applications in Photodynamic Therapy (PDT). This therapy is based on the preferential use of laser light and the presence of molecular oxygen in these cells. A thorough photothermal technique is possible to determine some physical parameters that help us to improve the PDT efficiency. Nowadays PDT is considered an effective method for diagnosis and treats some pre-malignant and malignant processes. PDT eliminates cancerous cells that accumulate the photosensitizer (Ps) which generate free radicals when this Ps is exposed to a laser beam with a suitable wavelength. The objective of this research is to improve

* Correspondence concerning this article should be addressed to: José Luis Jiménez Pérez, Ph.D., e-mail: jimenezp@fis.cinvestav.mx.

the photothermal treatment with nanoparticles and PpIX incorporated in the cells using the PDT.

INTRODUCTION

Metal nanoparticles have been proposed as targeted thermal agents for use in medical therapies and drug delivery [1–4] and could extend the precision of thermal effects below cellular dimensions [4]. Gold nanoparticles are leading candidate materials for these applications due to their biocompatibility and also because well-developed surface chemistries are available to functionalize Au nanoparticles for attachment to selected biological molecules or materials. Many research groups have studied how the environment of a nanoparticle affects the decay of the particle temperature [5–8], but these data, in most cases, have not been analyzed quantitatively to extract information about the thermophysical properties or microstructure of the material surrounding the nanoparticles. On the other hand, in the photodynamic therapy (PDT), porphyrins are currently used as photo-sensitizers of cancerous tumors; thus, it is important to measure their distribution in tissues, mainly in relation to the possible side effects after their injection into patients [9]. Among these porphyrins the protoporphyrin IX (PpIX), which is induced by δ-aminolevulinic acid (ALA) being accumulated in high concentrations in cancerous cells and low concentrations in normal cells [9], stands out. Thus, it is important to determine the thermal diffusivity of the nanoparticles and the surrounding liquid (PpIX and water) in order to know the heat transfer between the photosensitizers and nanoparticles with possible applications of treatment for cancerous tumors. The photothermal techniques, as PAS and TLS, offers some advantages in the field of photosensitization because one of the most distinctive features of this technique is its capability for the analysis of semitransparent or opaque samples, as well as its high sensitivity. For example TLS is a time-resolved method that can be used to measure, over a short time, the optical absorption coefficient and thermal diffusivity of a sample in an absolute sense [10]. Furthermore, it has been demonstrated that the dual-beam thermal-lens measurement is independent of scattered light [11,12]. TLS, therefore, is suitable for thermal-diffusivity measurements of the nanoparticles and surrounding liquid. The purpose of this work is to determine the physics parameters with different photothermal techniques by applications of PpIX solutions at different concentrations of gold metallic nanoparticles.

NRRT Determination

In this section, it was used the Photoacoustic Spectroscopy (PAS) to determine *in vitro* the NRRT of a PpIX standard solution and samples PpIX(1), PpIX(2) and PpIX(3) with Au nanoparticle concentrations of 0.001008, 0.00504 and 0.01008 mmol in 25 mL of water respectively.

Sample Preparation

Gold nanoparticles in aqueous solution were synthesized using ascorbic acid (AA) as a reducing agent [13]. The reduction of $HAuCl_4$ was carried out as follows: solutions of $HAuCl_4$ (0.033 mmol in 25 mL of water) and polyvinyl pyrrolidone (PVP, 25 mg in 20 mL of water) were prepared by dissolving the $HAuCl_4$ crystals and PVP in water. Both solutions were mixed to produce an Au (III) ion solution containing PVP. Then an aqueous solution of AA (0.033 mmol in 5 mL of water) was added to the resulting solution at room temperature. A colloidal solution containing metallic particles was formed after the addition of AA solution to the mixture solution. Three solutions of PpIX disodium salt (5 mL, 400 $\mu g \cdot mL^{-1}$, to 25% of HCl) were mixed at room temperature with 1, 2.5, and 5 mL of the colloidal Au solution to produce PpIX-Au nanocluster systems. The volume was adjusted to 10 mL with water and was placed in a quartz cuvette with 1 cm thick wall for the optical and thermal measurements. The experiments were performed at room temperature.

A Shimadzu UV-Vis 3101PC double-beam spectrophotometer was used to record the absorption spectra of the fluids. Particle sizes and size distribution were evaluated by TEM, using a JEOL-JEM200 microscope. For TEM observations, a drop of colloidal solution was spread on a carbon-coated copper micro-grid and dried subsequently in vacuum. Gold particles with an average size of 14.3 nm were measured.

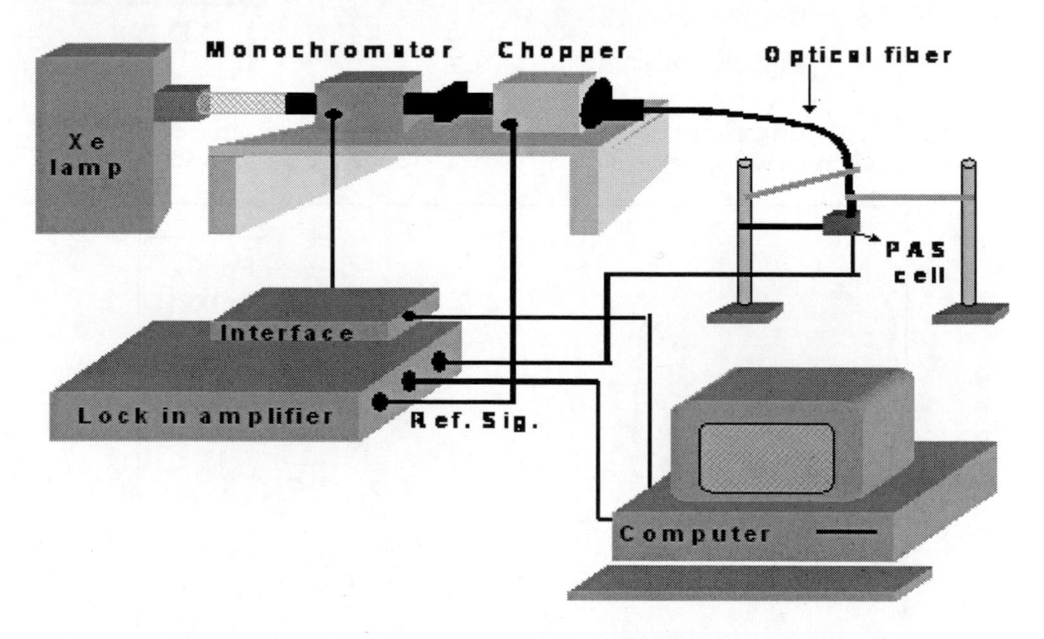

Figure 1. Experimental set-up used in Photoacoustic spectroscopy.

Pas Experimental Set-up

The experimental set-up consisted of a 1000-W xenon lamp, a monochromator, a variable frequency mechanical chopper, set at 17 Hz, and air filled homemade brass cell with an electric microphone (showed in Figure 1). The sample was placed into the PA cell. The PA signal from the microphone provided the input to the signal channel of a lock-in amplifier, displaying the PA signal amplitude and phase simultaneously. In the maximum absorption peak, observed from the UV-vis optical spectrum, at 404 nm, it was obtained the PA signal amplitude and phase as a function of the light modulation frequency, from 17 to 80 Hz.

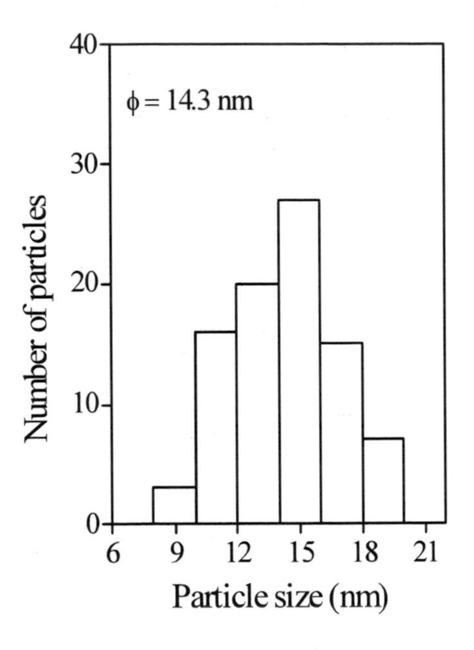

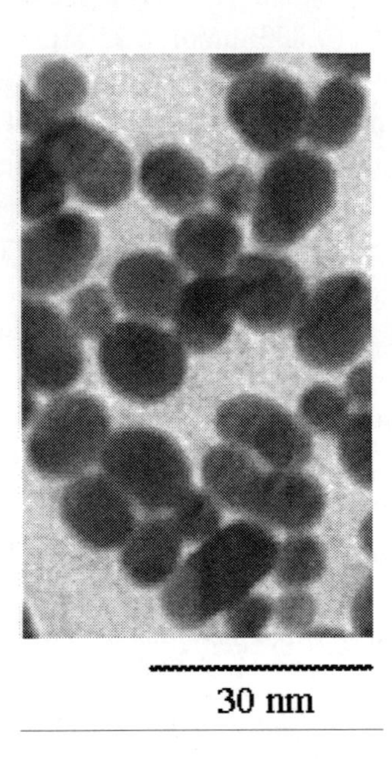

Figure 2. Particle size histogram and electron micrograph of Au nanoparticles prepared with concentration of metal ion of 0.096 mmol in 50ml of water. Average size φ is reported.

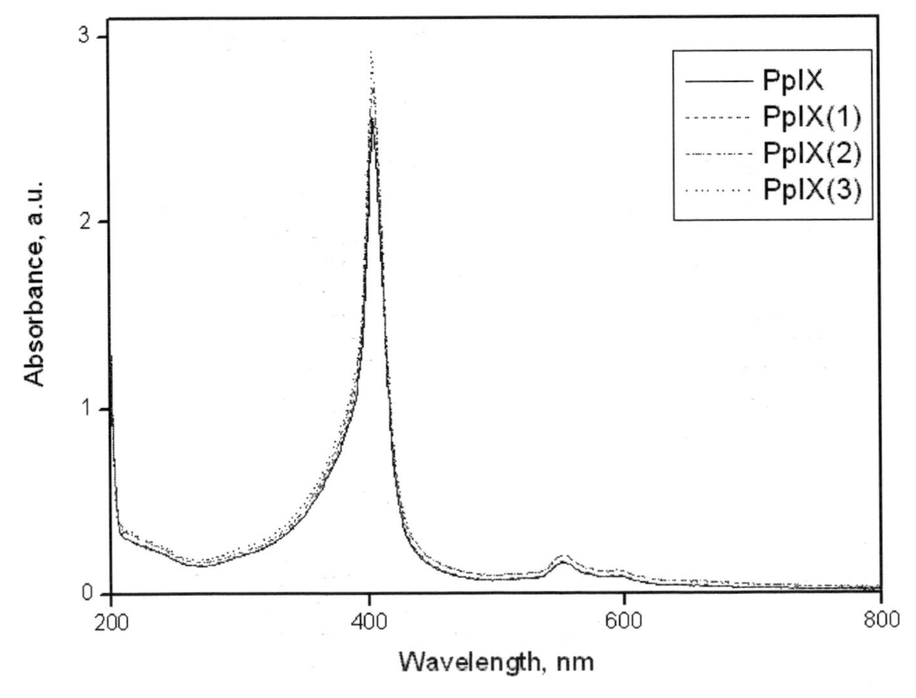

Figure 3. Optical absorption spectra of PpIX and PpIX containing Au nanoparticles prepared with different concentrations of metal ions.

From the TEM image and the corresponding size distribution of the Au nanoparticles (showed in Figure 2), it was found that the average size was around 14.3 nm. After finding the maximum absorption peak (showed in Figure 3) of the PpIX(1), PpIX(2) and PpIX(3) have a strong optical absorption band, with a maximum at 404 nm, which is known as the Soret band, characteristic of porphyrins [14] and also other characteristic peak at 580 nm. After finding the maximum absorption peak, the PpIX(1) sample was irradiated at this peak (404 nm) in the frequency range from 17 to 80 Hz. The PA signal amplitude, as function of the light modulation frequency (f), exhibits a $f^{-1.45}$ dependence (don't showed here), very close with the $f^{-1.5}$ predicted, from the thermal diffusion Rosencwaig and Gersho (R-G) model [15], for thermally thick sample, i.e. $l_s > \mu_s$, where l_s is the sample thickness and $\mu_s = (\alpha / \pi f)^{1/2}$, is the thermal diffusion length, with α being the sample thermal diffusivity.

By using the R-G theory modified to include the effect of a finite non radiative relaxation time (τ) it was found that, for thermally thick sample, the PA signal phase is given by [16]:

$$\Delta\phi = -\frac{3\pi}{4} - tg^{-1}(\omega\tau) + tg^{-1}\left(\frac{1}{1+\left(2\omega\tau_\beta\right)^{1/2}}\right) \tag{1}$$

Where $\tau_\beta = 1/\beta^2\alpha$, with β being the optical absorption coefficient. This dependency of the PA signal phase on the modulation frequency has been used by some authors to obtain the non radiative relaxation time τ in different radiationless process [16]. Deexcitations of exited states thorough nonradiative routes constitute the heat source for the photoacoustic effect. Since the relaxation of the triplet state is slow, the modulation of the triplet population will be delayed and lag in phase the modulation of other rapidly relaxing states [17]. We have performed the fitting of the experimental PA signal phase data in the Soret band, at 404 nm, where a maximum of PpIX molecules are carried to exited states, to obtain for each solution of PpIX the non radiative relaxation time τ as a fitting parameter in equation 1 (see Figure 4), obtaining: $\tau = 29 \pm 0.001$, $\tau = 84 \pm 0.001$ and $\tau = 62 \pm 0.009$ ms for PpIX(1), PpIX(2) and PpIX(3) respectively. These values are higher than the average value obtained for the standard PpIX ($\tau = 15.4$ ms) [17].

A complementary fluorescence analysis (showed in Figure 5) reveals that the fluorescence intensity of PpIX (2) is higher than the corresponding to PpIX. These results from the photoluminescence spectra are in agreement with the results from the photoacoustic experimental nonradiative relaxation times: for longer values of τ, meaning smaller non-radiative transition probabilities, the probability of radiative transitions increases, and so does the photoluminescence intensity, as it is observed in Figure 5 for PpIX(2).

The obtained average value of the nonradiative relaxation time agree in order of magnitude with lifetimes of triplet state of porphyrins, photosentitizers used in PDT [17] and also of chlorophylis, whose structure is similar to the porphyrins, both having tetrapyrrolic structure [18]. The increase of the non-radiative relaxation time in the PpIX with gold nanoparticles could be used in medical diagnostic applications and also in future studies in PDT.

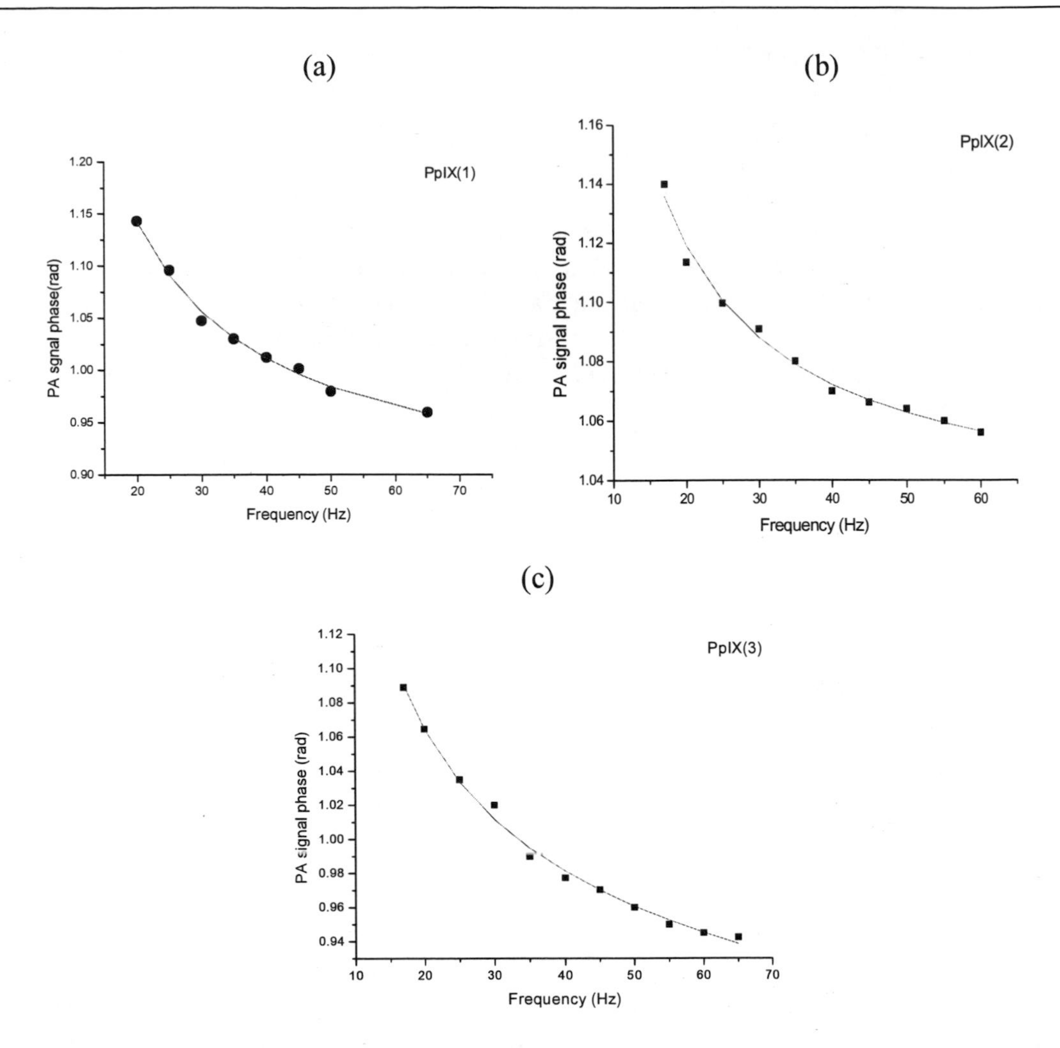

Figure 4. PA signal phase data as a function of the light modulation frequency for a) PpIX (1), b) PpIX (2) and c) PpIX (3). The solid line represents the best fit of equation (1) to the experimental data.

THERMAL CHARACTERIZATION

Thermal Lens Measurements

In the dual-beam thermal lens measurements, a sample is placed in a TEM_{00} Gaussian laser beam (excitation beam), and a temperature rise is produced by non-radiative decay processes following the optical energy absorption. Since the refractive index of the sample changes with temperature, a refractive index gradient is produced, creating a lens-like optical element, the so-called thermal lens. A weak TEM_{00} Gaussian laser beam (probe beam), which is co-linear with the excitation beam passing through the thermal lens, will be affected, resulting in a variation in its spot size and hence the intensity at the sample that can be obtained. A theoretical model for a continuous-wave (CW) laser-induced mode-mismatched dual-beam TLS has been developed, and the variation of the intensity in the center of the probe beam, caused by the thermal lens, can be expressed as [10,19]

$$I(t) = I(0)\left[1 - \frac{\theta}{2}\tan^{-1}\left(\frac{2mV}{\left[(1+2m)^2 + V^2\right]\frac{t_c}{2t} + 1 + 2m + V^2}\right)\right]^2 \quad (2)$$

where,

$$m = \left(\frac{\omega_{1p}}{\omega_e}\right)^2; \; V = \frac{Z_1}{Z_c}; \; \theta = -\frac{P_e A_e l_0}{k\lambda_p}\left(\frac{dn}{dT}\right)_p$$

and

$$t_c = \frac{\omega_e^2}{4D} \quad (3)$$

Here $I(0)$ is the initial intensity when t or θ is zero, P_e is the excitation beam power (W), A_e is the absorption coefficient (cm^{-1}), l_0 is the sample thickness, λp is the probe beam wavelength (cm), dn/dT is the refractive index change of the sample with temperature (K^{-1}), $Z_c = \pi\omega^2_{op}/\lambda$ is the confocal distance (cm), Z_l is the distance from the probe beam waist to the sample, $D = \kappa/(\rho c)$ is the thermal diffusivity of the sample ($cm^2 \cdot s^{-1}$), κ is the thermal conductivity ($J \cdot s^{-1} \cdot cm^{-1} \cdot K^{-1}$), ρ is the density of the sample ($g \cdot cm^{-3}$), c is the specific heat of the sample ($J \cdot g^{-1} \cdot K^{-1}$), and t_c is the characteristic thermal time constant (s). ω_e, Z_c, ω_{1p}, and ω_{0p} can be obtained from the spot-size measurements [10], and θ and t_c can be determined by fitting Eq.(2) to the measured time-resolved intensity signal data, $I(t)$. The thermal diffusivity, D, can be determined from t_c in Eq. (3). The mathematical expression in Eq. (2) is simple and convenient to use.

TLS Experimental Set-up

The experimental apparatus for time-resolved measurements of gold nanoparticles in water solution samples is show in Figure 6. The excitation laser is an Ar+ laser, at $\lambda = 514$ nm, which was focused by a converging lens ($\omega_e = 40$ μm), and the sample was placed at the focal plane lens. Exposure time of the sample to the excitation beam was controlled by means of a shutter, which was connected directly to the trigger of a digital oscilloscope. A He–Ne laser probe beam of 4 mW was focused with a lens. The probe beam was incident on the sample and carefully centered to pass through the thermal lens to maximize the thermal-lens signal. After passing through the sample, the probe beam was reflected by mirrors M3, M4, and M5 to a pinhole mounted before a photodiode or photodetector. A band-pass filter 1, at the He–Ne laser wavelength, was placed over the photodiode to prevent stray light from entering the photodetector. The spot size of the probe beam at the pinhole was 10 cm because of scattering by the sample, and the radius of the pinhole used here was 0.5 cm. The output of the photodiode was coupled to the digital oscilloscope. The parameters of the experimental setup such as ω_e, Z_c, ω_{0p}, and ω_{1p} were measured as described in reference [10].

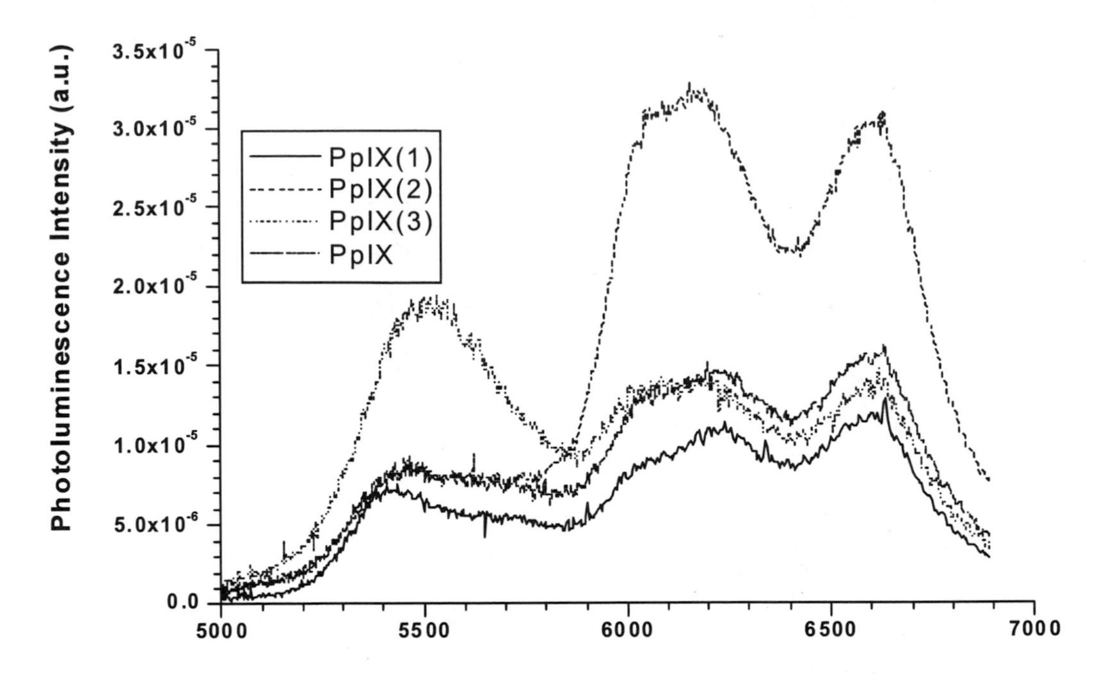

Figure 5. Analysis of the photoluminescence spectra measured at room temperature.

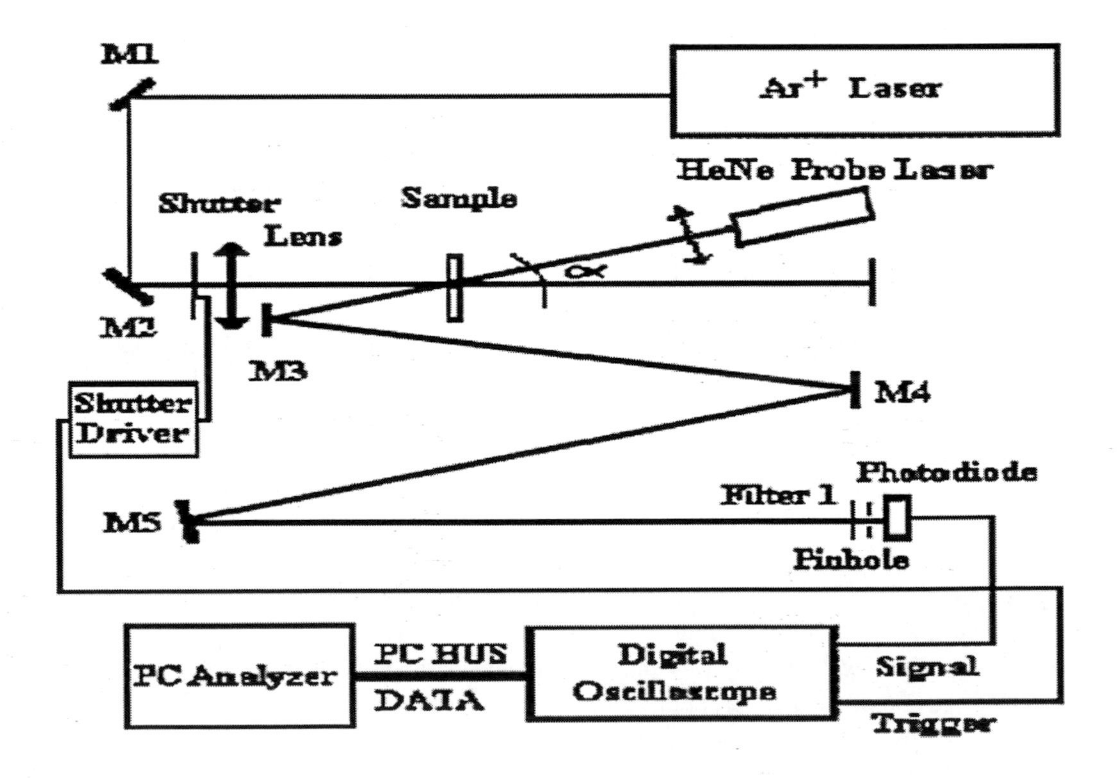

Figure 6. Schematic representation of the thermal lens (TL) experimental setup.

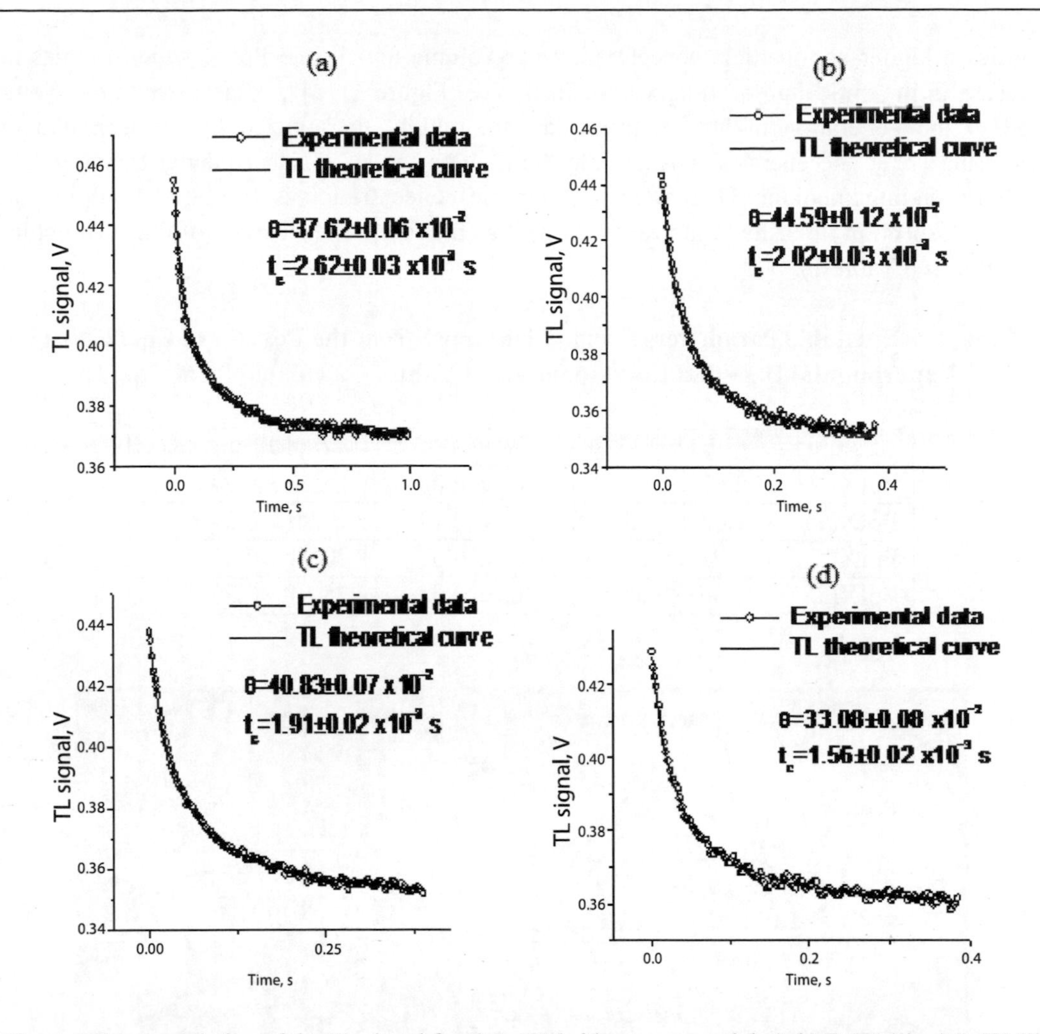

Figure 7. Time evolution of the TL signal for a) PpIX (without nanoparticles), b) PpIX (1), c) PpIX (2) and d) PpIX (3) with gold nanoparticles. Symbols represent the experimental data, and solid line represents the best fit of Eq. (2) to the experimental data.

Figure 7a shows the normalized time resolved thermal-lens signal of the PpIX solution without gold metallic nanoparticles; symbols (o) represent the experimental points and the solid line corresponds to the best fit of Eq. (1) to the experimental data with θ and tc as adjustable parameters. From this fit the values of $\theta = 0.37 \pm 0.06 \times 10^{-2}$ and $tc = 2.62 \pm 0.03 \times 10^{-3}$ s were obtained, which corresponds to the thermal diffusivity $D = 15.26 \pm 0.17 \times 10^{-4}$ $cm^2 \cdot s^{-1}$. This value is close to the thermal diffusivity of water ($D_{water} = 14 \times 10^{-4}$ $cm^2 \cdot s^{-1}$) [20].

Figure 7b shows the transient thermal lens signal for PpIX(1) sample. From the best fit of Eq. (2) to the experimental data, the thermal diffusivity of this sample was obtained. Similar TL signal evolution was obtained for PpIX(2), and PpIX(3) samples and their corresponding thermal diffusivities were obtained, see figures 7c and 7d respectively. Table 1 summarizes the thermal diffusivity values obtained from the fit of Eq. (2) to experimental data. It can be seen that there is an increase in the fluid thermal diffusivity when the Au particle concentration increases. A possible explanation for this increase in the thermal diffusivity, when the Au particle concentration increases, is due to the strong electrostatic interaction between the cationic PpIX and the negatively charged Au nanoparticles. This interaction implies a higher nanoparticle concentration per volume unit in the PpIX, which implies an increase in the optical absorption peak intensity (see Figure 3) [21]. A laser excitation would lead to the generation of hot electrons that are rapidly thermalized by electron–phonon scattering [22]. The energy deposited into the phonon modes is subsequently transferred to the surrounding medium. Then when the particle concentration is increased in PpIX, the optical absorption intensity is increased, as well as the thermal diffusivity of the surrounding medium (see Table 1).

Table 1. Adjustable Parameters t_c and θ, Obtained from the Best Fit of Eq. (2) to TL Experimental Data and Corresponding D Values Calculated from Eq. (2)

Sample	t_c (10^{-3} s)	θ x 10^{-2}	D (10^{-4} cm^2·s^{-1})
PpIX	2.62 ± 0.03	37.62 ± 0.06	15.26 ± 0.17
PpIX(1)	2.02 ± 0.03	44.59 ± 0.12	19.80 ± 0.29
PpIX(2)	1.91 ± 0.02	40.83 ± 0.07	20.94 ± 0.23
PpIX(3)	1.56 ± 0.02	33.08 ± 0.08	25.64 ± 0.32

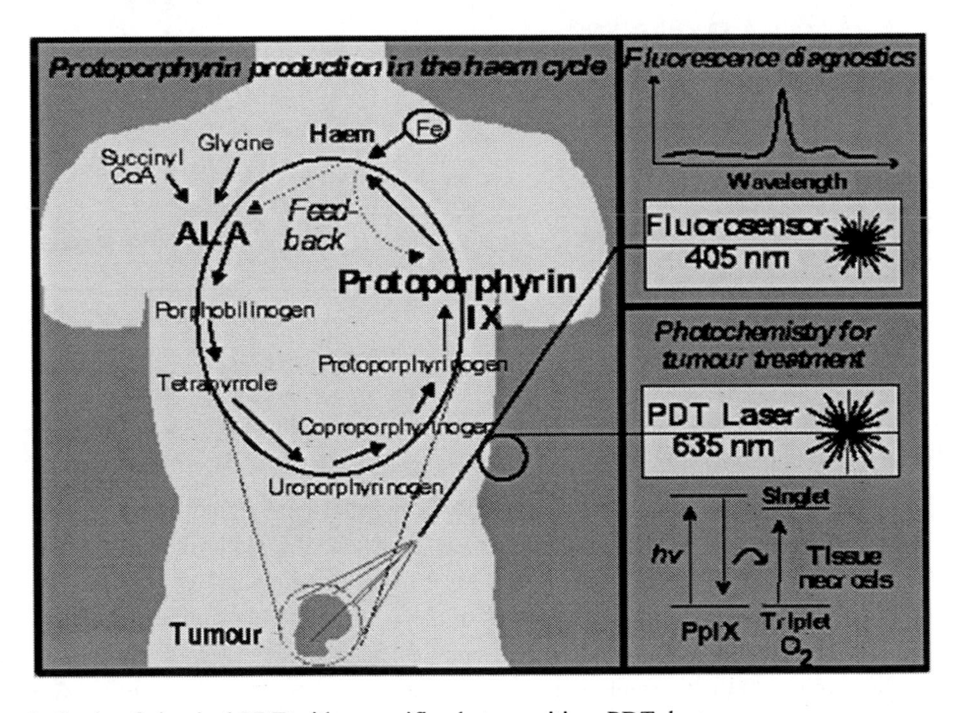

Figure 8. Cycle of classical PDT with a specific photosensitizer PDT drug.

Nanoparticles Incorporated into PpIX for Application in PDT

The effectiveness of photodynamic therapy (PDT) could be improved by the simultaneous use of Au-np and photosensitizes (Ps), emphasizing the high efficiency of the PDT to diagnose and to treat pre-malignant and malignant processes. It is based in the activation of a Ps, by means of light irradiation of a specific wave length that is absorbed by this one, on the Ps having relaxed, produces reactive oxygen which destroys cancerous cells (3) (showed Figure 8). In this section it was determined the efficiency of PDT using Au-np and protoporphyrin IX (PpIX) induced or not by the δ-aminolevulinic acid (ALA).

PDT Application

The PDT was applied to HeLa cells using a 1.7% Au-np solution and 20 μg/mL of PpIX as well as ALA at 40 μg/mL. The same concentrations of ALA and PpIX plus Au-np at 7.5% were applied to C33A cells. The cells were irradiated with an argon laser at 64.3 J/cm^2, and they were exposed 16 h to Au-np, 4h to ALA and 24 h to PpIX. Twenty four hours after irradiation cells viability was quantified by Alamar blue method.

Below 30 % Au-np doses the particles were not toxic *per se* in HeLa cells. When they were mix with the Ps it was found secure doses in HeLa cells of 1.7% Au-np + 20 μg/mL of ALA and 40μg/mL of PpIX respectively. In C33A cells both Ps were used at the same concentration while the Au-np was utilized at 7.5 %.

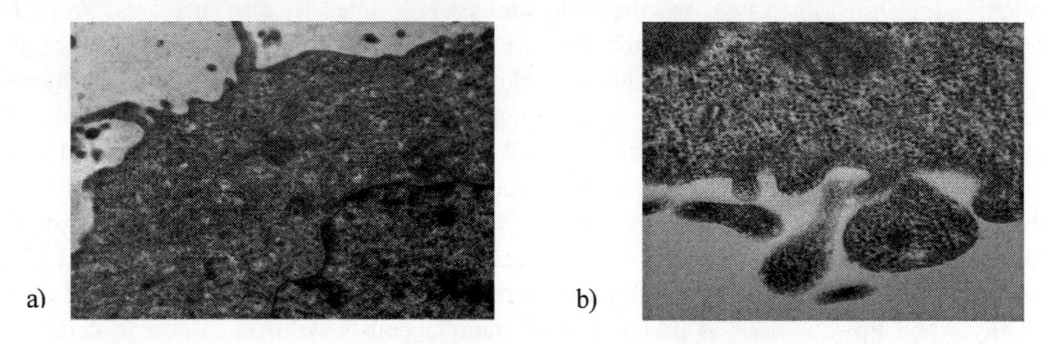

Figure 9. HeLa Cells without Au-np (a), exposed to 30 % Au-np during 16 h (b). Characterization by TEM. 100 000 X.

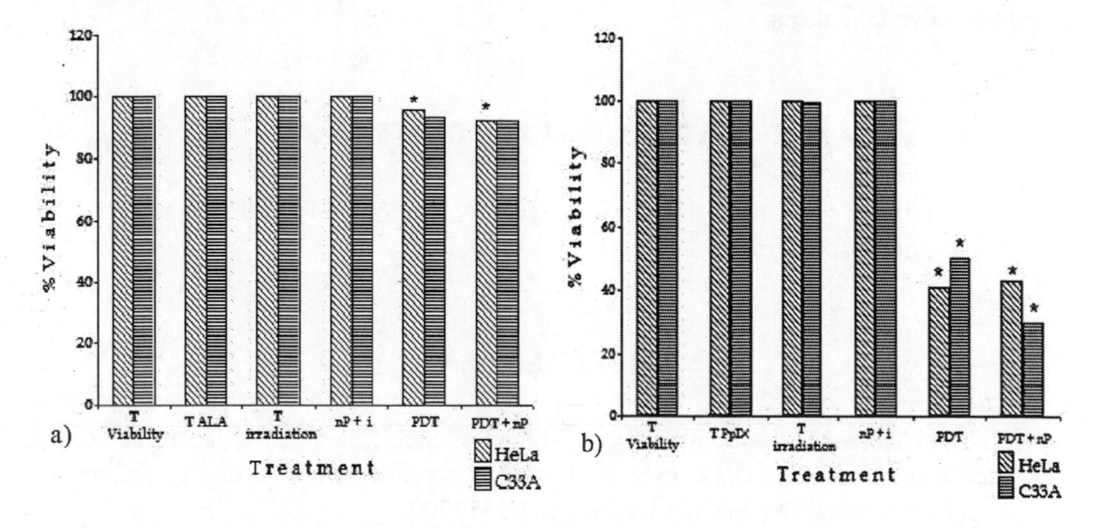

Figure 10. HeLa and C33A cells viability at 24 h exposed to PDT using PpIX (b) and ALA (a). *Significant difference in relation to the blank ($p < 0.001$).

From the TEM kinetic it was observed that the maximum incorporation time of Au-np to cells was 16 h (Figure 9). Also from PDT it was found the conditions of synthesis of hydrosoluble Au-np, and was characterized by transmission electronic microscopy (TEM) and UV-VIS spectroscopy. PDT was applied using different doses of Au-np and photosensitizers. The effectiveness of the therapy was determined by the Alamar blue method after 24 h of irradiation (Figure 10) [23].

Conclusion

The results show that the NRRT average value, obtained from each solution was: t = 29 ± 0.001, 84 ± 0.001 and 62 ± 0.009 ms for PpIX(1), PpIX(2) and PpIX(3), respectively. These values were compared with NRRT of triplet states reported in the literature for PpIX without Au nanoparticles, increasing the NRRT considerably. Photoluminescence results agree with the results from the photoacoustic experimental nonradiative relaxation times since for longer values of τ, meaning smaller non-radiative transition probabilities, then the probability of radiative transitions increases, and the photoluminescence intensity also increases. From TL the thermal diffusivity of PpIX and PpIX mixed with gold nanoparticles at different concentrations was obtained in aqueous solutions. The results show that the thermal diffusivity of PpIX mixed with gold nanoparticles increases with the Au particle concentration. The determination of this thermal parameter is very important in PDT in order to know the heat transfer between photosensitizers (such as porphyrins) and nanoparticles that are being studied in medical physics. From PDT study it was standardized the synthesis of Au-np between 30 and 50 nm. Also it was observed that PDT, when the ALA is simultaneously used with Au-np, did not increase the mortality of HeLa and C33 cells. Finally when PpIX is used as photosensitizer simultaneously with the Au-np in cells C33 increased in 20% the efficiency of PDT. Our investigations are devoted to improve the thermal treatments by porphyrins as photosensitizers used in cancerous tumor treatment and image photodynamic therapy.

Acknowledgments

The authors are thankful to the Mexican agencies, CONACYT, COFAA, and CGPI for financial support of this work.

References

[1] K. Hamad Schifferli, J.J. Scwartz, A.T. Santos, S.G. Zhang, J.M. Jacobson, Remote electronic control of DNA hybridization through inductive coupling to an attached metal nanocrystal antenna, *Nature 415*, 152-155 (2002).

[2] C. Loo, A. Lin, L. Hirsch, M.H. Lee, J. Barton, N. Halas, J. West, R. Drezck, Nanoshell-enabled photonics-based imaging and therapy of cancer, *Technol. Cancer Res.Treat. 3*, 33-40 (2004).

[3] D.P. O'Neal, L.R. Hirsch, N.J. Halas, J.D. Payne, J.L.West, Photo-thermal tumor ablation in mice using near infrared-absorbing nanoparticles, *Cancer Lett. 209*, 171-176 (2004).

[4] G. Huttmann, R. Birngruber, On the Possibility of High-Precision Photothermal Microeffects and the Measurement of Fast Thermal Denaturation of Proteins, *IEEE J. Sel. Top. Quant. Electronics 5*, 954-962 (1999).

[5] S. Link, A. Furube, M.B. Mohamed, T. Asahi, H. Masuhara, M.A. El-Sayed, Hot Electron Relaxation Dynamics of Gold Nanoparticles Embedded in MgSO4 Powder Compared To Solution: The Effect of the Surrounding Medium, *J. Phys. Chem. B 106*, 945-955 (2002).

[6] J.Y. Bigot, V. Halte, J.C. Merle, A. Daunois, Electron dynamics in metallic nanoparticles, *Chem. Phys. 251*, 181-203 (2000).

[7] J.Z. Zhang, Ultrafast Studies of Electron Dynamics in Semiconductor and Metal Colloidal Nanoparticles: Effects of Size and Surface, *Acc. Chem. Res. 30*, 423-429 (1997).

[8] M.B. Mohamed, T.S. Ahmadi, S. Link, M. Braun, M.A. El-Sayed, Hot electron and phonon dynamics of gold nanoparticles embedded in a gel matrix, *Chem. Phys. Lett. 343*, 55-63 (2001)

[9] J.C. Kennedy, R.H. Pottier, D.C. Pross, Photodynamic therapy with endogenous protoporphyrin IX: basic principle and present clinical experience, *J. Photochem. Photobiol. Biol. B. 6*, 143-148 (1990).

[10] J. Shen, R.D. Lowe, R.D. Snook, A model for CW laser induced mode-mismatched dual-beam thermal lens spectrometry, *Chem. Phys. 165*, 385-396 (1992).

[11] J. Shen, R.D. Snook, A radial finite model of thermal lens spectrometry and the influence of sample radius upon the validity of the radial infinity model, *J. Appl. Phys. 73*, 5286-5288 (1993).

[12] S.M. Brown, M.L. Baesso, J. Shen, R.D. Snook, Thermal diffusivity of skin measured by two photothermal techniques, *Anal. Chim. Acta. 282*, 711-719 (1993)

[13] J. Park, V. Privman, E. Matijevic, Model of Formation of Monodispersed Colloids, *J. Phys. Chem. B. 105*, 11630- 11635 (2001).

[14] S. Stolik, S.A. Tomás, E. Ramón Gallegos, A. Cruz-Orea, F. Sánchez-Sinencio, Determination of aminolevulinic-acid-induced protoporphyrin IX in mice skin *Rev. Sci. Instrum., 74*, 374-376 (2003).

[15] A. Rosencwaig, *Photoacoustic and Photoacoustic Spectroscopy*, R.E. Krieger Publishing Company, Inc., Malabar Florida, pp. 93-123, (1980).

[16] A. Torres-Filho, N.F. Leite, L.C.M. Miranda, N. Cella, H. Vargas, Photoacoustic investigation of iodine-doped polystyrene, *J. Appl. Phys., 66*, 97-102 (1989).

[17] V.H. Nieto-Cazares, E. Ramón-Gallegos, A. Cruz-Orea, *In vitro* determination of the non radiative relaxation time of triplet state in protoporphyrin IX, *J. Phys. IV, France 125*, 753-755 (2005).

[18] G. Renger, *Biophysics*, Springer-Verlag, Berlin, 515-542 (1983).

[19] J.F. Sánchez-Ramírez, J.L. Jiménez-Pérez, R. Carbajal-Valdez, A. Cruz-Orea, R. Gutierrez-Fuentes, J.L. Herrera-Pérez, Thermal diffusivity measurements in fluids

containing metallic nanoparticles using transient thermal lens, *Int. J. Thermophys. 27*, 1181-1188 (2006).

[20] R.C.Weast (ed.), *Handbook of Chemistry and Physics*, 67th Edn., Chemical Rubber Corp., Boca Raton, Florida, 1986–1987.

[21] R. Gutierrez-Fuentes, J.F. Sánchez Ramírez, J.L. Jiménez-Pérez, J. A. Pescador Rojas, E. Ramón-Gallegos, A. Cruz-Orea, Thermal Diffusivity Determination of Protoporphyrin IX Solution Mixed with Gold Metallic Nanoparticles, *Int. J. Thermophys., 28*, 1048-1055 (2007).

[22] N. Chandrasekharan, P.V. Kamat, J. Hu, G. Jones, II Dye-Capped Gold Nanoclusters: Photoinduced Morphological Changes in Gold/Rhodamine 6G Nanoassemblies, *J. Phys. Chem. B 104*, 11103-11109 (2000).

[23] E. Maldonado-Alvarado, E. Ramón-Gallegos, J. Tanatori-Cordova, F. J. Arenas-Huertero, M. E. Sánchez-Espindola, A. Reyes-Arellano, J.L. Jiménez-Pérez, A. Cruz-Orea, Eficiency of the Photodynamic Therapy using gold nanoparticles (np-Au) and PpIX induced and not induced, *AIP Conf. Proc., 1032*, 295-298 (2008).

In: New Approaches in the Treatment of Cancer
Editors: Carmen Mejia Vazquez et al. pp.139-172
ISBN 978-1-62100-067-9

Chapter VII

METALS IN CANCER TREATMENT

María Elena Bravo-Gómez and Lena Ruiz-Azuara*
Universidad Nacional Autónoma de México, México DF 04510, México

ABSTRACT

Bioinorganic chemistry offers many opportunities for medicinal chemistry research and the development of effective metal based chemotherapeutic agents. Metals have a large variety of coordination numbers and geometries, accessible redox states in physiological conditions and a wide range of thermodynamic and reactivity properties which can be successfully tuned by selection of suitable ligands. These characteristics can be used to develop new drugs with numerous advantages over the organic based drugs. Historically, research in this field has focus on platinum and DNA targeting; however, anticancer drug research may be expanded to include alternative metal compounds with different mode of action resulting in markedly different cytotoxic response profiles. The examples provided in this chapter were selected by the authors only to highlight some creative work in the field of anticancer metal based agents. The information about anticancer metal based drugs is organized in three main sections: platinum compounds, non platinum anticancer agents and essential metal based antitumor drugs. The latter section emphasizes the research on copper based agents Casiopeínas.

CHEMOTHERAPY

Paul Erhlich coined the term "chemotherapy" for the use of a chemical of known composition that treated parasites. From 1903 to 1915 devoted most of his attention to the development of chemotherapeutic agents, very much in the fashion used to identify anticancer drugs nowadays. He emphasized the value of animal models, using diseased ones to study the

* Correspondence concerning this article should be addressed to: Lena Ruiz-Azuara, Facultad de Química, Departamento de Química Inorgánica y Nuclear, Universidad Nacional Autónoma de México, Av. Universidad 3000, México DF 04510, México. Telephone and fax number: +52 55 56223529; E-mail address: ruizazuara@gmail.com

effects of drugs. Around 1900 such models existed for infectious diseases, shortly mice were infected with *tubercle bacillus* and *pneumococci*, mice and rats with trypanosomes, and rabbits with syphilis. Later on with the help of an organic chemist and the support of the pharmaceutical industry, Erhlich could synthesize a large series of arsenic compounds, finding that the number 606th was active, not only against trypanosome infections, but also against rabbit syphilis. This drug was called salvarsan (the savior of mankind) and was the first man-made chemical found to be effective to human parasitic diseases [1].

Chemotherapy of cancer started as the treatment of metastases. The ability to cure cancer depends on many variables due to its own etiology. The need for chemotherapy arose out of the appreciation that cancer is uncommonly a localized process, not amenable to control by purely local means [2]. The hypothesis that chemical compounds might be used in the treatment of cancer was not received with great enthusiasm even though the successful use of synthetic chemicals and natural products against parasitic, common bacterial infections and tuberculosis. It is important to mention that there are two types of drugs used for treatment of any disease, those that suppress the symptoms but do nothing to remove the cause of disease and those that cure. The use of drugs against malaria is considered the beginning of curative drug therapy. In each case, the possibility that chemotherapy could cure cancer was taken with great pessimism.

At the beginning of the 20th century Paul Erhlich took a more optimistic approach on this proposal earning to be considered the father of chemotherapy. He decided to give a step forward on this field, even his interest and optimism, in his laboratory dedicated to research on cancer had a sing over its stating *"Abandone all hope all you who enter here"*; but his effort was granted in 1898 when he discovered the first alkylating agent. It passed nearly 50 years before this observation was applied to the treatment of neoplastic diseases in humans. [1].

Cancer treatment research began at the turn of the century with three pieces of work [1-3]. The first was the development of cancer surgery leading Halsted, in 1894, to propose *en-block* resection as part of a cancer operation, particularly in a radical mastectomy. Around the same time, Roentgen discovered X-rays and gave physicians a second means of treating localized cancer. The third advance had its roots in the work of Paul Erhlich, who used rodent models for infectious diseases; his work was the base that led George Clowes, from Roswell Park Memorial Institute in Buffalo, to develop in the early 1900's inbred rodent lines that could carry transplanted rodent tumors. These models and others have since served as the testing ground for potential cancer chemotherapy agents [3-5].

METALS AND ITS COMPOUNDS USED IN MEDICINE

In medicine, up to these days there are several well known examples when metals have been used to treat or diagnose diseases. That is the case of silver compounds, applied as skin protector or after suffer burns; radioactive technetium compounds that used to improved the diagnostic of several diseases; salts of bismuth commonly used for the stomach or for diarrhea problems; gold complexes and copper salts successfully used for arthritis problems. In fact all these compounds can show toxic effects mainly related to the doses used; however, some of these so called toxic metals are fundamental for living beings, as trace elements or present as a drug. It is almost impossible to classify the metals under the terms toxic or non toxic, because the degree of "toxicity" may depend mainly of the exposition doses, in fact, physiological and toxic effects are a continuum (Figure 1). In this way of thinking, many toxic compounds used in a very low dose can be beneficial to some organisms and even present therapeutic effects in a narrow range of doses; whilst some considered non toxic, such as those present in living organisms (essential elements), can become dangerous and very toxic in high doses. Furthermore, an element can be beneficial or toxic depending on the speciation or its chemical form presented, the chemical nature of a molecule or ion is fundamental for the satisfactory further used of a compound. As a very good example of this is the importance of the speciation of selenium, that is an essential element, but some of its compounds are highly toxic, such as H_2Se.

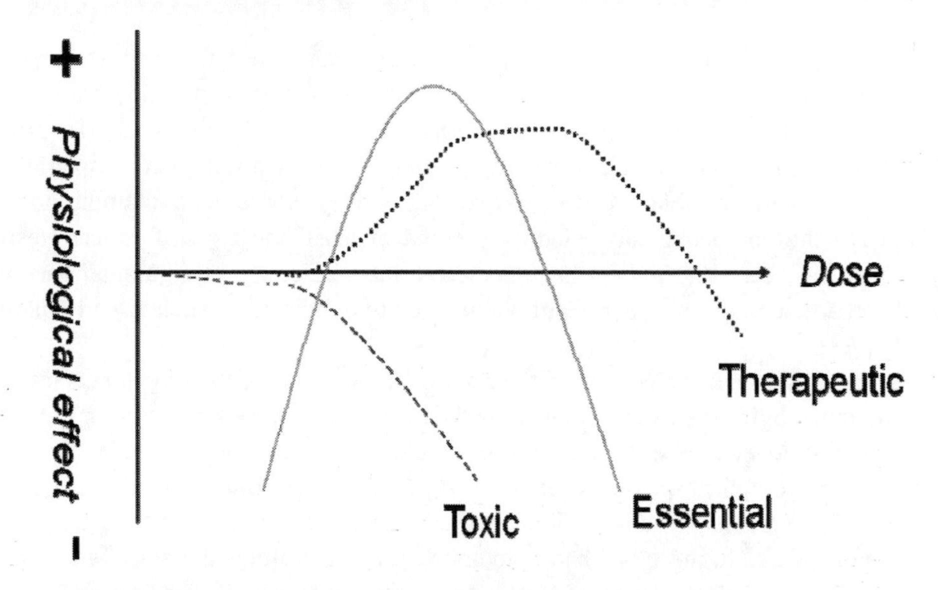

Figure 1. Bertrand diagram, adapted from G. Bertrand, 1912.[6].

Metal complexes important for our health are both endogenous (like those present in metalloproteins) and exogenous in origin. Exogenous metal complexes can be administered to our body desirably in a controlled way, as is the case of pharmaceuticals (drugs and diagnostic agents) or undesirably (uncontrolled) as by air or dietary pollutants. It is notable that some organic pharmaceutical agents or pollutants may be directed towards metal targets in the body, or requires metal binding to function (e.g. the anticancer agent bleomycin requires iron and dioxygen). The pharmacological activity of metal complexes depends on the metal, its ligands or both. Two factors, i.e. maximum thermodynamic stability and large degree of selectivity, are important in the design of metal complexes or ligands for medical application.

Metal ions not only posses much of the interesting reactivity and spectroscopy within the periodic table, but they also exhibit the most diverse binding modes and geometries among the elements. Carbon, the most important element in drug design, can generate inert, covalent bonds with connectivities from two to four, and with geometries about the carbon atom that range from linear to trigonal planar to tetrahedral. The types of geometries obtainable are fairly limited and, even so, this has allowed preparing an incredible number of different molecules based on carbon. By contrast, metal ions can create either labile or inert bonds with coordination numbers ranging from one to twelve, and with numerous geometries including linear, trigonal planar, tetrahedral, octahedral and many others. This simple fact suggests that metal ions can be used to construct therapeutic molecules that present shapes and structures that would be impossible or extremely difficult to achieve with carbon-based compounds. The judicious choice of ligands provides molecular reconnaissance in addition to the adequate tuning of reactivity and solubility properties, resulting in a very broad spectrum of therapeutic uses.

ANTICANCER METAL BASED DRUGS

Historically, several metal-containing agents have been tested for antitumor potential, from early transition metals to the main group of elements. The most prominent discovery in metal-containing therapeutics is the cisplatin (*cis*-diamminedichloroplatinum(II), *cis*-DDP, CDDP). From bioinorganic medicinal chemistry point of view, the success of cisplatin can be considered particularly notable because: *(i)* the drug is truly inorganic, containing no carbon atoms and *(ii)* the compound has effectively cured at least one type of cancer (testicular cancer). Over the years, researchers have dedicated huge efforts to design analogues which surpass the pharmacological properties of platinum compounds in use such as carboplatin and oxaliplatin [7,8].

Furthermore the selective control of their toxicity, the metal containing agents must have suitable pharmacologic properties which allow their use in clinic. Many antitumor compounds with high activity level and very interesting properties, have failed to reach the clinic phases because of their deficient physicochemical properties to pharmaceutical uses, *e.g.* low hydrosolubility, instability in aqua medium, and decomposition with the exposure to solvents, humidity, light or air. In the other hand, complexity in controlling the selective toxicity or their pharmacological properties have contributed to the reluctance of some researchers in the development of metal based drugs. Consequently, metal containing drugs are not studied beyond the tumor models *in vivo* despite the fact that metal complexes are often cytotoxic *in vitro* at a significantly lower dose than organic drugs [9]. Considering the compounds that are used on the clinic as antineoplastic agents, we can see that only 3 out of 48 are metal based drugs; only cisplatin (CDDP), carboplatin and oxaliplatin have reached worldwide clinical use [10]. Other critical factor about the therapeutic potential of a metal is the oxidation state; the reduction potential of most of the metals increases when the ionic radii decreases as consequence of a higher valence. However, toxicity does not seem to be directly related with a higher or lower oxidation state. For instance, the chromium (VI) compounds are more toxic than those of chromium (III), whereas the arsenite [As(III)] is more toxic than the arsenate [As(V)].

Therefore, the cytotoxic activity of a metal complex, which is close related with its antitumor activity, is controlled by the identity of the metal, its oxidation state and the properties of its coordination ligands; however, in many cases only one of them is the dominant factor. Despite all these variables, there are clear associations between structural similarity and cytotoxicity. In recent studies published by Ruili Huang *et al.* in 2005 [9], the cytotoxicity profiles of more than 1100 metalloid or metal based compounds with antitumor potential belonging to the National Cancer Institute data base were analyzed and classified. Molecular characteristics and reactivity of the compounds were analyzed according to the properties of their metals, the ligands attached and their capacity to inhibit tumor cell growth. The mechanisms of action for metal based compounds could be classified in four groups according to: *(i)* preference for binding to sulfhydryl groups (SH); *(ii)* chelators and metal complexes of chelators; *(iii)* generation of reactive oxygen species (ROS) and oxidative stress; and *(iv)* production of lipophilic ions.

Since the appearance of CDDP in the market, several research groups have started to search new anticancer metal based drugs mostly focused on those of platinum, especially analogs of cisplatin, and on DNA targeting [11]. Nowadays, inorganic chemistry offers many opportunities for medicinal chemistry, and the discovery of new metal-based drugs has moved on from serendipity to rational design. Recent progress in the field of cell biology and cancer research has resulted in the discovery of receptors and growth factors that are up-regulated in cancer cells and can be exploited as new targets for anticancer drug design. Research in metal-based anticancer drug design has several approaches; from classical drugs which molecular target is DNA, to alternative molecular targets such as thiol –containing proteins and redox processes [12]. In addition, there is an increasing interest in designing and developing drugs employing a pro-drug approach in order to activate the drugs selectively in the tumor by cellular processes or controlled external activation such a light activation [13,14].

The examples provided in this chapter are in no way meant to be comprehensive or necessarily reflect even the most significant new discoveries; however, they were selected by the authors to highlight some creative work in the field of anticancer metal based agents. Some of the examples, such cisplatin, have proved its clinical success and, some others have the potential for considerably impacting the future of the field.

PLATINUM COMPOUNDS

In history, it has often been the case of new discoveries at random and medicine has not been an exception; the first metal anticancer drug, cisplatin, was discovered without looking for it. Barnett Rosenberg in Michigan State University was interested in study the resemblance between the mitotic spindle of dividing cells and lines of magnetic force examining the effect of electric fields on growing cells. The study was made on bacterium *Escherichia Coli,* and platinum electrodes were used, over such conditions an inhibition of cell division was observed. Further studies to understand this fact led to the conclusion that $(NH_4)_2[PtCl_6]$ was formed and converted to $[PtCl_2(NH_3)_2]$, the later compound was first synthesized by Michele Peyrone in 1844. After this discovery, four platinum compounds were tested at the National Cancer Institute (NCI), $[PtCl_2(NH_3)_2]$, $[PtCl_2en]$, $[PtCl_4(NH_3)_2]$, $[PtCl_4en]$. The cisplatin went through all steps and entered to clinical trials in 1971 and probe to be active against a range of tumors, particularly testicular [15] and ovarium cancers. In spite of this activity several severe toxic side-effects were shown by cisplatin therapy, such as vomiting, nausea, ototoxicity, neuropathy, and the most important nephrotoxicity [16], lately this effect was found to be reduced by intravenous hydratation and the use of mannitol that induces diuresis [17]. The use of osmotic diuretic and hydratation could even allow increasing doses. The success of testicular and ovarium cancer treatment led to the approval of this compound as a drug at the FDA in 1978, and the British approval in 1979.

Nowadays cisplatin is wide used, its discovery opened the search of new drugs in the inorganic medicinal chemistry field and its use and effectiveness in cancer chemotherapy is by now well documented. However, cisplatin has several drawbacks such as toxicity and drug resistance. The natural course of events has led to many "second-generation" compounds based on the cisplatin structure in attempts to improve toxicity and/or expand the range of useful anticancer activity. Afterwards many more platinum compounds have been synthesized but most of them do not reach clinical trials. Tetraplatin did not progress beyond phase I due to neurotoxicity [18], only carboplatin and oxaliplatin have achieved clinical use in the late 90's [19]. The recent advance of research on the molecular mechanisms of drug action and the cellular mechanisms of the emergence of resistance to cisplatin assists the rational design of new classes of platinum antitumor drugs, though details of both mechanisms still remain elusive. DNA is believed to be the primary target for many metal-based drugs, for example, platinum-based anticancer drugs can form specific lesions on DNA that induce apoptosis. Information on DNA binding mode of platinum complexes, recognition and repair of DNA damage is instructive. Thus far, there is considerable evidence which points the therapeutic efficacy of platinum based compounds is determined by its molecular configuration which allows specific DNA binding mode. Cisplatin is transformed to the *trans* isomer in aqueous medium [20-22], losing its antitumor activity as consequence of the inability to cause irreversible intrastrand cross-links in nucleic acids as compared with the *cis* isomer [23,24]

Nevertheless, opposite to cisplatin, other platinum compounds with ligands in *trans* configuration have higher cytotoxicity when compared with their *cis* counterparts [25-28]. Newer novel platinum drugs break the cisplatin paradigm by binding to DNA in other ways different than cisplatin does [29], such as the trinuclear platinum complex BBR3464 [30], currently in Phase II clinical trials [31] (Figure 2). Also it is possible to design inert platinum (IV) pro-drugs which are non-toxic in the dark, but lethal when irradiated with certain wavelengths of light [14,32] to give highly reactive Pt(II) species which bind rapidly and stereospecifically to nucleotides, thereby forming known *cis*-platinum-nucleotide cross-links [33]. This gives rise to novel DNA lesions which are not as readily repaired as those induced by cisplatin, and provides the basis for a new type of photoactivated chemotherapy [29].

Since several not *cis* isomers but *trans* isomers and not neutral complexes but cation complexes have been found active *in vitro* and *in vivo*, the early empirical structure-activity relationships of cisplatin analogues should be reevaluated [34]. The hypothesis that platinum complexes which bind to DNA in a different manner will have different pharmacological properties has been tested, and now cationic multi-nuclear complexes and even *trans*-platinum complexes comprise unique classes of antitumor platinum-based agents with chemical and biological properties different from cisplatin.

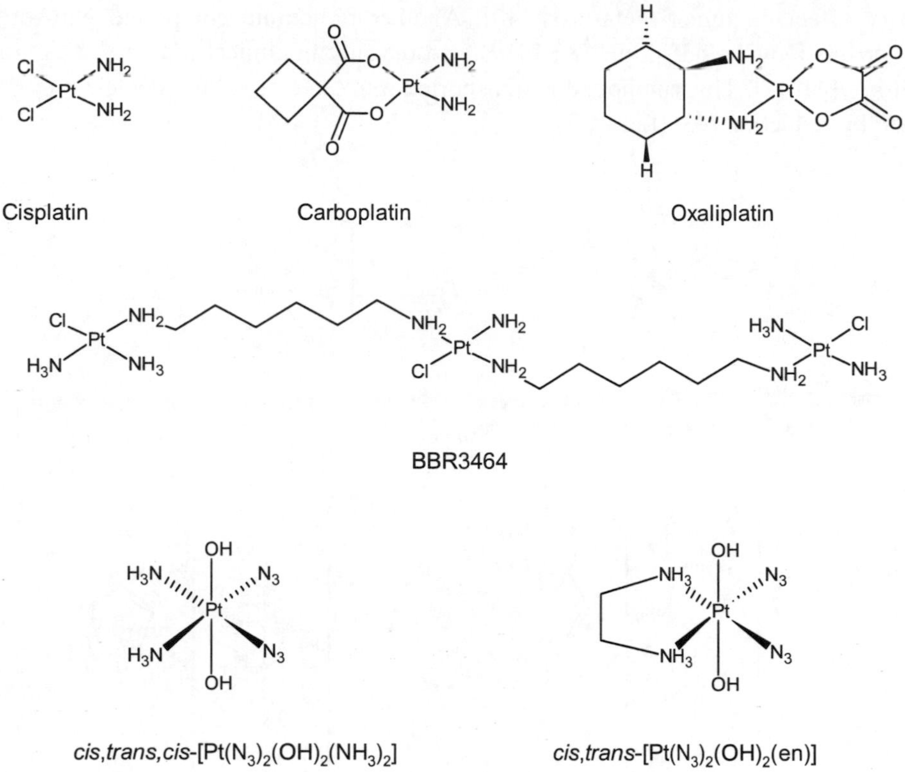

Cisplatin Carboplatin Oxaliplatin

BBR3464

cis,trans,cis-$[Pt(N_3)_2(OH)_2(NH_3)_2]$ *cis,trans*-$[Pt(N_3)_2(OH)_2(en)]$

Figure 2. Platinum anticancer agents.

NON PLATINUM ANTICANCER AGENTS

The search for new drugs in the field of bioinorganic chemistry was acquired by the groups working in coordination chemistry. A great effort was done in the synthesis of new compounds that may present activity against tumoral cells. In a parallel way, the *in vitro* and *in vivo* tests were standardized by the NCI (National Cancer Institute, U.S.). At first the most widely studied metals were does from the group of platinum, mainly palladium, [PdCl(2-benzylpyridine)(pyridine)], [PdCl(N,N-dimethylbenzylamine)(pyridine)] [35]. These studies were extended to the other noble metal elements as rhodium $[Rh_2(OOCCH_3)_4]$, $[Rh_2(OOCC_2H_5)_4]$ [36]; and ruthenium $[RuCl_2(NH_3)_4]$, $[RuCl_2(DMSO)_4]$ [37,38].

Ruthenium

Ruthenium (II) and (III) compounds are considered to be suitable candidates for anticancer drug design because they exhibit a similar spectrum of kinetics for their ligand substitution reactions as platinum (II); however, some of them exhibit significantly different properties to cisplatin. Especially noteworthy is the ruthenium complex *trans*-$[RuCl_4(Im)(DMSO)]$ImH (NAMI-A), currently in phase I clinical trials [39], which has promising activity against models of colorectal cancer, is redox activated and has a selective inhibitory effect on tumor metastasis [40]. Another ruthenium compound with promising future is *trans*-[$RuCl_4(Ind)_2$]IndH (KP1019) also recently in clinical trials showing no severe side effects [41-43]. This compound is transported into the cell via the trasferrin cycle and is activated by reduction [43] (Figure 3).

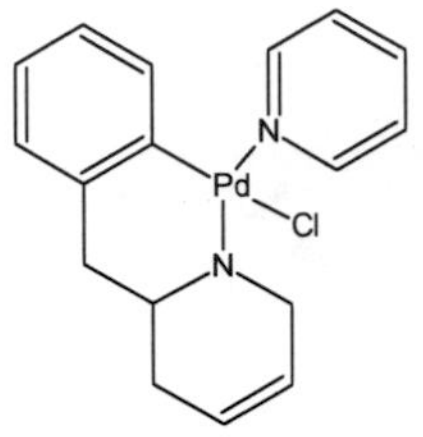

[PdCl(N,N-dimethylbenzylamine)(pyridine)]

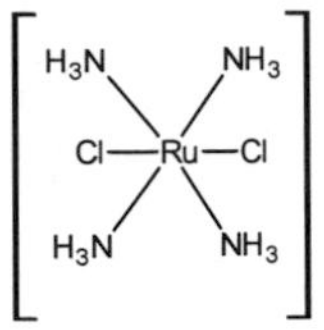

[$RuCl_2(NH_3)_4$]

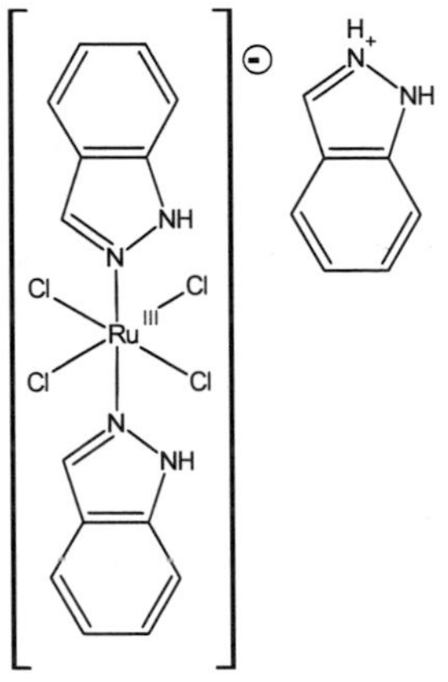

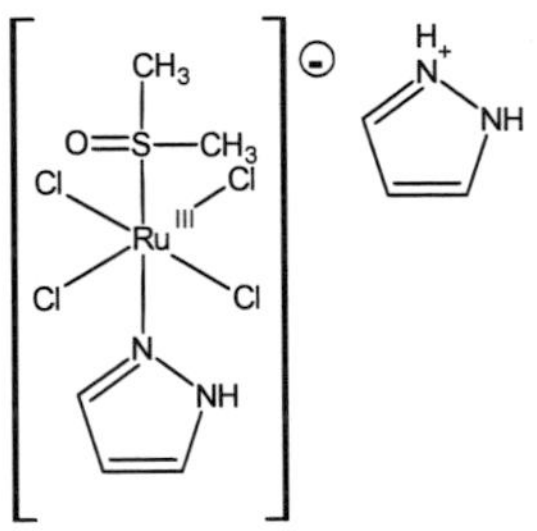

NAMI-A

KP1019

Figura 3. Palladium and Ruthenium anticancer agents.

Gold

One of the most known metals in the history of mankind is gold; it can be traced through the written history as a medicinal metal as far as prehistory. Its mystical properties as a metal associated to the sun were dismissed by modern medicine, due to the lack of known mechanism of action [44]. Even so, gold complexes are well-known pharmaceuticals, mainly for their application as antiarthritis drugs, such as (2,3,4,6-tetra-O-acetyl-β-1-D-glucopyanosato-S)(triethylphosphine) gold (I) (auronofin, Figure 4). Furthermore, auronofin was tested against HeLa cells in culture [45,46] and leukemia P388 [47], also this compound tested *in vivo* in mice with P388 line showed a significant increase life span [48]. Some tertiary phosphine gold (I) with thiosugar ligands [49-51], nucleotide ligands [52] and many others gold (I) based compounds have been synthesized and tested in several models. The tetrahedral Au(I) phosphine complexes display a wide spectrum of anticancer activity *in vivo* in cisplatin-resistant cell lines [53], some of them with good selectivity towards tumor cells [54,55]. Their cytotoxicity is mediated by inhibition of human glutathione reductase and thioredoxin reductase irreversibly [56]. Recently, cationic Au(I) complexes of N-heterocyclic carbenes have been designed to accumulate selectively in mitochondria of cancer cells, to cause cell death through a mitochondrial apoptotic pathway and to inhibit the activity of thioredoxin reductase (TrxR) [57].

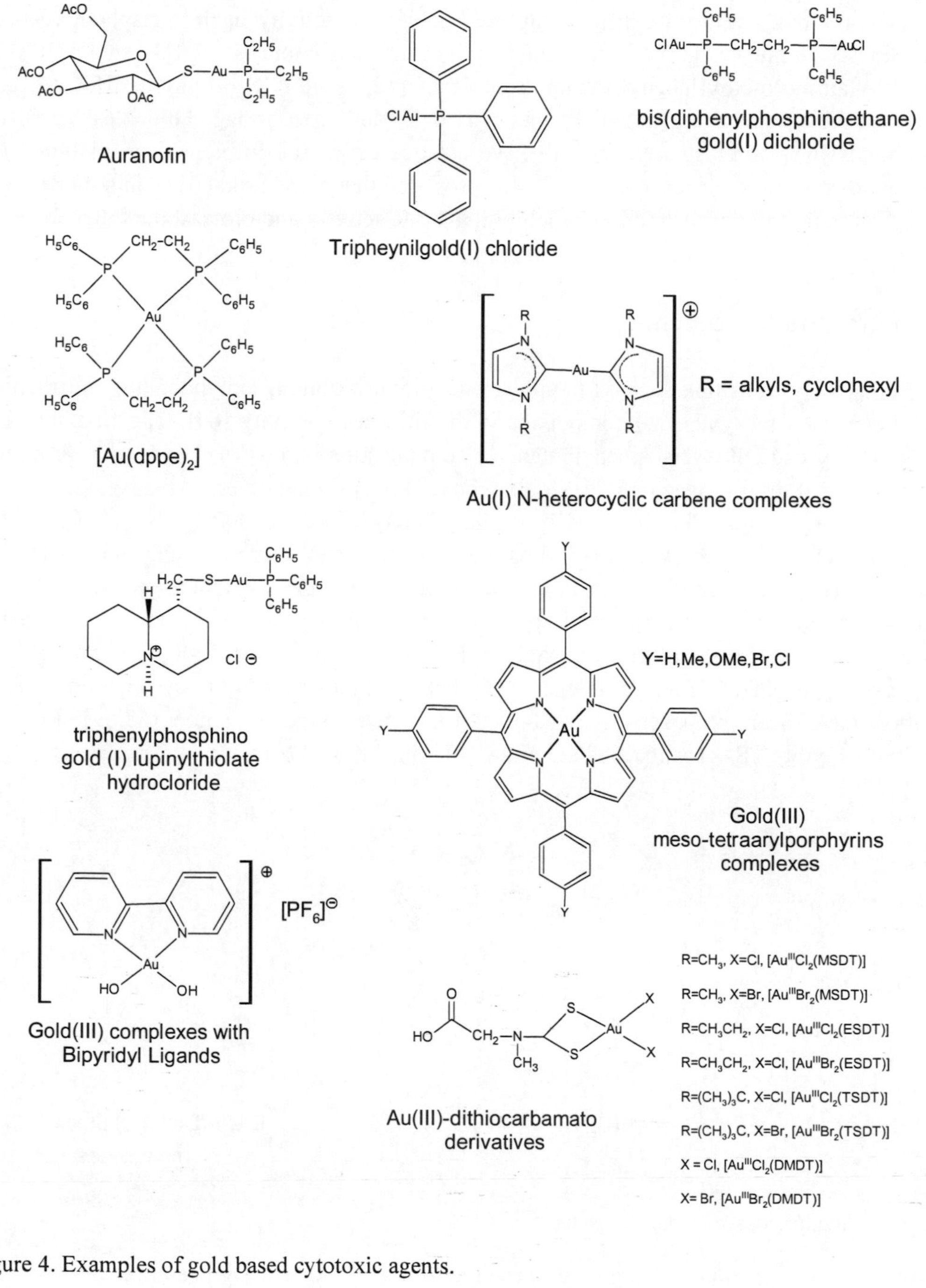

Auranofin

Tripheynilgold(I) chloride

bis(diphenylphosphinoethane) gold(I) dichloride

$[Au(dppe)_2]$

R = alkyls, cyclohexyl

Au(I) N-heterocyclic carbene complexes

triphenylphosphino gold (I) lupinylthiolate hydrocloride

Y=H,Me,OMe,Br,Cl

Gold(III) meso-tetraarylporphyrins complexes

$[PF_6]^{\ominus}$

Gold(III) complexes with Bipyridyl Ligands

Au(III)-dithiocarbamato derivatives

R=CH_3, X=Cl, $[Au^{III}Cl_2(MSDT)]$
R=CH_3, X=Br, $[Au^{III}Br_2(MSDT)]$
R=CH_3CH_2, X=Cl, $[Au^{III}Cl_2(ESDT)]$
R=CH_3CH_2, X=Cl, $[Au^{III}Br_2(ESDT)]$
R=$(CH_3)_3C$, X=Cl, $[Au^{III}Cl_2(TSDT)]$
R=$(CH_3)_3C$, X=Br, $[Au^{III}Br_2(TSDT)]$
X = Cl, $[Au^{III}Cl_2(DMDT)]$
X= Br, $[Au^{III}Br_2(DMDT)]$

Figure 4. Examples of gold based cytotoxic agents.

In the other hand, Gold (III) complexes have also been investigated searching for antitumor activity due to their resemblance in geometry and electronic properties to platinum (II), they are isoelectronic and their complexes are square-planar tetracoordinated (Figure 4). Gold (III) complexes are usually reduced and unstable at physiological conditions, but some interesting antitumor agents have been designed by the judicious choice of ligands that increase the stability of these complexes achieving activity against cisplatin resistant cell lines. Some examples are gold (III) dithiocarbamates [58], gold (III) 2-[(dimethylamino)methyl]phenyl (damp) complexes [12], gold (III) porphyrins [59,60], gold (III) complexes with bipyridyl ligands [61,62], and *oxo*-bridged binuclear gold(III) compounds [63]. Interestingly, they all have a mode of action different from platinum (II) compounds despite their resemblance. It was proposed that some gold (III) compounds might exert their activity in mitochondria by inhibiting TrxR activity and proteasome [58].

Titanium and Vanadium

Some early-transition such as titanium, vanadium, niobium, molybdenum, and rhenium have been used to synthesize compounds with anticancer activity [64]. The titanium drug budotitane [*cis*-diethoxybis(-phenylbutane-1,3-dionato)titanium (IV)] was the first non-platinum metal drug to reach clinical trials (phase I) [65]. Some other derivatives of titanium with promising antiproliferative activity are $[Ti(C_5H_5)_2Cl_2]$[66], and $[Ti(C_5H_5)_2(O_2C(S)C_6H_4$-1,2] (Figure 5) [66,67], which are less nephrotoxic than cisplatin, and the budotitane derivative Bis(β-diketone)titanium(IV). The therapeutic target of budotitane derivatives is gastrointestinal tumors, but the mode of action of titanium anticancer compounds remains unknown. The activation of H_2O_2 to yield $^{\cdot}OH$ through Fenton reaction, formation of TiO_2 after hydrolysis of titanium complexes and photoproduction of H_2O_2 by TiO_2 in aqueous solution have been proposed as feasible part of their mode of action [68,69]. Recently titanium silicalite TS-1 has reached the phase II clinical trials [70].

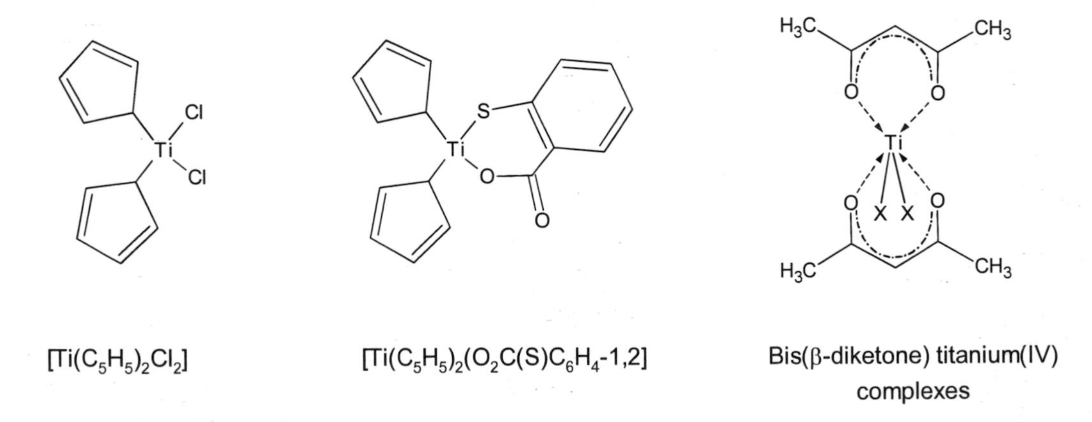

Figure 5. Titanium based cytotoxic agents.

Also some vanadium analogues to these titanium complexes have been prepared and their antitumor activities have been reviewed extensively [71,72]. Vanadium compounds seem to exert their antitumor effects mainly trough inhibition of cellular protein tyrosine phosphatases (PTPs) and/or activation of protein tyrosine kinases leading to apoptosis; in addition, they can generate ROS by Fenton-like reactions [9]. Some examples of vanadium compounds with promising antiproliferative activity are peroxovanadate (V) complexes [73]; bisperoxovanadium (V) complexes [74]; vanadyl-1,10-phenanthroline complex, $[VO(phen)^{2+}]$ [75]; vanadium (IV) with cyclopentadienyl moieties ($C5H5^{-}=Cp^{-}$), vanadocenes (VCp_2) [76,77]; amino acid complexes of vanadium (III) particularly L-cysteine [78]. It is worth mentioning that these selected examples of vanadium compounds cover all three common oxidation states of vanadium, i.e., V(III), V(IV), and V(V), they also exhibit activity against a wide range of tumor types. The anticarcinogenic effects of vanadium, in combination to its low toxicity, suggest vanadium as a candidate antineoplastic agent against human cancer [69].

TIN

Also some metals, from the main group have been used to synthesize compounds that may have antitumor activity, as cisplatin analogues. After it was shown in 1972 that triphenyltin acetate (but not the corresponding chloride) retarded tumor growth in mice [79,80] a huge number of organotin derivatives have been prepared and tested *in vitro* and *in vivo*, against different panels of human cancer cell lines [81,82]. Organotins exhibit significant *in vitro* antiproliferative activity which, in some cases, is higher than the corresponding activity of cisplatin or other drugs used for clinical treatment in cancer chemotherapy. Also organotin complexes have been tested *in vivo* with encouraging results [83,84]. Although the mechanism of this antiproliferative activity is not well established, it has been suggested that organotin(IV) compounds wield antiproliferative effects through several probable mechanisms such as binding to thiol groups of the proteins [9,83,85]; inhibition of macromolecular synthesis, mitochondrial energy metabolism, and reduction of DNA synthesis, as well as direct interaction with the cell membrane and cytosolic Ca^{2+} overload [86-88]; promotion of oxidative and its consequent DNA damage *in vivo* [84]; and even direct interaction with DNA [89].

Many research have been performed in organotin (IV) complexes with oxygen donor ligands such as carboxilates [82,89,90], α-aminoacids [82,91,92] and their derivatives, oxamates [93] and others; also antiproliferative activity of complexes with sulfur donor ligands like thione/thiol [94,95] and dithiocarbamates [96] have been widely studied in the past five years [82] (Figure 6). The organotin moiety (R), the ligand (L), the number of tin atoms and the number of free coordination positions offered appear to play an important role in their antiproliferative action of the compounds [82]. While the organotin moiety is crucial for cytotoxicity, the ligand plays a key role in transporting and addressing the molecule to the target, resisting untimely exchanges with biomolecules and tuning solubility which is a frequent issue for organotin derivatives. Sulfur-containing ligands (which may represent widely differing chemical structures) appear particularly suitable to fulfill this task overall because they are more stable than those organotin coordinated by oxygen or nitrogen containing ligands [90]. Finally the most active compounds are four- or five-coordinated with free coordination positions around Sn(IV) [82].

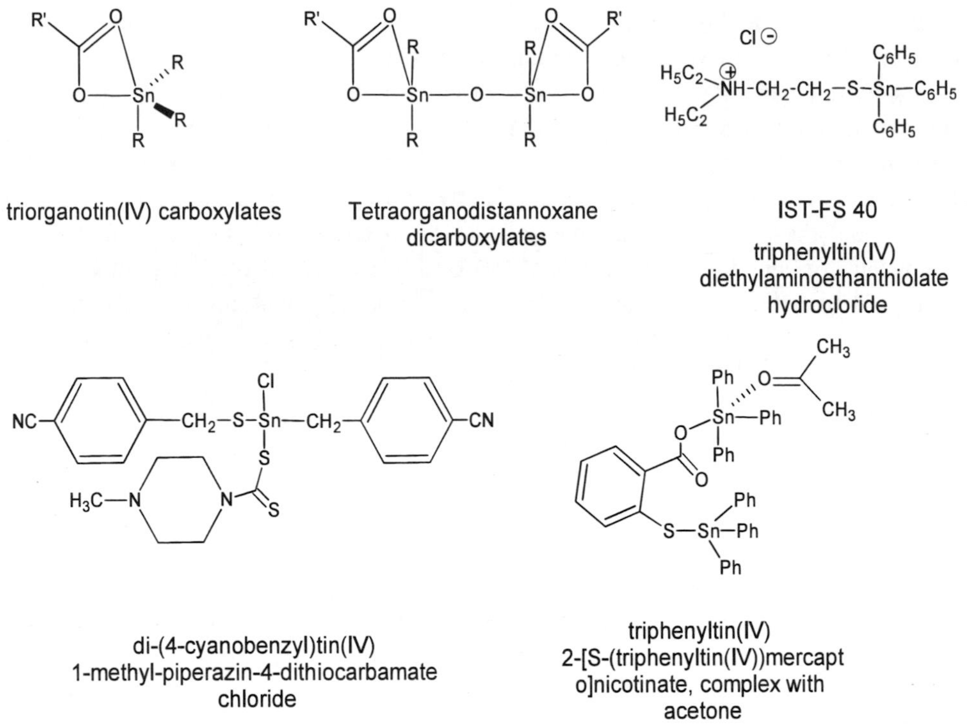

triorganotin(IV) carboxylates

Tetraorganodistannoxane dicarboxylates

IST-FS 40

triphenyltin(IV) diethylaminoethanthiolate hydrocloride

di-(4-cyanobenzyl)tin(IV) 1-methyl-piperazin-4-dithiocarbamate chloride

triphenyltin(IV) 2-[S-(triphenyltin(IV))mercapto]nicotinate, complex with acetone

Figure 6. Tin based cytotoxic agents.

The potential of organotin compounds as anti-cancer drugs are actually being studied widely. They are very efficacious and perhaps curative against a select number of neoplasias; however, they suffer from a variety of deficiencies, from notably severe systemic toxicity to a tendency to elicit drug resistance [97].

ESSENTIAL METAL BASED ANTITUMOR DRUGS

Despite research on some other non essential metals with antitumor properties was developed for several groups with success [24]; another innovator approach is the use of compounds based on essential metals. Actually, since many years a lot of researches have actively investigated essential metal complexes as antitumor agents based on the assumption proposal that endogenous metals may be less toxic [98].

In the course of many years, the use of essential metals in cancer therapy was limited to the activation of drugs as bleomicyne, by iron and copper [99,100]; or the employ of chelators which may act by depleting iron and other necessary nutrients in cell proliferation, and consequently, limiting tumor growth [101-103]. Currently, there is remarkable antitumor research on essential metals as iron [9,103-108], cobalt [9,109-111], manganese [9,109,112-115], and copper [116-118]. In the coming sections, we want to focus and highlight the research on copper and its complexes as antitumor agents, mostly those named Casiopeínas®.

Copper

In recent years, several families of copper complexes have been studied as potential antitumor agents [116-118]. Although only a little understanding of the molecular basis of their mechanism of action has been documented, copper complexes have attracted attention based on modes of action different from that of cisplatin (covalent binding to DNA) [117]. Therefore, copper complexes may provide, at least in principle, a broader spectrum of antitumor activity, may have relatively lower side effects than platinum-based drugs, and are suggested to be able to overcome inherited or acquired resistance of cisplatin [118].

Copper is found in all living organisms and is a crucial trace element in redox chemistry, growth and development [119-125]. It is important for the function of several enzymes and proteins involved in energy metabolism, respiration, and DNA synthesis, notably cytochrome oxidase, superoxide dismutase, ascorbate oxidase, and tyrosinase. The major functions of copper-biological molecules involve oxidation-reduction reactions in which they react directly with molecular oxygen to produce free radicals. Therefore, copper requires tightly regulated homeostatic mechanisms [121,122,124,126] to ensure adequate supplies without any toxic effects [127-129]. Overload or deficiency of copper is associated, respectively, with Wilson disease (WD) [130-134] and Menkes disease (MD) [133,135-139], which are of genetic origin.

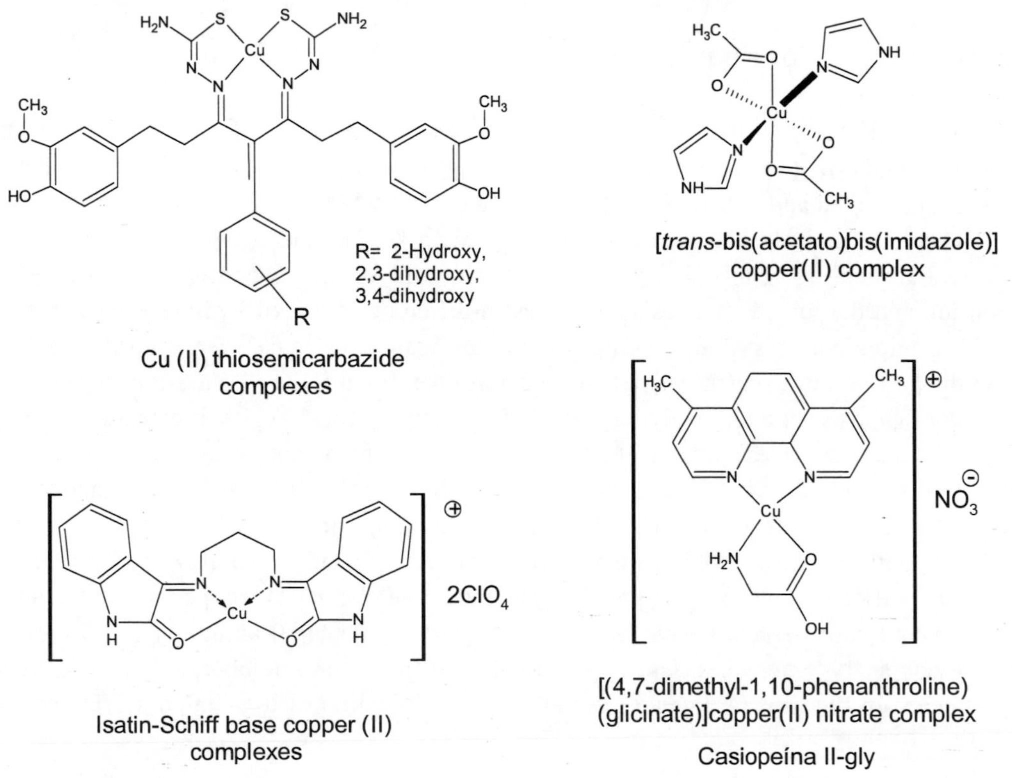

R= 2-Hydroxy, 2,3-dihydroxy, 3,4-dihydroxy

Cu (II) thiosemicarbazide complexes

[*trans*-bis(acetato)bis(imidazole)] copper(II) complex

Isatin-Schiff base copper (II) complexes

[(4,7-dimethyl-1,10-phenanthroline)(glicinate)]copper(II) nitrate complex

Casiopeína II-gly

Figure 7. Some copper based antitumor agents.

Up to now, a great variety of copper complexes have been tested as cytotoxic agents and showed antitumor activity in several *in vitro* tests (on cultured cancer cell lines) and few *in vivo* experiments (on murine tumor models). Some representative examples of copper complexes with anti-cancer activity are thiosemicarbazone complexes [140-143]; conjugates schiff base complexes [144-147]; imidazole, benzimidazole, pyrazole and triazole complexes [148-152]; phospine complexes [151]; and phenanthroline and bipyridine complexes [153-158] (Figure 7). According to the well established coordination chemistry of copper, frequently enriched by the flexible Cu(I/II) redox behavior, there still exist an enormous prospect in the design of more potent and less toxic copper based antitumor drugs. Most of the compounds reported in literature belong to the family of copper (II) complexes showing either five-coordinate environments comprising distorted square pyramidal or trigonal bipyramidal geometries or distorted six-coordinate octahedral arrays. The majority of these agents are mononuclear species, but there are few distinctive examples of dimeric compounds exhibiting remarkable antitumor activity [116,117]. Not many, but noteworthy examples of tetrahedral copper (I) complexes having soft tertiary phosphines or aromatic amines (*e.g. phen, bpy*) as donor ligands, display antiproliferative activity in the sub-micromolar range. The mode of action of copper complexes is miscellaneous and different from cisplatin; it includes DNA interaction, mitochondrial toxicity and ROS generation [9,116,117]. Among the most representative copper complexes with antitumor potential are Casiopeínas.

Research in Casiopeinas®

The Cu (II) complexes named Casiopeínas are among a series of mixed chelate copper (II) compounds of general formula $[Cu(N\text{-}N)(O\text{-}O)]NO_3$ or $[Cu(N\text{-}N)(O\text{-}N)]NO_3$[1] and they have been patented and registered under the name of CASIOPEÍNAS® [159-163] (Figure 8).

Design of the molecules was based in three main factors, the compound should contain an essential metal for diminish toxicity; chelates that favor the *cis*-configuration around the metal ion and the mixed chelates should present different degree of hydrophobicity to favor the absorption and distribution properties. The ligands selected were substituted 2,2'-bipyridines (*bpy*) and substituted 1,10-phenanthrolines (*phen*), they both are nitrogen-donor bidentate ligands with a relatively high affinity for copper [166-168]; their extended aromatic ring system allows these ligands to bind to DNA by intercalative and non-intercalative interactions either as free ligands or in metal complexes [9,169]. α-L-amino acids were chosen as secondary ligands due to their affinity for (*bpy)* and (*phen)*copper(II) complexes [170,171] and their low toxicity. Finally *salal* and *acac* ligands have also good affinity for (*phen*)copper(II) complexes [170] and might modulate the redox properties of the metal center. These considerations have led to the study of the potential antitumor activity of this type of copper(II) complexes. Our hypothesis is that the nature, number and position of the substituents on the diimine ligands, and also the modification of α-L-amino acidate or O-O

[1] N-N= 1,10-phenanthroline, 4,7-diphenyl, 1,10-phenanthroline, 4,7-dimethyl, 1,10-phenanthroline, 2,2′-bipyridine or 4,4′-dimethyl-2,2′-bipyridine, O-O= acetylacetonate or salicylaldehidate (Cas III family). When N-N= 1,10-phenanthroline, 4,7-diphenyl, 1,10-phenanthroline N-O= (aminoacidate) valine, serine or glycine (Cas I family). When N-N= 4,7-dimethyl, 1,10-phenanthroline N-O= (aminoacidate) valine, serine or glycine (Cas II family). For N-N= 4,4′-dimethyl-2,2′-bipyridine N-O= (aminoacidate) valine, serine, glycine or methionine (Cas IV family).

donor will have an effect either on the selectivity or on the degree of biological activity shown by the ternary copper(II) complexes. This effect would be due to the modification of physicochemical properties of the complexes, *e.g.* the redox behavior of metal center or the water solubility of the complex.

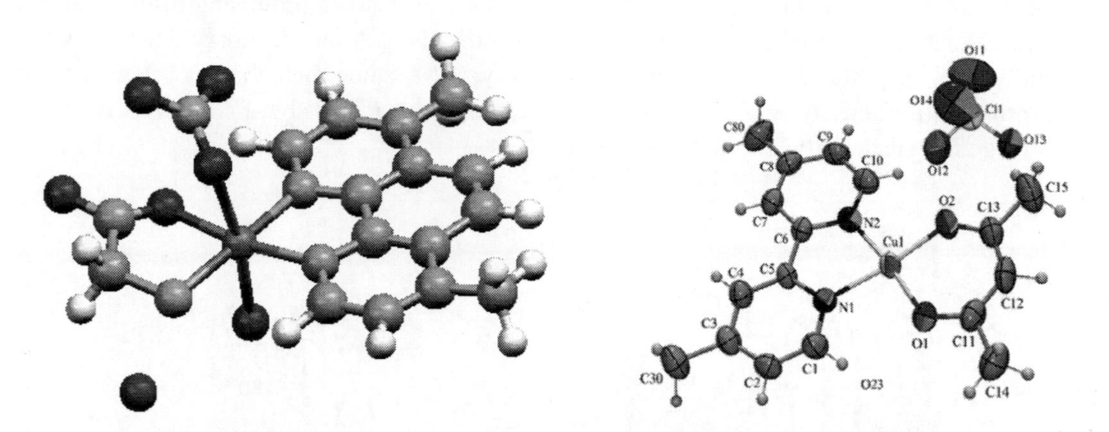

Figure 8. Structures of Casiopeína II-gly [164] (left) and Casiopeína III-ia [165] (right).

They have been fully characterized by all analytical methods, and structures have been solved by X-ray diffraction techniques [164,172-180]. The chemical and structural data reported so far shows that the copper (II) center in this type of ternary complexes is placed in a slightly distorted square planar geometry [164,165,172-174,176-179]. Stability formation constants for mixed-ligand complexes with 1,10-phenanthroline as primary ligand shows an enhancement compared to statistical expectations when the secondary ligand is an O-O donor [170]. There is no experimental data for stability constants for ternary Cu complexes with substituted phenanthrolines due, probably, to their low solubility. However, the effect on the strength of the interaction between Cu(x-*phen*) and oxygen donor bidentate ligands caused by the substituent on the phenanthroline was studied by Gasque et al.[181] through the variations on the Cu-O stretching frequencies and its relationship with phenanthroline pKa, the study suggests that an increase in phenanthroline basicity weakness Cu-O bonds in this type of compounds. The higher stability of this compounds also correlate well with local softness providing an explanation of the particular reactivity behavior [182].

Biologic Evaluation and Structure-activity Relationships

These compounds have been tested in several models *in vitro*, as *in vivo*, showing antiproliferative [183], cytotoxic [184], cytostatic [185], genotoxic [184-186] and antitumor activities [153,154,187] with promising results. It is noteworthy, the antiproliferative activity has been also observed on cisplatin-resistant murine cell lines without difference in susceptibility to induce apoptosis between cisplatin sensitive and resistant cells [188]. According with QSAR studies the presence of the central fused aromatic ring in the *phen* containing complexes is necessary to preserve the antiproliferative activity. IC_{50} has a strong relationship with half-wave potential ($E_{1/2}$) of copper center; being the most active complexes those which are weaker oxidants. The change of secondary ligand from *acac* to *gly* has less influence on biological activity than the changes on the diimine ligand [155].

Regardless antitumor activity *in vivo,* it has been tested mainly on murine model (L1210, S180. B16 and Lw1) where ILS (increase life span) is determined according to National Cancer Institute screening panel finding promising results (Figure 9). Additionally, some of these compounds has been tested *in vivo* in murine glioma C6 [154] and xenograft tumor models as colon carcinoma HCT-15 [153]. Every study has shown promising results and has revealed that the substitution on diimina ligand and the changes on secondary ligand as well, modify the magnitude of the biological activity. The same behavior is observed on antiproliferative activity on human tumor cell lines tested *in vitro* (Table 1) [155,183,189] and on the genotoxic activity [184,185].

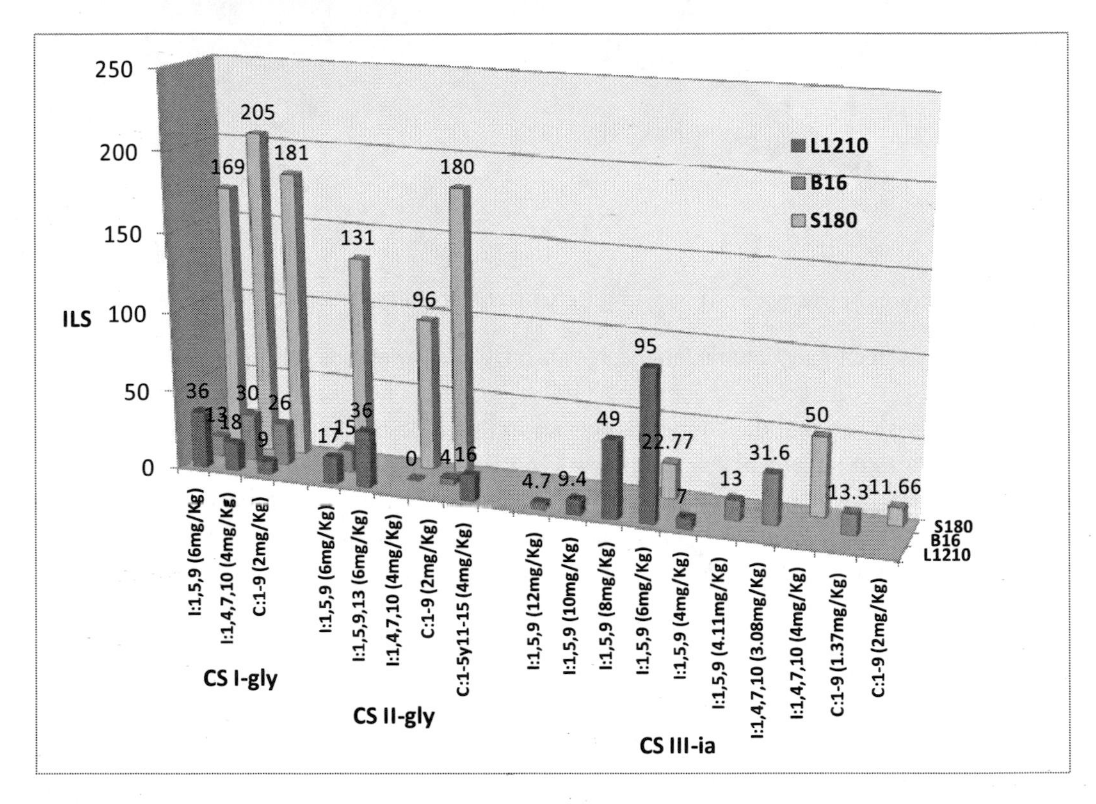

Figure 9. Antitumor activity in vivo tested according to National Cancer Institute (NCI) screening panel on murine models Sarcoma S180 (S180), Melanoma B16 (B16), and Leukemia L1210 (L1210). Activity is reported as Increase Life Span (ILS) for the complexes [Cu(4,7-diphenyl-1,10-phenanthroline)(glycinate)]NO_3 (CS I-gly), [Cu (4,7-dimethyl-1,10-phenanthroline)(glycinate)]NO_3 (CS II-gly), and [Cu(4,4'-dimetil-2,2'-bypiridine)(acetylacetonate)]NO_3 (CS III-ia). I: 1,5,9 = intermittent dose days 1,5,9; I: 1,4,7,10 = intermittent dose days 1,4,7,10; C:1-9 = chronic dose from day 1 to day 9.

Mode of Action

The mode of action of Casiopeínas® remains to be satisfactorily elucidated; however, there is evidence that supports these compounds are able to inhibit cell proliferation and produce cell dose-dependent death by apoptosis in several tumor models as medulloblastoma [189], HCT-15 [153] and murine glioma C6 [154]. The apoptosis takes place through mechanisms dependent and independent of caspase activation [154,188] and might be the result of one or several signals which lead to this final effect. These signals could be mediated by generation of ROS [184], by the observed mitochondrial toxicity [154,190,191], or both, and might play, alone or cooperatively, an important role in the regulation of cell death induced by this type of complexes.

Table 1. Antiproliferative activity on human tumor cell lines tested in vitro. IC50 (μM) on HeLa, SiHa, MCF-7 and HCT-15, the values are given as the mean of 3 independent experiments ± SE. (Bravo-Gomez et al, 2009 [155])

No	Compound	IC50			
		HeLa	SiHa	MCF-7	HCT-15
1	[Cu(2,2'-bipyridine)(acetylactonate)]NO_3	42 ± 3.1	40.5 ± 2.0	103.7 ± 9.6	67.3 ± 1.6
2	[Cu(4,4'-dimethyl-2,2'-bipyridine)(acetylacetonate)]NO_3	18.2 ± 2.7	14.5 ± 1.5	15.9 ± 1.8	40.5 ± 4.6
3	[Cu(1,10-phenanthroline)(acetylacetonate)]NO_3	10.7 ± 0.9	6.8 ± 0.9	8.1 ± 0.5	7.3 ± 0.7
4	[Cu(4-methyl-1,10-phenanthroline)(acetylacetonate)]NO_3	1.6 ± 0.1	3.4 ± 0.5	5.6 ± 0.7	6.0 ± 0.9
5	[Cu(5-methyl-1,10-phenanthroline)(acetylacetonate)]NO_3	6.2 ± 0.7	3.2 ± 0.2	4.4 ± 0.5	2.6 ± 0.4
6	[Cu(4,7-dimethyl-1,10-phenanthroline)(acetylacetonate)]NO_3	1.4 ± 0.1	0.96 ± 0.09	4.9 ± 0.6	2.1 ± 0.1
7	[Cu(5,6-dimethyl-1,10-phenanthroline)(acetylacetonate)]NO_3	3.4 ± 0.5	1.7 ± 0.2	3.9 ± 0.4	1.9 ± 0.3
8	[Cu(3,4,7,8-tetramethyl-1,10-phenanthroline)(acetylacetonate)]NO_3	1.9 ± 0.2	1.2 ± 0.1	2.2 ± 0.3	1.4 ± 0.2
9	[Cu(5-phenyl-1,10-phenanthroline)(acetylacetonate)]NO_3	3.9 ± 0.3	3.0 ± 0.3	3.9 ± 0.4	2.5 ± 0.3
10	[Cu(4,7-diphenyl-1,10-phenanthroline)(acetylacetonate)]NO_3	4.2 ± 0.6	3.2 ± 0.5	2.2 ± 0.3	3.2 ± 0.4
11	[Cu(5-chloro-1,10-phenanthroline)(acetylacetonate)]NO_3	4.5 ± 0.5	8.8 ± 0.6	9.8 ± 0.5	12.9 ± 0.5
12	[Cu(5-nitro-1,10-phenanthroline)(acetylacetonate)]NO_3	21.3 ± 2.6	10.2 ± 1.1	14.7 ± 1.4	35.0 ± 2.4
13	[Cu(1,10-phenanthroline)(glycinate)]NO_3	13.9 ± 1.3	27.3 ± 2.2	9.6 ± 1.1	21.2 ± 2.5
14	[Cu(4-methyl-1,10-phenanthroline)(glycinate)]NO_3	8.7 ± 0.7	10.2 ± 1.0	7.7 ± 0.6	5.1 ± 0.5
15	[Cu(5-methyl-1,10-phenanthroline)(glycinate)]NO_3	6.2 ± 0.6	5.7 ± 0.6	4.7 ± 0.2	3.7 ± 0.4
16	[Cu(4,7-dimethyl-1,10-phenanthroline)(glycinate)]NO_3	5.5 ± 0.7	5.5 ± 0.8	4.6 ± 0.4	2.0 ± 0.2
17	[Cu(5,6-dimethyl-1,10-phenanthroline)(glycinate)]NO_3	5.3 ± 0.1	3.1 ± 0.3	4.4 ± 0.3	2.1 ± 0.1
18	[Cu(3,4,7,8-tetramethyl-1,10-phenanthroline)(glycinate)]NO_3	1.8 ± 0.0	1.4 ± 0.2	2.6 ± 0.2	1.8 ± 0.4
19	[Cu(4,7-diphenyl-1,10-phenanthroline)(glycinate)]NO_3	5.1 ± 0.2	6.6 ± 0.9	4.1 ± 0.4	7.6 ± 0.7
20	[Cu(5-chloro-1,10-phenanthroline)(glycinate)]NO_3	14.3 ± 0.5	13.9 ± 1.3	23.2 ± 2.3	22.3 ± 1.6
21	[Cu(5-nitro-1,10-phenanthroline)(glycinate)]NO_3	44.8 ± 1.5	17.9 ± 2.2	28.64 ± 3.4	47.3 ± 6.5
	CDDP	5.1 ± 0.4	5.4 ± 0.5	5.6 ± 0.8	21.8 ± 2.4

Nowadays, mitochondrial toxicity is considered a possible therapeutic target and a good strategy in cancer therapy [192]. Inhibition of respiration and ATP synthesis was observed in mitochondria after the administration of these complexes as result of damage in several different mitochondrial sites in a dose dependent manner, which compromises the energy dependent processes in cells [193]. Casiopeína II-gly inhibits the enzymes 2-oxoglutrarate deshydrogenase (2-OGDH) [191], succinate deshydrogenase (SDH) [191] and piruvate deshydrogenase (PDH) [190] probably by direct interaction with sulfhydryl groups in these enzymes or with coenzyme A, interfering in this way with normal mitochondrial functions [191]. This compound, in higher doses than 15 nmol (mg protein)$^{-1}$ induces the stimulation of basal respiration, followed of strong inhibition, which correlates with mitochondrial swelling dependent of potassium channels activation and the consequent cytochrome *c* releasing [191]. This final event is an apoptotic signal which activates caspase 9 and apoptosis protease-activating factor-1 [194]. Likewise, Casiopeínas cause the loss of mitochondrial membrane potential in meduloblastoma [189], and glioma C6 [154]. Casiopeínas IIgly and III-ia inhibit the rates of state 3 and uncoupled respiration in mithocondria, being the first one about 10 times more potent than the second one [191]. Mitochondria from liver, kidney and hepatoma AS-30D showed a similar sensitivity towards CasIIgly, whereas heart mitochondria were more resistant. The data suggested that Casiopeínas disrupt several different mitochondrial sites, bringing about inhibition of respiration and ATP synthesis, which could compromise energy-dependent processes such as cellular duplication [191].

In the other hand, some researchers have observed that the inhibition of cell proliferation [154,184] and DNA degradation [154,184,195] in the presence of reducing agents are simultaneous to ROS generation. Lipid peroxidation [154] and reduced glutathione depletion [196] have been observed as well as result of Casiopeínas administration. These effects suggest that oxidation to DNA and other cellular components could also be the stress signal that triggers by itself cell death by apoptosis. Although copper normally participates in ROS generation by Fenton reaction, there is no direct evidence yet about Casiopeínas capability to catalyze this reaction *in vitro* or *in vivo*. However, the cytotoxicity increment when reducing agents are added to cell culture and, the decrease of this effect by addition of hydroxyl radical ($^{\cdot}OH$) trapping agent DMSO, lead to think that this reaction is reasonably possible [196].

On the other hand, there also exists the possibility of direct interaction of complexes with DNA by intercalative and non intercalative interactions as expected for these complexes due to the planar aromatic moiety of its diimine ligands [9,169,175]. Literature reports that the activation of Poli(ADP-ribose) polymerase -1 (PARP-1), as result of DNA damage, induces apoptosis inductor factor release (AIF) and its nuclear translocation leading to cell death caspase-independent [197]. This could explain observations on murine glioma C6 [154] and human ovarian carcinoma CH1 [188] where the apoptosis takes place by caspases-independent mechanisms. Likewise, these compounds have shown good biological activity on tumoral cell line HCT-15 [153], which has inactive p53. It is well known that cellular lines with inactive p53 are resistant to mitochondrial drugs [198]. Because the DNA damage induced by some chemotherapeutics enhances the apoptotic function of p73, it has been proposed that apoptotic signal comes from p73 [199].

Nevertheless, the cellular targets could be others beyond mitochondria and DNA; the administration *in vivo* of complexes of this family produces severe damage in erythrocytes which is expressed as hemolytic anemia [200]. These cells are lack the two mentioned main cellular targets; therefore it is reasonably to conclude that other cellular targets are also involved. In summary, at the molecular level, the evidence points to several biological targets of damage mediated by quite heterogeneous mechanisms working simultaneously. QSAR studies support, at least in part, the modes of action proposed for the cytotoxicity of these complexes [155]. Although the knowledge about the behavior of these complexes in biological systems points to a complex network of mechanisms of toxicity, it seems that the DNA intercalation and ROS production are the two dominant factors involved [155].

Toxicity

Cytotoxicity raises preoccupation about their selectivity towards tumor cells; that is why several comparative studies have been performed in different cell lines, normal and transformed. Casiopeína II-gly has shown inhibition *in vitro* on HeLa and hepatoma AS-30D cell line, without disrupt the viability of non tumor cell lines as lymphocytes at equivalent level doses [193,201]. Opposite to this effect, inhibition of cell respiration and the loss of mitochondrial potential are similar in liver, kidney and AS-30 D cells employing 1-10 nmol $(\text{mg protein})^{-1}$ *in vitro* concentrations [191], which leads to reasonably conclude that adverse reactions could exist resulting of administration of these complexes *in vivo*.

Regardless the *in vivo* toxicity in mice and rats, these compounds have a LD_{50} higher than cisplatin and shows different degrees of toxicity as result of changes in their structures with a strong relationship with cytotoxicity [155]. Casiopeína III-ia at i.p. doses of 6.74 μmol/Kg and 13.5 μmol/Kg q.d. 4x 6 causes adhesions and inflammation at peritoneal surface of mice *nu/nu*, the latter effect is consequence of chronic irritation. In the other hand, the i.v. administration of Casiopeína II-gly causes hemolytic anemia accompanied by leukocytosis and neutrophilia, an inflammation response to the increased erythrocyte destruction and morphological changes in spleen [200]. All hematological effects are dose-dependent and reversible after 15 days whit a single dose of 5 mg/Kg. The type of damage is compatible with ROS and it is similar to those produced by toxicity associated to copper [128,129,202].

The principal adverse effects of these complexes are respiratory and cardiovascular toxicity. In the other hand, Casipeina II-gly and Casiopeína III-ia induce diminution in cardiac work and O_2 consumption in isolated perfused rat hearts with glucose + octanoate. The half-maximal inhibitory concentrations are 4 and 4.6 μM, respectively. These effects are attributable to the strong inhibition of energetic metabolism mentioned above. Remarkably, Casiopeínas were less toxic than adriamycin, a well-known potent cardiotoxic and antineoplastic drug, which has a wide clinical use [190]. The 99 lethal dose in an acute toxicity study in dogs was calculated to be 200 mg/m^2 for Casiopeína III-ia and 160 mg/m^2 for Casiopeína II-gly [203]. At these high doses both compounds causes tachypnoea, drop in arterial blood pressure, tachycardia followed by bradycardia and finally cardiac arrest no later than 25 minutes post-administration. Probably the lung edema is caused by a joined toxicity to the lung capillary bed, and particularly to the heart. The analysis by transmission electron microscopy shows structural disarrangement of cardiac muscle fibers, swelling and loss of mitochondrial crests [203]. The same effects have been observed on mitochondrion HCT-15 cells *in vitro* [153].

Conclusions

The platinum anticancer drug cisplatin has made a major contribution to the treatment of testicular and ovarian cancer. This chance discovery has been the stimulus for research into other metal-based drugs offering many opportunities to medicinal bioinorganic chemistry research. Nowadays, the discovery of metal-based drugs has moved on from chance discovery to rational drug design. The role of bioinorganic chemistry in both, the development of medicinal inorganic agents and in the understanding of the underlying mechanism of disease, clearly indicates that the field of 'metals in medicine' will continue to make contributions to advancements in human health in the 21st century. Herein, some new discoveries were highlighted as ways in which inorganic and bioinorganic chemistry might contribute to improving cancer therapy in the decades to come.

Recent progress in the field of cell biology has resulted in the discovery of receptors and growth factors that are up-regulated in cancer cells. These provide new targets for anticancer drug design, which results in the development of innovative non-platinum metal-based antitumor agents, whose activity do not rely on direct DNA damage and may involve proteins and enzymes as targets. Current research addressing the problems associated with platinum drugs has focused in the exploration of other transition metal-based therapeutics that have different modes of action and pro-drug activation strategies in an effort to overcome some of the disadvantages associated with cisplatin therapy such as side-effects, limited spectrum of activity and resistance.

Among this new generation of innovator chemotherapeutics with mechanisms different from cisplatin, we found those based on essential metals. Until a few years ago, very little was known about essential metals compounds and their capacity to induce apoptosis; currently, remarkable research on this field is performed, being copper-based drugs an example of high relevance. One of the most promising designs in the field of copper-based antitumor agents is the group of complexes named Casiopeínas ®. These compounds can act by miscellaneous mechanisms besides DNA binding, providing, at least in principle, a new class of chemotherapeutic with broader spectrum of activity.

Taken all together, the cytotoxic activity of a metal complex is found to be dictated by both, the metal speciation and the organic components (ligands) that are bound to the metal and, in many cases, one could be the dominating factor over the other. Target specificity can be achieved by finding the right metal–ligand combination. Toxicity and antitumor activity may be tuned by selection of the most suitable ligands which allow controlling thermodynamics and kinetics of ligand substitution, reactivity, and recognition of target sites.

References

[1] Marshall, E.K., *Historical perspectives in chemotherapy, in Advances in Chemotherapy*, Goldin, A. and Hawking, I.F., Editors. 1964, Academic Press: New York, N.Y.

[2] De Vita, V.T., Cell Kinetics and the Chemotherapy of Cancer. *Cancer Chemother Rep*: Part 3, 1971. 2: p. 23-33.

[3] DeVita, V.T., Jr., Human models of human diseases; breast cancer and the lymphomas. *Int J Radiat Oncol Biol Phys*, 1979. 5(10): p. 1855-67.

[4] DeVita, V.T., Jr., The evolution of therapeutic research in cancer. *N Engl J Med*, 1978. 298(16): p. 907-10.

[5] De Vita, V.T., Henney, J.E., y Hubbard, S.M., Estimations of the Numerical and Economic Impact of Chemotherapy in the Treatment of Cancers., in *Cancer Achievements, Challenges and Prospects for the 1980's.*, Burchenal, J.M. and Oettgen, M.S., Editors. 1981, Grune Stratton: New York. p. 857-880.

[6] Bertrand, G., On the role of trace substances in agriculture. 8th *Int Congr Appl Chem* 1912. 28: p. 30-40.

[7] Lippert, B., ed. *30 Years of Cisplatin-Chemistry and Biochemistry of a Leading Anticancer Drug*. 1999, Verlag Helvetica Chimica Acta, Wiley-VCH: Zürich.

[8] Kelland, L.R. y Farrell, N., eds. *Platinum-Based Drugs in Cancer Therapy*. 2000, Humana Press Inc.

[9] Ruili Huang, A.W., David G. Covell., Anticancer metal compounds in NCI's tumor-screening database: putative mode of action. *Biochem Pharmacol,* 2005. 69: p. 1009-1039.

[10] Kelland, L., The resurgence of platinum-based cancer chemotherapy. *Nat Rev Cancer,* 2007. 7(8): p. 573-84.

[11] Clarke, M.J. y Sadler, P.J., eds. Metallopharmaceuticals. Vol. 1. 1999, Springer: Dublin.

[12] Fricker, S.P., Metal based drugs: from serendipity to design. *Dalton Trans*, 2007(43): p. 4903-17.

[13] van Rijt, S.H. y Sadler, P.J., Current applications and future potential for bioinorganic chemistry in the development of anticancer drugs. *Drug Discovery Today,* 2009.

[14] Ronconi, L. y Sadler, P.J., Using coordination chemistry to design new medicines. *Coord Chem Rev*, 2007. 251: p. 1633-1648.

[15] Higby, D.J., Wallace, H.J., Jr., Albert, D., y Holland, J.F., Diamminodichloroplatinum in the chemotherapy of testicular tumors. *J Urol,* 1974. 112(1): p. 100-4.

[16] Goldstein, R.S. y Mayor, G.H., Minireview. The nephrotoxicity of cisplatin. *Life Sci,* 1983. 32(7): p. 685-90.

[17] Hayes, D.M., Cvitkovic, E., Golbey, R.B., Scheiner, E., Helson, L., y Krakoff, I.H., High dose cis-platinum diammine dichloride: amelioration of renal toxicity by mannitol diuresis. *Cancer*, 1977. 39(4): p. 1372-81.

[18] Schilder, R.J., LaCreta, F.P., Perez, R.P., Johnson, S.W., Brennan, J.M., Rogatko, A., Nash, S., McAleer, C., Hamilton, T.C., Roby, D., y et al., Phase I and pharmacokinetic study of ormaplatin (tetraplatin, NSC 363812) administered on a day 1 and day 8 schedule. *Cancer Res*, 1994. 54(3): p. 709-17.

[19] Wong, E. y Giandomenico, C.M., Current status of platinum-based antitumor drugs. *Chem Rev*, 1999. 99(9): p. 2451-66.

[20] Greene, R.F., Chatterji, D.C., Hiranaka, P.K., y Gallelli, J.F., Stability of cisplatin in aqueous solution. *Am J Hosp Pharm*, 1979. 36(1): p. 38-43.

[21] LeRoy, A.F., Some quantitative data on cis-dichlorodiammineplatinum(II) species in solution. *Cancer Treat Rep*, 1979. 63(2): p. 231-3.

[22] Repta, A.J., Long, D.F., y Hincal, A.A., cis-Dichlorodiammineplatinum(II) stability in aqueous vehicles: an alternate view. *Cancer Treat Rep*, 1979. 63(2): p. 229-31.

[23] Kleinwachter, V. y Zaludova, R., Reaction of cis and trans isomers of platinum(II) diamminedichloride with purine, adensine and its derivatives in dilute solutions. *Chem Biol Interact*, 1977. 16(2): p. 207-22.

[24] Fricker, S.P., Metal Compounds in Cancer Therapy. 1994, London: Chapman & Hall. 1-31.

[25] Montero, E.I., Diaz, S., Gonzalez-Vadillo, A.M., Perez, J.M., Alonso, C., y Navarro-Ranninger, C., Preparation and characterization of novel trans-[PtCl(2)(amine)(isopropylamine)] compounds: cytotoxic activity and apoptosis induction in ras-transformed cells. *J Med Chem*, 1999. 42(20): p. 4264-8.

[26] Brabec, V., Kasparkova, J., Vrana, O., Novakova, O., Cox, J.W., Qu, Y., y Farrell, N., DNA modifications by a novel bifunctional trinuclear platinum phase I anticancer agent. *Biochem*, 1999. 38(21): p. 6781-90.

[27] Farrell, N., Kelland, L.R., Roberts, J.D., y Van Beusichem, M., Activation of the trans geometry in platinum antitumor complexes: a survey of the cytotoxicity of trans complexes containing planar ligands in murine L1210 and human tumor panels and studies on their mechanism of action. *Cancer Res*, 1992. 52(18): p. 5065-72.

[28] Aris, S.M., Gewirtz, D.A., Ryan, J.J., Knott, K.M., y Farrell, N.P., Promotion of DNA strand breaks, interstrand cross-links and apoptotic cell death in A2780 human ovarian cancer cells by transplatinum planar amine complexes. *Biochem Pharmacol*, 2007. 73(11): p. 1749-57.

[29] Pizarro, A.M. y Sadler, P.J., Unusual DNA binding modes for metal anticancer complexes. *Biochimie*, 2009. 91(10): p. 1198-211.

[30] Farrell, N. y Spinelli, S., Dinuclear and trinuclear platinum anticancer agents, in Uses of Inorganic Chemistry in Medicine, Farrell, N., Editor. 1999, Royal Society of Chemistry. p. 124-134.

[31] Hensing, T.A., Hanna, N.H., Gillenwater, H.H., Gabriella Camboni, M., Allievi, C., y Socinski, M.A., Phase II study of BBR 3464 as treatment in patients with sensitive or refractory small cell lung cancer. *Anticancer Drugs*, 2006. 17(6): p. 697-704.

[32] Mackay, F.S., Woods, J.A., Heringova, P., Kasparkova, J., Pizarro, A.M., Moggach, S.A., Parsons, S., Brabec, V., y Sadler, P.J., A potent cytotoxic photoactivated platinum complex. *Proc Natl Acad Sci U S A*, 2007. 104(52): p. 20743-8.

[33] Muller, P., Schroder, B., Parkinson, J.A., Kratochwil, N.A., Coxall, R.A., Parkin, A., Parsons, S., y Sadler, P.J., Nucleotide cross-linking induced by photoreactions of platinum(IV)-azide complexes. *Angew Chem Int Ed Engl,* 2003. 42(3): p. 335-9. International Patent Application WO 03/017993.

[34] Chikuma, M., Sato, T., y Komeda, S., [Current status of and future perspectives for platinum antitumor drugs]. *Yakugaku Zasshi*, 2008. 128(3): p. 307-16.

[35] Higgins, J.D., 3rd, Neely, L., y Fricker, S., Synthesis and cytotoxicity of some cyclometallated palladium complexes. *J Inorg Biochem*, 1993. 49(2): p. 149-56.

[36] Fricker, S.P., in Metal Ions in Biology and Medicine, Collery, P., Poirier, L.A., Manfait, M., and Etienne, J.-C., Editors. 1990, Jonh Libbey Eurotext: Paris. p. 452-56.

[37] Sava, G., Pacor, S., Zorzet, S., Alessio, E., y Mestroni, G., Antitumour properties of dimethylsulphoxide ruthenium (II) complexes in the Lewis lung carcinoma system. *Pharmacol Res*, 1989. 21(5): p. 617-28.

[38] Sava, G., Pacor, S., Bregant, F., Ceschia, V., y Mestroni, G., Metal complexes of ruthenium: antineoplastic properties and perspectives. *Anticancer Drugs*, 1990. 1(2): p. 99-108.

[39] Rademaker-Lakhai, J.M., van den Bongard, D., Pluim, D., Beijnen, J.H., y Schellens, J.H., A Phase I and pharmacological study with imidazolium-trans-DMSO-imidazole-tetrachlororuthenate, a novel ruthenium anticancer agent. *Clin Cancer Res*, 2004. 10(11): p. 3717-27.

[40] Bergamo, A. y Sava, G., Ruthenium complexes can target determinants of tumour malignancy. *Dalton Trans*, 2007(13): p. 1267-72.

[41] Galanski, M., Arion, V.B., Jakupec, M.A., y Keppler, B.K., Recent developments in the field of tumor-inhibiting metal complexes. *Curr Pharm Des*, 2003. 9(25): p. 2078-89.

[42] Lentz, F., Drescher, A., Lindauer, A., Henke, M., Hilger, R.A., Hartinger, C.G., Scheulen, M.E., Dittrich, C., Keppler, B.K., y Jaehde, U., Pharmacokinetics of a novel anticancer ruthenium complex (KP1019, FFC14A) in a phase I dose-escalation study. *Anticancer Drugs*, 2009. 20(2): p. 97-103.

[43] Hartinger, C.G., Jakupec, M.A., Zorbas-Seifried, S., Groessl, M., Egger, A., Berger, W., Zorbas, H., Dyson, P.J., y Keppler, B.K., KP1019, a new redox-active anticancer agent--preclinical development and results of a clinical phase I study in tumor patients. *Chem Biodivers*, 2008. 5(10): p. 2140-55.

[44] Higby, G.J., Gold in medicine: a review of its use in the West before 1900. *Gold Bull,* 1982. 15(4): p. 130-40.

[45] Simon, T.M., Kunishima, D.H., Vibert, G.J., y Lorber, A., Inhibitory effects of a new oral gold compound on HeLa cells. *Cancer*, 1979. 44(6): p. 1965.

[46] Simon, T.M., Kunishima, D.H., Vibert, G.J., y Lorber, A., Cellular antiproliferative action exerted by auranofin. *J Rheumatol Suppl*, 1979. 5: p. 91-7.

[47] Simon, T.M., Kunishima, D.H., Vibert, G.J., y Lorber, A., Screening trial with the coordinated gold compound auranofin using mouse lymphocyte leukemia P388. *Cancer Res,* 1981. 41(1): p. 94-7.

[48] Mirabelli, C.K., Johnson, R.K., Sung, C.M., Faucette, L., Muirhead, K., y Crooke, S.T., Evaluation of the in vivo antitumor activity and in vitro cytotoxic properties of auranofin, a coordinated gold compound, in murine tumor models. *Cancer Res*, 1985. 45(1): p. 32-9.

[49] Mirabelli, C.K., Johnson, R.K., Hill, D.T., Faucette, L.F., Girard, G.R., Kuo, G.Y., Sung, C.M., y Crooke, S.T., Correlation of the in vitro cytotoxic and in vivo antitumor activities of gold(I) coordination complexes. *J Med Chem*, 1986. 29(2): p. 218-23.

[50] Snyder, R.M., Mirabelli, C.K., y Crooke, S.T., Cellular association, intracellular distribution, and efflux of auranofin via sequential ligand exchange reactions. *Biochem Pharmacol,* 1986. 35(6): p. 923-32.

[51] Berners-Price, S.J., Girard, G.R., Hill, D.T., Sutton, B.M., Jarrett, P.S., Faucette, L.F., Johnson, R.K., Mirabelli, C.K., y Sadler, P.J., Cytotoxicity and antitumor activity of some tetrahedral bis(diphosphino)gold(I) chelates. *J Med Chem*, 1990. 33(5): p. 1386-92.

[52] Agrawal, K.C., Bears, K.B., Marcus, D., y Jonassen, H.B., Gold triphenylphosphines complexes as a new class of potential antitumor agents. . *Proc. Am. Assoc. Cancer Res.*, 1978. 69: p. 110.

[53] Barnard, P.J. y Berners-Price, S.J., Targeting the mitochondrial cell death pathway with gold compounds. *Coord Chem Rev*, 2007. 251: p. 1889-1902.

[54] Humphreys, A.S., Filipovska, A., Berners-Price, S.J., Koutsantonis, G.A., Skelton, B.W., y White, A.H., Gold(I) chloride adducts of 1,3-bis(di-2-pyridylphosphino)propane: synthesis, structural studies and antitumour activity. *Dalton Trans*, 2007(43): p. 4943-50.

[55] Rackham, O., Nichols, S.J., Leedman, P.J., Berners-Price, S.J., y Filipovska, A., A gold(I) phosphine complex selectively induces apoptosis in breast cancer cells: implications for anticancer therapeutics targeted to mitochondria. *Biochem Pharmacol,* 2007. 74(7): p. 992-1002.

[56] Powis, G. y Kirkpatrick, D.L., Thioredoxin signaling as a target for cancer therapy. *Curr Opin Pharmacol,* 2007. 7(4): p. 392-7.

[57] Hickey, J.L., Ruhayel, R.A., Barnard, P.J., Baker, M.V., Berners-Price, S.J., y Filipovska, A., Mitochondria-targeted chemotherapeutics: the rational design of gold(I) N-heterocyclic carbene complexes that are selectively toxic to cancer cells and target protein selenols in preference to thiols. *J Am Chem Soc,* 2008. 130(38): p. 12570-1.

[58] Aldinucci, D., Ronconi, L., y Fregona, D., Groundbreaking gold(III) anticancer agents. *Drug Discov* Today, 2009.

[59] Li, W., Xie, Y., Sun, R.W., Liu, Q., Young, J., Yu, W.Y., Che, C.M., Tam, P.K., y Ren, Y., Inhibition of Akt sensitises neuroblastoma cells to gold(III) porphyrin 1a, a novel antitumour drug induced apoptosis and growth inhibition. *Br J Cancer,* 2009. 101(2): p. 342-9.

[60] To, Y.F., Sun, R.W., Chen, Y., Chan, V.S., Yu, W.Y., Tam, P.K., Che, C.M., y Lin, C.L., Gold(III) porphyrin complex is more potent than cisplatin in inhibiting growth of nasopharyngeal carcinoma in vitro and in vivo. *Int J Cancer*, 2009. 124(8): p. 1971-9.

[61] Casini, A., Cinellu, M.A., Minghetti, G., Gabbiani, C., Coronnello, M., Mini, E., y Messori, L., Structural and solution chemistry, antiproliferative effects, and DNA and protein binding properties of a series of dinuclear gold(III) compounds with bipyridyl ligands. *J Med Chem*, 2006. 49(18): p. 5524-31.

[62] Marcon, G., Carotti, S., Coronnello, M., Messori, L., Mini, E., Orioli, P., Mazzei, T., Cinellu, M.A., y Minghetti, G., Gold(III) complexes with bipyridyl ligands: solution chemistry, cytotoxicity, and DNA binding properties. *J Med Chem*, 2002. 45(8): p. 1672-7.

[63] Gabbiani, C., Casini, A., Messori, L., Guerri, A., Cinellu, M.A., Minghetti, G., Corsini, M., Rosani, C., Zanello, P., y Arca, M., Structural characterization, solution studies, and DFT calculations on a series of binuclear gold(III) oxo complexes: relationships to biological properties. *Inorg Chem*, 2008. 47(7): p. 2368-79.

[64] Kopf-Maier, P., Complexes of metals other than platinum as antitumour agents. *Eur J Clin Pharmacol,* 1994. 47(1): p. 1-16.

[65] Keppler, B.K., Friesen, C., Vongerichten, H., y E., V., Budotitane, a new tumor-inhibiting titanium compound: preclinical and clinical development. *Met Complexes Cancer Chemother*, 1993: p. 297-323.

[66] Kalirai, B.S., Foulon, J.-D., Hamor, T.A., Jones, C.J., Paul D. Beer, y Fricker, S.P., Some substitution reactions of ligands coordinated to the bis(cyclopentadienyl)titanium moiety, the X-ray crystal structure of Ti(η5-C5H5)2(OPh)2 and an assessment of the

anti-tumour activity of some cyclopentadienyl titanium compounds. *Polyhedron*, 1991. 10(16): p. 1847-1856.

[67] Kopf-Maier, P. y Martin, R., Subcellular distribution of titanium in the liver after treatment with the antitumor agent titanocene dichloride. A study using electron spectroscopic imaging. *Virchows Arch B Cell Pathol Incl Mol Pathol,* 1989. 57(4): p. 213-22.

[68] Melendez, E., Titanium complexes in cancer treatment. *Crit Rev Oncol Hematol,* 2002. 42(3): p. 309-15.

[69] Kostova, I., Titanium and Vanadium Complexes as Anticancer Agents. *Anticancer Agents Med Chem*, 2009. 9(8): p. 827-842.

[70] Imamura, H., Furukawa, H., Kishimoto, T., Nakae, S., Inoue, K., Tsukahara, Y., Imano, M., Yamazaki, K., Okano, S., Morimoto, T., Sugihara, S., y Shimokawa, T., Phase II study of 2-week TS-1 administration followed by 1-week rest for gastric cancer. *Hepatogastroenterol*, 2007. 54(79): p. 2167-71.

[71] Evangelou, A.M., Vanadium in cancer treatment. *Crit Rev Oncol Hematol,* 2002. 42(3): p. 249-65.

[72] Thompson, K.H. y Orvig, C., Coordination chemistry of vanadium in metallopharmaceutical candidate compounds. *Coordination Chemistry Reviews*, 2001. 219(221): p. 1033-1053.

[73] Djordjevic, C. y Wampler, G.L., Antitumor activity and toxicity of peroxo heteroligand vanadates(V) in relation to biochemistry of vanadium. *J Inorg Biochem,* 1985. 25(1): p. 51-5.

[74] Sam, M., Hwang, J.H., Chanfreau, G., y Abu-Omar, M.M., Hydroxyl radical is the active species in photochemical DNA strand scission by bis(peroxo)vanadium(V) phenanthroline. *Inorg Chem*, 2004. 43(26): p. 8447-55.

[75] Sakurai, H., Tamura, H., y Okatani, K., Mechanism for a new antitumor vanadium complex: hydroxyl radical-dependent DNA cleavage by 1,10-phenanthroline-vanadyl complex in the presence of hydrogen peroxide. *Biochem Biophys Res Commun*, 1995. 206(1): p. 133-7.

[76] Navara, C.S., Benyumov, A., Vassilev, A., Narla, R.K., Ghosh, P., y Uckun, F.M., Vanadocenes as potent anti-proliferative agents disrupting mitotic spindle formation in cancer cells. *Anticancer Drugs,* 2001. 12(4): p. 369-76.

[77] D'Cruz, O.J. y Uckun, F.M., Vanadocene-mediated in vivo male germ cell apoptosis. *Toxicol Appl Pharmacol*, 2000. 166(3): p. 186-95.

[78] Evangelou, A., Karkabounas, S., Kalpouzos, G., Malamas, M., Liasko, R., Stefanou, D., Vlahos, A.T., y Kabanos, T.A., Comparison of the therapeutic effects of two vanadium complexes administered at low dose on benzo[a]pyrene-induced malignant tumors in rats. *Cancer Lett*, 1997. 119(2): p. 221-5.

[79] Crowe, A.J., Smith, P.J., y Atassi, G., Investigations into the antitumour actitvity of organotin compounds. 2. Diorganotin dihalide and dipseudohalide complexes. *Inorg Chimica Acta*, 1984. 93(4): p. 179-184.

[80] Crowe, A.J., The chemotherapeutic properties of tin compounds. *Drugs Fut.*, 1987. 12(3): p. 255-275.

[81] Gielen, M. y Tiekink, E.R.T., Tin compounds and their therapeutic potential, in Metallotherapeutic Drugs and Metal-Based Diagnostic Agents. The Use of Metals in Medicine, Gielen, M. and Tiekink, E.R.T., Editors. 2005, J. Wiley & Sons. p. 421-439.

[82] Hadjikakou, S.K. y Hadjiliadis, N., Antiproliferative and anti-tumor activity of organotin compounds. *Coord Chem Rev*, 2009. 253: p. 235-249.
[83] Khan, M.I., Musa Kaleem Baloch, Ashfaq, M., y Stoter, G., In vivo toxicological effects and spectral studies of new triorganotin (IV)-N-maleoyltranexamates. *J Organometal Chem*, 2006. 691(11): p. 2556-2562.
[84] Liu, H.G., Wang, Y., Lian, L., y Xu, L.H., Tributyltin induces DNA damage as well as oxidative damage in rats. *Environ Toxicol*, 2006. 21(2): p. 166-71.
[85] Keppler, B.K., in Metal Complexes in Cancer Chemother, Keppler, B.K., Editor. 1993, VCH, Weinheim: New York.
[86] Aw, T.Y., Nicotera, P., Manzo, L., y Orrenius, S., Tributyltin stimulates apoptosis in rat thymocytes. *Arch Biochem Biophys*, 1990. 283(1): p. 46-50.
[87] Viviani, B., Rossi, A.D., Chow, S.C., y Nicotera, P., Triethyltin interferes with Ca2+ signaling and potentiates norepinephrine release in PC12 cells. *Toxicol Appl Pharmacol*, 1996. 140(2): p. 289-95.
[88] Viviani, B., Rossi, A.D., Chow, S.C., y Nicotera, P., Organotin compounds induce calcium overload and apoptosis in PC12 cells. *Neurotoxicology*, 1995. 16(1): p. 19-25.
[89] Gielen, M., An Overview of Forty Years Organotin Chemistry Developed at the Free Universities of Brussels ULB and VUB. *J. Braz. Chem. Soc.*, 2003. 14(6): p. 870-877.
[90] Pellerito, L. y Nagy, L., Organotin(IV)n+ complexes formed with biologically active ligands: equilibrium and structural studies, and some biological aspects. *Coord Chem Rev*, 2002. 224(111-50.).
[91] Tian, L., Qian, B., Sun, Y., Zheng, X., Yang, M., Li, H., y Liu, X., Synthesis, structural characterization and cytotoxic activity of diorganotin(IV) complexes of N-(5-halosalicylidene)--amino acid. *App Organometal Chem*, 2005. 19(8): p. 980-987.
[92] Khan, M.I., Musa Kaleem Baloch, y Ashfaq, M., In vivo toxicological effects and spectral studies of organotin(IV) N-maleoylglycinates. *App Organometal Chem*, 2005. 19(1): p. 132-139.
[93] Li, Q., Guedes da Silva, M.F.C., y Pombeiro, A.J.L., Diorganotin(IV) Derivatives of Substituted Benzohydroxamic Acids with High Antitumor Activity. *Chem - A Eur J*, 2004. 10(6): p. 1456-1462.
[94] Xanthopoulou, M.N., Hadjikakou, S.K., Hadjiliadis, N., Milaeva, E.R., Gracheva, J.A., Tyurin, V.Y., Kourkoumelis, N., Christoforidis, K.C., Metsios, A.K., Karkabounas, S., y Charalabopoulos, K., Biological studies of new organotin(IV) complexes of thioamide ligands. *Eur J Med Chem*, 2008. 43(2): p. 327-35.
[95] Xanthopoulou, M.N., Hadjikakou, S.K., Hadjiliadis, N., Kubicki, M., Skoulika, S., Bakas, T., Baril, M., y Butler, I.S., Synthesis, structural characterization, and biological studies of six- and five-coordinate organotin(IV) complexes with the thioamides 2-mercaptobenzothiazole, 5-chloro-2-mercaptobenzothiazole, and 2-mercaptobenzoxazole. *Inorg Chem*, 2007. 46(4): p. 1187-95.
[96] Yin, H.D. y Xue, S.C., Synthesis and characterization of organotin complexes with dithiocarbamates and crystal structures of (4-NCC6H4CH2)2Sn(S2CNEt2)2 and (2-ClC6H4CH2)2 Sn(Cl)S2CNBz2. *App Organometal Chem*, 2006. 20(4): p. 283-289.
[97] Tabassum, S. y Pettinari, C., Chemical and biotechnological developments in organotin cancer chemotherapy. *J Organometal Chem*, 2006. 691(8): p. 1761-1766.

[98] Ruiz-Ramírez, L., Gracia-Mora, I., Moreno-Esparza, R., Díaz, D., Gasque, L., Mayet, L., Ortiz, V., y Lomelí, C., The antitumor activity of several transition metal complexes. *J Inorg Biochem*, 1991. 43(2-3): p. 615.

[99] Burger, R.M., Drlica, K., y Birdsall, B., The DNA cleavage pathway of iron bleomycin. Strand scission precedes deoxyribose 3-phosphate bond cleavage. *J Biol Chem,* 1994. 269(42): p. 25978-85.

[100] Dorr, R.T., Bleomycin pharmacology: mechanism of action and resistance, and clinical pharmacokinetics. *Semin Oncol*, 1992. 19(2 Suppl 5): p. 3-8.

[101] Buss, J.L., Greene, B.T., Turner, J., Torti, F.M., y Torti, S.V., Iron chelators in cancer chemotherapy. *Curr Top Med Chem*, 2004. 4(15): p. 1623-35.

[102] Pahl, P.M. y Horwitz, L.D., Cell permeable iron chelators as potential cancer chemotherapeutic agents. *Cancer Invest*, 2005. 23(8): p. 683-91.

[103] Bernhardt, P.V., Sharpe, P.C., Islam, M., Lovejoy, D.B., Kalinowski, D.S., y Richardson, D.R., Iron chelators of the dipyridylketone thiosemicarbazone class: precomplexation and transmetalation effects on anticancer activity. *J Med Chem,* 2009. 52(2): p. 407-15.

[104] Kovjazin, R., Eldar, T., Patya, M., Vanichkin, A., Lander, H.M., y Novogrodsky, A., Ferrocene-induced lymphocyte activation and anti-tumor activity is mediated by redox-sensitive signaling. *FASEB J*, 2003. 17(3): p. 467-9.

[105] Mishra, L., Said, M.K., Itokawa, H., y Takeya, K., Antitumor and antimicrobial activities of Fe(II)/Fe(III) complexes derived from some heterocyclic compounds. *Bioorg Med Chem*, 1995. 3(9): p. 1241-5.

[106] Tabbi, G., Cassino, C., Cavigiolio, G., Colangelo, D., Ghiglia, A., Viano, I., y Osella, D., Water stability and cytotoxic activity relationship of a series of ferrocenium derivatives. ESR insights on the radical production during the degradation process. *J Med Chem*, 2002. 45(26): p. 5786-96.

[107] Wong, E.L., Fang, G.S., Che, C.M., y Zhu, N., Highly cytotoxic iron(II) complexes with pentadentate pyridyl ligands as a new class of anti-tumor agents. *Chem Commun (Camb)*, 2005(36): p. 4578-80.

[108] Yuasa, M., Oyaizu, K., Horiuchi, A., Ogata, A., Hatsugai, T., Yamaguchi, A., y Kawakami, H., Liposomal surface-loading of water-soluble cationic iron(III) porphyrins as anticancer drugs. *Mol Pharm*, 2004. 1(5): p. 387-9.

[109] Shrivastav, A., Singh, N.K., y Singh, S.M., Synthesis, characterization and antitumor studies of Mn(II), Fe(III), Co(II), Ni(II), Cu(II) and Zn(II) complexes of N-salicyloyl-N'-o-hydroxythiobenzhydrazide. *Bioorg Med Chem*, 2002. 10(4): p. 887-95.

[110] Jung, M., Kerr, D.E., y Senter, P.D., *Bioorganometallic chemistry--synthesis and antitumor activity of cobalt carbonyl complexes.* Arch Pharm (Weinheim), 1997. 330(6): p. 173-6.

[111] Sathisha, M.P., Shetti, U.N., Revankar, V.K., y Pai, K.S., Synthesis and antitumor studies on novel Co(II), Ni(II) and Cu(II) metal complexes of bis(3-acetylcoumarin)thiocarbohydrazone. *Eur J Med Chem*, 2008. 43(11): p. 2338-46.

[112] Kasugai, N., Murase, T., Ohse, T., Nagaoka, S., Kawakami, H., y Kubota, S., Selective cell death by water-soluble Fe-porphyrins with superoxide dismutase (SOD) activity. *J Inorg Biochem*, 2002. 91(2): p. 349-55.

[113] Moeller, B.J., Batinic-Haberle, I., Spasojevic, I., Rabbani, Z.N., Anscher, M.S., Vujaskovic, Z., y Dewhirst, M.W., A manganese porphyrin superoxide dismutase

mimetic enhances tumor radioresponsiveness. *Int J Radiat Oncol Biol Phys*, 2005. 63(2): p. 545-52.
[114] Shrivastav, A., Singh, N.K., Tripathi, P., George, T., Dimmock, J.R., y Sharma, R.K., Copper(II) and manganese(III) complexes of N'-[(2-hydroxy phenyl) carbonothioyl] pyridine-2-carbohydrazide: novel therapeutic agents for cancer. *Biochimie*, 2006. 88(9): p. 1209-16.
[115] Xu, Z.D., Liu, H., Wang, M., Xiao, S.L., Yang, M., y Bu, X.H., Manganese(II) complex of 6,7-dicycanodipyridoquinoxaline with antitumor activities: synthesis, crystal structure and binding with DNA. *J Inorg Biochem*, 2002. 92(3-4): p. 149-55.
[116] Tisato, F., Marzano, C., Porchia, M., Pellei, M., y Santini, C., Copper in diseases and treatments, and copper-based anticancer strategies. *Med Res Rev*, 2009.
[117] Marzano, C., Pellei, M., Tisato, F., y Santini, C., Copper complexes as anticancer agents. *Anticancer Agents Med Chem*, 2009. 9(2): p. 185-211.
[118] Wang, T. y Guo, Z., Copper in medicine: homeostasis, chelation therapy and antitumor drug design. *Curr Med Chem*, 2006. 13(5): p. 525-37.
[119] Barceloux, D.G., *Copper.* J Toxicol Clin Toxicol, 1999. 37(2): p. 217-30.
[120] Cousins, R.J., Absorption, transport, and hepatic metabolism of copper and zinc: special reference to metallothionein and ceruloplasmin. *Physiol Rev*, 1985. 65(2): p. 238-309.
[121] Linder, M., The Biochemistry of Copper. 1991, New York: Plenum.
[122] Linder, M.C. y Hazegh-Azam, M., Copper biochemistry and molecular biology. *Am J Clin Nutr*, 1996. 63(5): p. 797S-811S.
[123] Sandstead, H.H., Requirements and toxicity of essential trace elements, illustrated by zinc and copper. *Am J Clin Nutr*, 1995. 61(3 Suppl): p. 621S-624S.
[124] Turnlund, J.R., *Copper*, in Modern Nutrition in Health and Disease, Shils, M.E., Olson, J.A., Shike, M., and Ross, A.C., Editors. 1999, Lippincott Williams and Wilkins: Baltimore, MD.
[125] Olivares, M. y Uauy, R., Copper as an essential nutrient. *Am J Clin Nutr*, 1996. 63(5): p. 791S-6S.
[126] Harris, E.D., Copper transport: an overview. *Proc Soc Exp Biol Med*, 1991. 196(2): p. 130-40.
[127] Gaetke, L.M. y Chow, C.K., Copper toxicity, oxidative stress, and antioxidant nutrients. *Toxicology*, 2003. 189(1-2): p. 147-63.
[128] Hill, R., Copper toxicity II. *Br Vet J*, 1977. 133(4): p. 365-73.
[129] Hill, R., Copper toxicity. I. *Br Vet J*, 1977. 133(3): p. 219-24.
[130] Brewer, G.J., Wilson disease and canine copper toxicosis. *Am J Clin Nutr,* 1998. 67(5 Suppl): p. 1087S-1090S.
[131] Bull, P.C., Thomas, G.R., Rommens, J.M., Forbes, J.R., y Cox, D.W., The Wilson disease gene is a putative copper transporting P-type ATPase similar to the Menkes gene. *Nat Genet*, 1993. 5(4): p. 327-37.
[132] Harada, M., Kumemura, H., Sakisaka, S., Shishido, S., Taniguchi, E., Kawaguchi, T., Hanada, S., Koga, H., Kumashiro, R., Ueno, T., Suganuma, T., Furuta, K., Namba, M., Sugiyama, T., y Sata, M., Wilson disease protein ATP7B is localized in the late endosomes in a polarized human hepatocyte cell line. *Int J Mol Med*, 2003. 11(3): p. 293-8.
[133] Tanzi, R.E., Petrukhin, K., Chernov, I., Pellequer, J.L., Wasco, W., Ross, B., Romano, D.M., Parano, E., Pavone, L., Brzustowicz, L.M., y et al., The Wilson disease gene is a

copper transporting ATPase with homology to the Menkes disease gene. *Nat Genet*, 1993. 5(4): p. 344-50.

[134] Yamaguchi, Y., Heiny, M.E., y Gitlin, J.D., Isolation and characterization of a human liver cDNA as a candidate gene for Wilson disease. *Biochem Biophys Res Commun*, 1993. 197(1): p. 271-7.

[135] Chelly, J., Tumer, Z., Tonnesen, T., Petterson, A., Ishikawa-Brush, Y., Tommerup, N., Horn, N., y Monaco, A.P., Isolation of a candidate gene for Menkes disease that encodes a potential heavy metal binding protein. *Nat Genet,* 1993. 3(1): p. 14-9.

[136] Lutsenko, S., Petrukhin, K., Cooper, M.J., Gilliam, C.T., y Kaplan, J.H., N-terminal domains of human copper-transporting adenosine triphosphatases (the Wilson's and Menkes disease proteins) bind copper selectively in vivo and in vitro with stoichiometry of one copper per metal-binding repeat. *J Biol Chem*, 1997. 272(30): p. 18939-44.

[137] Mercer, J.F., Livingston, J., Hall, B., Paynter, J.A., Begy, C., Chandrasekharappa, S., Lockhart, P., Grimes, A., Bhave, M., Siemieniak, D., y et al., Isolation of a partial candidate gene for Menkes disease by positional cloning. *Nat Genet,* 1993. 3(1): p. 20-5.

[138] Murata, Y., Kodama, H., Abe, T., Ishida, N., Nishimura, M., Levinson, B., Gitschier, J., y Packman, S., Mutation analysis and expression of the mottled gene in the macular mouse model of Menkes disease. *Pediatr Res*, 1997. 42(4): p. 436-42.

[139] Vulpe, C., Levinson, B., Whitney, S., Packman, S., y Gitschier, J., Isolation of a candidate gene for Menkes disease and evidence that it encodes a copper-transporting ATPase. *Nat Genet,* 1993. 3(1): p. 7-13.

[140] Bisceglie, F., Baldini, M., Belicchi-Ferrari, M., Buluggiu, E., Careri, M., Pelosi, G., Pinelli, S., y Tarasconi, P., Metal complexes of retinoid derivatives with antiproliferative activity: synthesis, characterization and DNA interaction studies. *Eur J Med Chem*, 2007. 42(5): p. 627-34.

[141] Garcia-Tojal, J., Pizarro, J.L., Garcia-Orad, A., Perez-Sanz, A.R., Ugalde, M., Alvarez Diaz, A., Serra, J.L., Arriortua, M.I., y Rojo, T., Biological activity of complexes derived from thiophene-2-carbaldehyde thiosemicarbazone. Crystal structure of [Ni(C(6)H(6)N(3)S(2))(2)]. *J Inorg Biochem*, 2001. 86(2-3): p. 627-33.

[142] Garcia-Tojal, J., Garcia-Orad, A., Diaz, A.A., Serra, J.L., Urtiaga, M.K., Arriortua, M.I., y Rojo, T., Biological activity of complexes derived from pyridine-2-carbaldehyde thiosemicarbazone. Structure of. *J Inorg Biochem*, 2001. 84(3-4): p. 271-8.

[143] Afrasiabi, Z., Sinn, E., Padhye, S., Dutta, S., Newton, C., Anson, C.E., y Powell, A.K., Transition metal complexes of phenanthrenequinone thiosemicarbazone as potential anticancer agents: synthesis, structure, spectroscopy, electrochemistry and in vitro anticancer activity against human breast cancer cell-line, T47D. *J Inorg Biochem,* 2003. 95(4): p. 306-14.

[144] Ambike, V., Adsule, S., Ahmed, F., Wang, Z., Afrasiabi, Z., Sinn, E., Sarkar, F., y Padhye, S., Copper conjugates of nimesulide Schiff bases targeting VEGF, COX and Bcl-2 in pancreatic cancer cells. *J Inorg Biochem*, 2007. 101(10): p. 1517-24.

[145] Zhong, X., Wei, H.L., Liu, W.S., Wang, D.Q., y Wang, X., The crystal structures of copper(II), manganese(II), and nickel(II) complexes of a (Z)-2-hydroxy-N'-(2-

oxoindolin-3-ylidene) benzohydrazide--potential antitumor agents. *Bioorg Med Chem Lett*, 2007. 17(13): p. 3774-7.

[146] Cerchiaro, G., Aquilano, K., Filomeni, G., Rotilio, G., Ciriolo, M.R., y Ferreira, A.M., Isatin-Schiff base copper(II) complexes and their influence on cellular viability. *J Inorg Biochem*, 2005. 99(7): p. 1433-40.

[147] Filomeni, G., Cerchiaro, G., Da Costa Ferreira, A.M., De Martino, A., Pedersen, J.Z., Rotilio, G., y Ciriolo, M.R., Pro-apoptotic activity of novel Isatin-Schiff base copper(II) complexes depends on oxidative stress induction and organelle-selective damage. *J Biol Chem*, 2007. 282(16): p. 12010-21.

[148] Tamura, H., Imai, H., Kuwahara, J., y Sugiura, Y., A new antitumor complex bis(acetato)bis(imidazole)copper(II). *J. Am. Chem. Soc.*, 1987. 109(22): p. 6870-6871.

[149] Raptopoulou, C.P., Paschalidou, S., Pantazaki, A.A., Terzis, A., Perlepes, S.P., Lialiaris, T., Bakalbassis, E.G., Mrozinski, J., y Kyriakidis, D.A., Bis(acetato)bis(1-methyl-4,5-diphenylimidazole)copper(II): preparation, characterization, crystal structure, DNA strand breakage and cytogenetic effect. *J Inorg Biochem*, 1998. 71(1-2): p. 15-27.

[150] Devereux, M., McCann, M., Shea, D.O., Kelly, R., Egan, D., Deegan, C., Kavanagh, K., McKee, V., y Finn, G., Synthesis, antimicrobial activity and chemotherapeutic potential of inorganic derivatives of 2-(4'-thiazolyl)benzimidazole[thiabendazole]: X-ray crystal structures of [Cu(TBZH)2Cl]Cl.H2O.EtOH and TBZH2NO3 (TBZH=thiabendazole). *J Inorg Biochem*, 2004. 98(6): p. 1023-31.

[151] Marzano, C., Pellei, M., Colavito, D., Alidori, S., Lobbia, G.G., Gandin, V., Tisato, F., y Santini, C., Synthesis, characterization, and in vitro antitumor properties of tris(hydroxymethyl)phosphine copper(I) complexes containing the new bis(1,2,4-triazol-1-yl)acetate ligand. *J Med Chem*, 2006. 49(25): p. 7317-24.

[152] Chen, R., Liu, C.S., Zhang, H., Guo, Y., Bu, X.H., y Yang, M., Three new Cu(II) and Cd(II) complexes with 3-(2-pyridyl)pyrazole-based ligand: syntheses, crystal structures, and evaluations for bioactivities. *J Inorg Biochem*, 2007. 101(3): p. 412-21.

[153] Carvallo-Chaigneau, F., Trejo-Solis, C., Gomez-Ruiz, C., Rodriguez-Aguilera, E., Macias-Rosales, L., Cortes-Barberena, E., Cedillo-Pelaez, C., Gracia-Mora, I., Ruiz-Azuara, L., Madrid-Marina, V., y Constantino-Casas, F., Casiopeina III-ia induces apoptosis in HCT-15 cells in vitro through caspase-dependent mechanisms and has antitumor effect in vivo. *Biometals*, 2008. 21(1): p. 17-28.

[154] Trejo-Solis, C., Palencia, G., Zuniga, S., Rodriguez-Ropon, A., Osorio-Rico, L., Luvia, S.T., Gracia-Mora, I., Marquez-Rosado, L., Sanchez, A., Moreno-Garcia, M.E., Cruz, A., Bravo-Gomez, M.E., Ruiz-Ramirez, L., Rodriguez-Enriquez, S., y Sotelo, J., Cas IIgly induces apoptosis in glioma C6 cells in vitro and in vivo through caspase-dependent and caspase-independent mechanisms. *Neoplasia*, 2005. 7(6): p. 563-74.

[155] Bravo-Gomez, M.E., Garcia-Ramos, J.C., Gracia-Mora, I., y Ruiz-Azuara, L., Antiproliferative activity and QSAR study of copper(II) mixed chelate [Cu(N-N)(acetylacetonato)]NO3 and [Cu(N-N)(glycinato)]NO3 complexes, (Casiopeinas). *J Inorg Biochem*, 2009. 103(2): p. 299-309.

[156] Devereux, M., McCann, M., O'Shea, D., O'Connor, M., Kiely, E., McKee, V., Naughton, D., Fisher, A., Kellett, A., Walsh, M., Egan, D., y Deegan, C., Synthesis, Superoxide Dismutase Mimetic and Anticancer Activities of Metal Complexes of 2,2-Dimethylpentanedioic Acid(2dmepdaH(2)) and 3,3-

Dimethylpentanedioic acid(3dmepdaH(2)): X-Ray Crystal Structures of [Cu(3dmepda)(bipy)](2). 6H(2)O and [Cu(2dmepda)(bipy)(EtOH)](2). 4EtOH (bipy = 2,2'Bipyridine). *Bioinorg Chem Appl*, 2006: p. 80283.

[157] Deegan, C., Coyle, B., McCann, M., Devereux, M., y Egan, D.A., In vitro anti-tumour effect of 1,10-phenanthroline-5,6-dione (phendione), [Cu(phendione)3](ClO4)2.4H2O and [Ag(phendione)2]ClO4 using human epithelial cell lines. *Chem Biol Interact,* 2006. 164(1-2): p. 115-25.

[158] Deegan, C., McCann, M., Devereux, M., Coyle, B., y Egan, D.A., In vitro cancer chemotherapeutic activity of 1,10-phenanthroline (phen), [Ag2(phen)3(mal)]x2H2O, [Cu(phen)2(mal)]x2H2O and [Mn(phen)2(mal)]x2H2O (malH2=malonic acid) using human cancer cells. *Cancer Lett*, 2007. 247(2): p. 224-33.

[159] Ruiz-Azuara, L.,Preparation of new mixed copper aminoacidate complexes from phenylate phenathrolines to be used as "anticancerigenic" agents. 07/628,628: Re 35,458. 1992, USA

[160] Ruiz-Azuara, L.,Copper amino acidate diimine nitrate compounds and their methyl derivatives and a process for preparing them. 07/628,628: 5,576,326. 1996, United States Patent

[161] Ruiz-Azuara, L.,Procedimiento para la obtención de complejos metálicos como agentes anticancerígenos. 172248. 1990, México

[162] Ruiz-Azuara, L.,Process to obtain new mixed copper aminoacidate complexes from phenylatephenanthroline to be used as anticancerigenic agents. 07/628,843: RE 35,458, Feb. 18 (1997). 1992, United States Patent

[163] Ruiz-Azuara, L.,Procedimiento para la obtención de complejos metálicos como agentes anticancerígenos. 18802. 1993, México

[164] Solans, X., Ruíz-Ramírez, L., Martínez, A., Gasque, L., y Moreno-Esparza, R., Mixed chelate complexes. II. Structures of L-alaninato(aqua)(4,7-diphenyl-1,10-phenanthroline)copper(II) nitrite monohydrate and aqua(4,7-dimethyl-1,10-phenanthroline)(glycinato)(nitrato)copper(II) monohydrate. *Acta Cryst C,* 1993. 49: p. 890-893.

[165] Tovar-Tovar, A., Ruiz-Ramirez, L., Campero, A., Romerosa, A., Moreno-Esparza, R., y Rosales-Hoz, M.J., Structural and reactivity studies on 4,4'-dimethyl-2,2'-bipyridine acetylacetonate copper(II) nitrate (CASIOPEINA III-ia®) with methionine, by UV-visible and EPR techniques. *J Inorg Biochem*, 2004. 98(6): p. 1045-1053.

[166] McBryde, W.A.E., Brisbin, D.A., y Irving, H., The stability of metal complexes of 1,10-phenanthroline and its analogues. Part III. 5-Methyl-1,10-phenanthroline. *J. Chem. Soc.*, 1962: p. 5245-5253.

[167] Mellor, H.I.a.D.H., The stability of Metal complexes of 1,10-phenanthroline and its analogues. Part II. 2-methyl- and 2,9-dimethyl-phenanthroline. *J Chem Soc,* 1962: p. 5237 - 5245.

[168] Mellor, H.I.a.D.H., The stability of Metal complexes of 1,10-phenanthroline and its analogues. Part I. 1,10-Phenanthroline and 2,2'-bipyridyl. *J Chem Soc*, 1962: p. 5222-5237.

[169] Chikira, M., Tomizawa, Y., Fukita, D., Sugizaki, T., Sugawara, N., Yamazaki, T., Sasano, A., Shindo, H., Palaniandavar, M., y Antholine, W.E., DNA-fiber EPR study of the orientation of Cu(II) complexes of 1,10-phenanthroline and its derivatives bound to

DNA: mono(phenanthroline)-copper(II) and its ternary complexes with amino acids. *J Inorg Biochem*, 2002. 89(3-4): p. 163-73.

[170] Gasque, L., Moreno-Esparza, R., y Ruiz-Ramírez, L., Stability of Ternary Copper and Nickel Complexes with 1,10-phenanthroline. *J Inorg Biochem*, 1992. 48: p. 121-127

[171] Kwik, W.L., Ang, K.P., y Chen, G., Complexes of (2,2′-bipyridyl) copper(II) and (1,10-phenanthroline) copper(II) with some amino acids. *J Inorg Nuclear Chem*, 1980. 42(2): p. 303-313.

[172] Alvarez-Larena, A., Briansó-Penalva, J.L., Piniella, J.F., Moreno-Esparza, R., Ruiz-Ramírez, L., y Ferrer-Sueta, G., Aqua(glycinato)(3,4,7,8-tetramethyl-1,10-phenanthroline)copper(II) Nitrate. Acta Cryst. C, 1995. 51: p. 852-854.

[173] Gasque, L., Moreno-Esparza, R., Ruiz-Ramírez, L., y Medina-Dickinson, G., Aqua(4,7-diphenyl-1,10-phenanthroline)(salicylaldehydato)copper(II) nitrate monohydrate. *Acta Cryst. C*, 1999. 55: p. 1065-1067

[174] Gasque, L., Moreno-Esparza, R., Ruiz-Ramírez, L., y Medina-Dickinson, G., (5,6-Dimethyl-1,10-phenanthroline)(nitrato)(salicylaldehydato)copper(II). Acta Cryst. C, 1999. 55: p. 1063-1065

[175] Moreno-Esparza, R., Escalante-Tovar, S., y Ruiz-Ramirez, L., DNA-planar copper complexes interaction, - stacking vs H bond. Acta Cryst. A, 2002. A58 (Supplement): p. C18

[176] Moreno-Esparza, R., Molins, E., Briansó-Penalva, J.L., Ruiz-Ramírez, L., y Redón, R., Aqua(1,10-phenanthroline)(L-serinato)copper(II) Nitrate. *Acta Cryst. C,* 1995. 51: p. 1505-1508

[177] Solans, X., Ruiz-Ramírez, L., Gasque, L., y Briansó, J.L., Structure of (1,10-phenanthroline)(salicylaldehydato)copper(II) nitrate. *Acta Cryst. C*, 1987. 43: p. 428-430

[178] Solans, X., Ruiz-Ramirez, L., Martinez, A., Gasque, L., y Brianso, J.L., Structures of chloro(glycinato)(1,10-phenanthroline)copper(II) monohydrate (I) and aqua(1,10-phenanthroline)(L-phenylalaninato)copper(II) nitrate monohydrate (II). *Acta Cryst C*, 1988. 44 (Pt 4): p. 628-31.

[179] Solans, X., Ruíz-Ramírez, L., Martínez, A., Gasque, L., y Moreno-Esparza, R., *Mixed chelate complexes. III.* Structures of (L-alaninato)(aqua)(2,2'-bipyridine)copper(II) nitrate monohydrate and aqua(2,2'-bipyridine)(L-tyrosinato)copper(II) chloride trihydrate. *Acta Cryst. C*, 1992. 48: p. 1785-1788

[180] Venkatraman, R., Zubkowski, J.D., y Valente, E.J., Aqua(1,10-phenanthroline)(L-prolinato)copper(II) nitrate monohydrate. *Acta Cryst. C,* 1999. 55: p. 1241-1243

[181] Gasque, L., Medina, M., Ruiz-Ramírez, L., y Moreno-Esparza, R., Cu-O stretching frequency correlation with phenanthroline pKa values in mixed copper complexes. *Inorg Chimica Acta*, 1999. 288: p. 106-111.

[182] Martinez, A., Salcedo, R., Sansores, L.E., Medina, G., y Gasque, L., A density functional study of the reactivity and stability of mixed copper complexes. Is hardness the reason? *Inorg Chem*, 2001. 40(2): p. 301-6.

[183] Gracia-Mora, I., Ruiz-Ramírez, L., Gómez-Ruiz, C., Tinoco-Méndez, M., Márquez-Quiñones, A., Romero-De Lira, L., Marín-Hernández, A., Macías-Rosales, L., y Bravo-Gómez, M.E., Knigth's Move in the Periodic Table, From Copper to Platinum, Novel Antitumor Mixed Chelate Copper Compounds, Casiopeinas, Evaluated by an in Vitro Human and Murine Cancer Cell Line Panel. *Metal-Based Drugs* 2001. 8(1): p. 19-28.

[184] Alemon-Medina, R., Brena-Valle, M., Munoz-Sanchez, J.L., Gracia-Mora, M.I., y Ruiz-Azuara, L., Induction of oxidative damage by copper-based antineoplastic drugs (Casiopeinas). *Cancer Chemother Pharmacol*, 2007. 60(2): p. 219-28.

[185] Sánchez-Bartéz, F. Tesis Maestro en Ciencias Químicas "Determinación de la capacidad genotóxica, citotóxica y citostática de las Casiopeínas Igli, IIgli y III-ia en linfocitos, médula ósea de ratón y linfocitos humanos en cultivo.". Asesor: Ruiz-Azuara, L. Universidad Nacional Autónoma de México, 2006.

[186] Ruiz-Ramírez, L., de la Rosa, M.E., Gracia-Mora, I., Mendoza, A., Pérez, G., Ferrer-Sueta, G., Tovar, A., Breña, M., Gutierrez, P., Cruces Martínez, M.P., Pimentel, E., y Natarajan, A.T., Casiopeinas, metal-based drugs a new class of antineoplastic and genotoxic compounds. *J Inorg Biochem*, 1995. 59(2-3): p. 207.

[187] Lena Ruiz-Ramírez, Isabel Gracia-Mora, Ma.Esther de la Rosa, Hector Sumano, Celedonio Gómez, Francisco Arenas, Eusebio Gómez, Emilio Pimentel, y Cruces, M., Cytostatic, mutagenic, antineoplastic activities and preliminar toxicity of copper (II) new drugs: Casiopeinas I, II, III. *J Inorg Biochem*, 1993. 51(1-2): p. 406.

[188] De Vizcaya-Ruiz, A., Rivero-Muller, A., Ruiz-Ramirez, L., Kass, G.E., Kelland, L.R., Orr, R.M., y Dobrota, M., Induction of apoptosis by a novel copper-based anticancer compound, casiopeina II, in L1210 murine leukaemia and CH1 human ovarian carcinoma cells. *Toxicol In Vitro*, 2000. 14(1): p. 1-5.

[189] Mejia, C. y Ruiz-Azuara, L., Casiopeinas IIgly and IIIia Induce Apoptosis in Medulloblastoma Cells. *Pathol Oncol Res*, 2008.

[190] Hernandez-Esquivel, L., Marin-Hernandez, A., Pavon, N., Carvajal, K., y Moreno-Sanchez, R., Cardiotoxicity of copper-based antineoplastic drugs casiopeinas is related to inhibition of energy metabolism. *Toxicol Appl Pharmacol,* 2006. 212(1): p. 79-88.

[191] Marin-Hernandez, A., Gracia-Mora, I., Ruiz-Ramirez, L., y Moreno-Sanchez, R., Toxic effects of copper-based antineoplastic drugs (Casiopeinas) on mitochondrial functions. *Biochem Pharmacol,* 2003. 65(12): p. 1979-89.

[192] Dias, N. y Bailly, C., Drugs targeting mitochondrial functions to control tumor cell growth. *Biochem Pharmacol*, 2005. 70(1): p. 1-12.

[193] Rodriguez-Enriquez, S., Vital-Gonzalez, P.A., Flores-Rodriguez, F.L., Marin-Hernandez, A., Ruiz-Azuara, L., y Moreno-Sanchez, R., Control of cellular proliferation by modulation of oxidative phosphorylation in human and rodent fast-growing tumor cells. *Toxicol Appl Pharmacol*, 2006. 215(2): p. 208-17.

[194] Budihardjo, I., Oliver, H., Lutter, M., Luo, X., y Wang, X., Biochemical pathways of caspase activation during apoptosis. *Annu Rev Cell Dev Biol*, 1999. 15: p. 269-90.

[195] Rivero-Muller, A., De Vizcaya-Ruiz, A., Plant, N., Ruiz, L., y Dobrota, M., Mixed chelate copper complex, Casiopeina IIgly, binds and degrades nucleic acids: a mechanism of cytotoxicity. *Chem Biol Interact,* 2007. 165(3): p. 189-99.

[196] Alemon-Medina, R., Munoz-Sanchez, J.L., Ruiz-Azuara, L., y Gracia-Mora, I., Casiopeina IIgly induced cytotoxicity to HeLa cells depletes the levels of reduced glutathione and is prevented by dimethyl sulfoxide. *Toxicol In Vitro*, 2008. 22(3): p. 710-5.

[197] Yu, S.W., Wang, H., Poitras, M.F., Coombs, C., Bowers, W.J., Federoff, H.J., Poirier, G.G., Dawson, T.M., y Dawson, V.L., Mediation of poly(ADP-ribose) polymerase-1-dependent cell death by apoptosis-inducing factor. *Science*, 2002. 297(5579): p. 259-63.

[198] Bunz, F., Hwang, P.M., Torrance, C., Waldman, T., Zhang, Y., Dillehay, L., Williams, J., Lengauer, C., Kinzler, K.W., y Vogelstein, B., Disruption of p53 in human cancer cells alters the responses to therapeutic agents. *J Clin Invest*, 1999. 104(3): p. 263-9.

[199] Costanzo, A., Merlo, P., Pediconi, N., Fulco, M., Sartorelli, V., Cole, P.A., Fontemaggi, G., Fanciulli, M., Schiltz, L., Blandino, G., Balsano, C., y Levrero, M., DNA damage-dependent acetylation of p73 dictates the selective activation of apoptotic target genes. *Mol Cell,* 2002. 9(1): p. 175-86.

[200] De Vizcaya-Ruiz, A., Rivero-Muller, A., Ruiz-Ramirez, L., Howarth, J.A., y Dobrota, M., Hematotoxicity response in rats by the novel copper-based anticancer agent: casiopeina II. *Toxicol*, 2003. 194(1-2): p. 103-13.

[201] Peláez-Sánchez, F.M. Tesis "Cinética de inhibición y recuperación de la proliferación celular de líneas tumorales y linfocitos humanos tratados con Casiopeína® IIgly y Casiopeína III-ia". Asesor: Gracia-Mora, I. and Bravo-Gomez, M.E. Universidad Nacional Autónoma de México, 2008.

[202] Asano, R., Kaseda, M., y Hokari, S., [The effect of copper and copper . o-phenanthroline complex on cattle erythrocytes.]. *Nippon Juigaku Zasshi*, 1983. 45(1): p. 77-83.

[203] Leal-Garcia, M., Garcia-Ortuno, L., Ruiz-Azuara, L., Gracia-Mora, I., Luna-Delvillar, J., y Sumano, H., Assessment of acute respiratory and cardiovascular toxicity of casiopeinas in anaesthetized dogs. *Basic Clin Pharmacol Toxicol,* 2007. 101(3): p. 151-8.

In: New Approaches in the Treatment of Cancer
Editors: Carmen Mejia Vazquez et al. pp.173-201
ISBN 978-1-62100-067-9

Chapter VIII

GENE THERAPY FOR CANCER TREATMENT

***Irma Alicia Martínez-Dávila*[1] *and Iván Delgado Enciso*[2,3,*]**
[1]Royal Free Hospital, Medical School, University College London, London, UK
[2]School of Medicine, University of Colima, México
[3]Instituto Estatal de Cancerología, Colima, México

ABSTRACT

Gene therapy is a new tool used in combating different diseases. It began to be intensely used in research projects in 1989 and important advances have been made in this therapy since then. The majority of gene therapy clinical trials are focused on cancer and so it was no coincidence that the first commercial gene treatment in 2003 was for a neoplasia. Nevertheless, some unfavorable events have been observed in the use of this therapy resulting in its strict surveillance and in the promotion of creating safer therapeutic regimens. Currently there are a wide variety of gene therapy proposals involving a large number of antitumor molecular mechanisms that will conceivably pave the way for highly effective treatment options. Despite the significant advances that have been made in gene therapy in the fight against cancer, its efficacy, safety and commercial availability are still limited. These limitations are expected to gradually be overcome.

INTRODUCTION

Cancer is a disease characterized by an accelerated and uncontrolled growth of cells that have the capacity to spread throughout the body and affect vital organ function. When detected at a late stage, cancer is generally fatal, therefore intensifying the search for new medication to help patients. Gene therapy appears to be an adequate antineoplastic strategy

* Correspondence concerning this article should be addressed to: Iván Delgado Enciso, School of Medicine, Universidad de Colima, Av. Universidad 333, Colonia Las Viboras, CP 28040, Colima, Col., Mexico. ivan_delgado_enciso@ucol.mx.

that currently plays an important role in research projects and has a promising future in clinical oncological practice.

DEFINITION OF GENE THERAPY

Gene therapy is the treatment or prevention of a disease that is carried out through the insertion of nucleotide sequences (DNA or RNA) into the cell. Genes that carry the information necessary to create a protein within the cell are usually introduced (figure 1) [1]. The purpose of this transference of genetic material or of genes is to reestablish a cellular function that had been abolished or become defective, to introduce a new function or to interfere in an existing function. A simple example would be the use of gene therapy in treating a disease caused by a defective gene in a patient's cells. This defective gene would produce a defective protein incapable of carrying out a certain function. With gene therapy, a normal gene could be introduced into the patient's cells that would produce the adequate protein and thus cure the disease. However, it is presently very difficult to substitute the function of a defective gene by replacing it with a new gene. Very few projects have successfully achieved this and there have been adverse effects that can be very serious [2].

The present development of gene therapy is directed towards somatic cells rather than germ cells. This ensures that genetic transference only affects the individual and not his or her offspring [3]. Different gene therapy strategies are based on a combination of three key elements: the genetic material to be transferred, the transference method and the type of target cell.

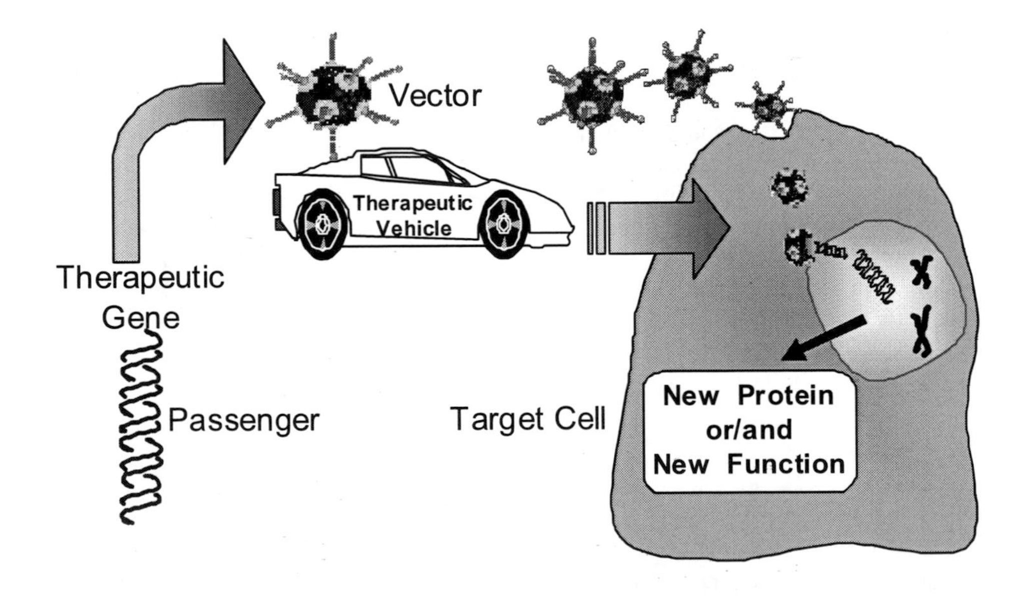

Figure 1. Gene therapy is based on the idea that genes or foreign sequences can be inserted into cells through "vehicles" or vectors. A vector acts as a carrier vehicle to deliver a therapeutic passenger into the target cell.

GENETIC MATERIAL TO BE TRANSFERRED

The majority of nucleotide sequences are genes, that is, sequences that will produce a functional protein within a cell. The therapeutic gene must carry out a function that helps fight a disease. In the case of disease caused by a defective (mutated) gene the intention is to introduce a normal gene. If new tissue is to be created a growth factor gene is inserted. In the case of cancer, the goal is to eliminate neoplastic cells or restrict their growth.

The following are the most common altered functions of cancerous cells: 1) uncontrolled accelerated growth capacity, 2) the spreading to and invasion of vital organs, 3) accelerated angiogenesis and 4) immune system evasion to avoid being eliminated [4]. Anticancer therapeutic genes will have to block these abilities of malignant cells or create cytotoxic effects that directly cause malignant cell death.

Over 220 different genes have been introduced into cells in human gene therapy trials [2]. The ones most commonly used against cancer are those that encode antigens or cytokines used to stimulate an immune response, tumor-suppressor genes (pro-apoptotic), suicide genes (that produce a direct toxic effect), anti-angiogenic genes and to a much lesser degree, antisense or short interfering RNA [2]. The latter two have the capacity to interfere and block the production of a chosen gene. Other very frequently used genes are the growth factor genes. Not used to fight cancer, they are almost all being aimed at cardiovascular diseases [2]. Once inside the cell, the genes or therapeutic sequences must become activated so that production of therapeutic proteins or interfering RNA molecules may begin. Genes are controlled by regulating sequences called promoters that allow this to take place. It can be said that a therapeutic gene will always be accompanied by a promoter that controls its "activation" or expression (see Targeting Gene Therapy to Cancer section).

TRANSFERENCE METHOD

Functional gene sequences are placed in vectors that serve as vehicles for transporting the sequences to the interior of the cell. Vectors types can be viral or non-viral [5]. The nucleotide sequence or therapeutic gene is inserted into the non-viral vector or into the genome of the viral vector using molecular biology and genetic manipulation techniques.

There are various types of non-viral vectors: 1) Naked DNA, which is generally a circular DNA (such as bacterial plasmid) that is injected directly into the tissues, 2) DNA surrounded by in cationic lipids which help it pass through the cellular membrane due to the membrane's liposoluble component, 3) DNA that is condensed in particles (or surrounded by them) that can be nanoparticles and 4) oligonucleotides (generally antisense RNA) to inactivate the genes involved in the disease process. Naked DNA is the most popular non-viral system used in clinical trials, followed by cationic lipid/DNA complexes [2]. This type of vector is not inserted into the cell with much efficiency and so its distribution is limited and relatively low levels of therapeutic protein are produced. Therefore it is used for inserting genes that can, with very little activity, produce significant responses - as is the case with growth factors in muscle. When dealing with cancer, elevated levels of therapeutic protein production are generally needed, as well as a wide vector distribution in cancerous tissue. Therefore the use of non-viral vectors is limited when working with cancer. Non-viral vectors would be useful in antineoplastic therapies that do not require large quantities of therapeutic protein or in which the gene does not act directly on the cancer as is the case in immune system stimulation by vaccines or immunotherapy.

Viral vectors are the most commonly used vectors to fight cancer [2]. In a general sense their order of importance when used against cancer is first adenovirus, followed by poxvirus, herpes simplex virus, retrovirus and adeno-associated virus. These viral vectors have been used in multiple clinical trials in humans presenting with different diseases. However, a large variety of other viruses may also be used as vectors. Each vector has different characteristics in relation to its tropism, activity duration, its integration or non-integration into cellular chromosomes and immunogenicity, to mention a few. Therefore it is very important to be aware of the behavior of the different types of viral vectors.

In gene therapy against cancer, the therapeutic gene is generally required to carry out its mission for only a certain amount of time. The toxic gene does not need to be active in a patient for his or her entire life. A very intense but transitory (weeks) effect is required to eliminate the greatest number of cancerous cells in which the vector and therapeutic gene also disappear after a period of time in order to limit their adverse effects. Of course in the case of immune system stimulation against cancer beneficial effects may be observed for years [6]. Retroviruses and adeno-associated viruses are capable of integrating or inserting their genomes into cellular chromosomes [7]. When this takes place, the therapeutic gene will remain active as long as the cell lives and it will be replicated and passed on to the cell descendants. This is ideal for correcting diseases in which a defective gene is substituted and therapeutic gene activity is sought after for the entire life of the patient, but it is not recommended for cancer treatment. The vector best suited for carrying out a proposed therapeutic idea may be selected for each gene therapy strategy. Even new vectors or combined fragments of different types of vectors to produce a chimera may be created.

Adenovirus

The most widely used vectors in gene therapy against cancer are adenoviruses. They make up a DNA genome virus family of at least 51 different serotypes. Type 5 is the most frequently used as a vector [8]. These viruses commonly cause diseases of the respiratory tract, primarily the upper tract. They may also cause gastroenteritis, conjunctivitis or cystitis, although the majority of these pathologies are self-limited and therefore not considered very dangerous. However, they may cause infections that spread in immunocompromised patients [7]. Adenoviruses enter the cells through the interaction of viral proteins (fiber protein) with cellular receptors (Coxsackie and adenovirus receptor –CAR- and integrins). The viruses enter through clathrin-coated pits and vesicles, after which the membranes of these vesicles (endosomes) are degraded in the cytoplasm leaving the viral particles in a free state. The particles are quickly transported toward the nucleus where only the DNA and a few proteins pass into its interior [8]. Once inside the nucleus, the adenoviral DNA begins to replicate. A gene therapy adenoviral vector will begin its activity of initiating the processes that culminate in therapeutic protein production. The DNA of these viruses does not integrate into the cellular chromosomes and so its activity is transitory (generally weeks).

Adenoviruses can infect a large variety of cellular types whether or not they are in active cellular division. This makes their use in gene therapy against cancer advantageous since they can be used in many different neoplasms regardless of their primary origin or the velocity of their growth. Adenoviruses are easily introduced into epithelium which makes them ideal for treating carcinomas. On the other hand, adenoviral vectors are not very useful in neoplasms of hematopoietic origin because it is difficult to introduce them into the majority of hematopoietic cells [8].

Adenoviral vector gene therapy can eliminate neoplastic cells through selective replication and/or through pro-apoptotic, anti-angiogenic, immunogenic or suicide gene expression [5]. Adenoviral vectors can be replication-deficient and be used exclusively for transporting genes, they may have a preferential replication in neoplastic cells and cause tumor lysis or they may combine these two mechanisms. Another advantage of adenoviruses is the immune response they trigger to fight against infected neoplastic cells. These vectors are capable of generating a significant antitumor response in immunocompetent individuals, even in the absence of replication or therapeutic gene expression [9]. In immunocompetent murine models of cancer, intratumorally injected adenoviruses have been shown to set an acute inflammatory response in motion, resulting in an improved therapeutic response [10]. However this characteristic turns into a limitation when multiple doses are required at different periods since the vector would be eliminated more rapidly in subsequent applications and/or its toxicity (principally hepatic) at high vector doses would be strengthened [11,12]. However, if the immune response against the adenovirus is to be reduced, multiple strategies have been devised to achieve that [13].

Finally, it is worth mentioning that the so-called helper-dependent adenovirus vectors have been developed, which are completely devoid of all viral protein-coding sequences. These modifications have significantly reduced the immunogenicity of adenoviral vectors and have enhanced their safety. In addition, they possess a considerably larger capacity to transfer large DNA or multiple genes and mediate longer high-level gene expression [14].

The adenovirus vector system has shown real promise in treating cancer and it is not surprising that the first gene therapy product to be licensed to treat cancer uses an adenovirus.

Poxviruses

Poxviruses represent a heterogeneous group of DNA viruses that have been utilized to transport a multitude of foreign genes. Vaccinia virus is the prototypical recombinant poxvirus [15]. Vaccinia virus has been used as a vaccine for smallpox for more than 150 years and there is great experience in its clinical use. Poxviruses can infect a broad range of cells, have a genome that can accommodate large DNA inserts (multiple genes), replicate entirely in the cytoplasm of the host cell with high efficiency (with rapid cell-to-cell spread), do not have the possibility of chromosomal integration and elicit strong immune responses. These factors make them especially well-suited as vaccines for the prevention and treatment of human immunodeficiency virus (HIV) and cancer [16-18]. Vaccinia virus has been used as (1) a delivery vehicle for anti-cancer genes, (2) a vaccine carrier for tumor-associated antigens and immunoregulatory molecules in cancer immunotherapy, and (3) an oncolytic agent that selectively replicates in and lyses cancer cells [19].

Certain highly attenuated, host-restricted, non- or poorly replicating poxvirus strains have been developed as vectors for transporting therapeutic genes. Two of the most promising poxvirus vectors for human use are the vaccinia virus Ankara (MVA) and the Copenhagen derived NYVAC strains (both Orthopoxviruses) [20]. Certain avipoxviruses are also used, such as ALVAC (derived from the canarypox virus) and TROVAC (derived from fowlpox viruses) [21].

However, news strains of Vaccinia virus with great replicative capacity are beginning to be used for treating cancer [22]. These vectors selectively replicate in and lyses cancer cells, and at the same time are able to transport therapeutic genes. Initial preclinical and clinical results show that products from this therapeutic class can systemically target cancers in a highly selective and potent fashion using a multi-pronged action mechanism [23]. JX-594 vector is an example of this and is a targeted oncolytic poxvirus designed to selectively replicate in and destroy cancer cells with cell-cycle abnormalities and epidermal growth factor receptor (EGFR)-Ras pathway activation [24].

Herpes Simplex Virus

Herpes simplex viruses (HSV) belong to the subfamily of Alphaherpesvirinae, which cause infections in humans. Herpes viruses consist of a relatively large linear DNA genome of double-stranded [7]. Type 1 virus is the virus most frequently used as a vector for gene therapy. Herpes simplex begins its life cycle by binding heparan sulfate, a proteoglycan found on the surface of many cell types. It subsequently interacts with one of several cellular receptors closer to the cell surface and fusion with the cell membrane occurs. Once inside the cell, the virus travels along the host cytoskeleton to the nucleus, where its replication begins or where its therapeutic gene expression begins if it is a vector.

HSV is highly infectious, so HSV vectors are efficient vehicles for the delivery of exogenous genetic material to cells. They do not have the possibility of integrating into cellular chromosomes. Latent infection with wild-type virus results in episomal viral persistence in sensory neuronal nuclei for the duration of the host lifetime. Transduction with replication-defective vectors causes a latent-like infection in both neural and non-neural tissue; the vectors are non-pathogenic, unable to reactivate and persist long-term. The latency can be exploited in vector design to achieve long-term stable therapeutic gene expression in the nervous system [25].

Non-neurotropic viral gene transfer vectors (e.g., adenovirus, adeno-associated virus, and lentivirus) do not spread very far in the nervous system, and consequently these vectors transduce brain regions mostly near the injection site in adult animals. This indicates that numerous, well-spaced injections with these vectors would be required to achieve widespread transduction in a large brain. In contrast, HSV-1 is a promising vector for widespread gene transfer to the brain owing to the innate ability of the virus to spread through the nervous system [26].

HSV vectors are ideal for the neural system and thanks to their natural tropism their usefulness is even greater since they are capable of entering a broad range of tissues because of the wide expression pattern of cellular receptors recognized by the virus. These vectors are also capable of targeting non-dividing as well as dividing tumor cells [27]. Vectors derived from HSV-1 may be replication-deficient (utilized to carry long sequences of foreign DNA) or like adenoviral or Vaccinia vectors may be capable of selectively replicating themselves and lysing cancerous cells. Defective and non-integrative vectors derived from HSV-1 known as amplicons also exist [28]. They carry no viral genes in the vector genome and therefore are not toxic to the infected cells or pathogenic for the transduced organisms, making them safer to use [28]. In addition, the large transgenic capacity of amplicons, which allows delivery of ≤ 150 Kbp of foreign DNA, makes these vectors some of the most powerful, interesting and versatile gene delivery platforms [29].

HSV vectors have been used as transporters of anti-angiogenic agents, immune enhancing proteins, pro-drug activating enzymes, and apoptosis-inducing factors, as well as inhibitory RNA for tumor-associated messages. Similar to adenoviruses, HSV-1 derived vectors themselves appear to have intrinsic immune-enhancing properties which can be considered an advantage in cancer treatment [27].

Retroviruses

Retroviral genetic material is in the form of RNA. When a retrovirus infects a host cell, it will introduce its RNA together with some enzymes (reverse transcriptase and integrase) into the cell. This RNA molecule from the retrovirus must produce a DNA copy from its RNA molecule before it can be integrated into the cell chromosomes [30]. The genetic material of the virus is then inserted into the cell genome and becomes part of the genetic material of the host cell. If this host cell later divides, its descendants will all contain the new genes inserted by the virus.

One of the problems of using retroviruses in gene therapy is that the integrase enzyme can insert the genetic material of the virus into any arbitrary location in the cell genome. If the insertion of viral genetic material occurs in the middle of or very near a cellular gene, the function of that gene is respectively blocked or over-stimulated [30]. If that gene is important for proliferation regulation, uncontrolled cell division can occur along with a potential cancer risk. This problem has been resolved by modifying retroviruses to direct the site of integration to specific chromosomal sites. Gene therapy trials using retroviral vectors have demonstrated a great potential for curing diseases such as X-linked severe combined immunodeficiency (X-SCID), but the appearance of leukemia as a consequence of its use in patients treated in the French X-SCID gene therapy trial has also been documented [2].

Retrovirus use has been suggested for anti-tumor immunotherapy in cancer. Lentiviral vectors, a type of retrovirus, have been carefully examined as gene transfer vehicles for modification of dendritic cells and have been demonstrated to induce potent T cell mediated immune responses that can control tumor growth [31]. In contrast to all other retroviruses, lentivirus can infect cell types independently of whether or not they are in active cell division. The use of lentiviral vectors for transferring RNA molecules that interfere with protein production necessary for neoplastic cell proliferation is also being studied [32,33]. However, these vectors are not widely used as antitumor agents.

Adeno-associated Virus

Adeno-associated viruses from the parvovirus family are small viruses with a genome of single stranded DNA. They can infect dividing and non-dividing cells. Wild type adeno-associated viruses can insert genetic material at a specific site on chromosome 19 with almost 100% certainty [7,34]. Because they can integrate into cellular chromosomes they are useful principally in treating diseases that require gene activity for long periods of time. However, some modified adeno-associated viral vectors which do not contain any viral genes but only the therapeutic gene, do not integrate into the cellular genome. They are mainly used for muscle and eye diseases, although they are beginning to be used to deliver genes to the brain. An important aspect of this is that people treated with adeno-associated viral vectors will not build up an immune response to remove the virus. This is very good when therapeutic gene activity is required for long periods of time or when multiple applications over a period of time are required because an immune response that would eliminate the vector in future applications is not created.

Although this vector is not used very often in gene therapy against cancer because of its safety profile shown in clinical trials for other kinds of diseases [34,35], its usefulness in the transport of immunostimulatory gene or pro-apoptotic genes in neoplastic cells is beginning to be explored [36].

Other Vectors and the Ideal Vector

New viruses or naked vector designs appear every year. New proteins or other molecules for bringing different vectors together to facilitate their entrance into cells are being looked for. Different viral strains have been suggested as potential vector backbones, including baculoviruses, Newcastle disease virus, reovirus, vesicular stomatitis virus, polio virus, Sindbis virus, picornavirus, mumps and measles virus and many of them are progressing to clinical trials [37].

Other types of vectors currently being researched include nonviral biological agents (bacteria, bacteriophage, virus-like particles or VLPs, erythrocyte ghosts, and exosomes). Exploiting the natural properties of these biological entities for specific gene delivery applications will complement the established techniques for gene therapy applications. A detailed description of these vectors has been recently published [38].

To decide which vector is ideal, different factors must be taken into consideration. When a vector for gene therapy is designed, researchers carry out the genetic changes necessary for the vector to perform a particular function or activity. Each type of vector has very special biological characteristics. Depending on the activity or function to be carried out, the most adequate vector is chosen to successfully achieve its purpose. Virus toxicity, tropism, the amount of vector entering the cells, whether it integrates into chromosome cells or not, replication capacity and velocity, if it unleashes an immune response, the facility with which it can be genetically manipulated and produced in the laboratory, etc., are all factors that are taken into consideration. The vector meeting all the particular requirements of a certain therapeutic strategy will be the ideal vector for that activity. A vector characteristic that is an advantage for a certain therapeutic strategy can be a disadvantage if used in a different strategy. Vectors are improved every year and are adapting more and more to therapeutic necessities. Just as with any vehicle, the ideal vehicle or vector is always waiting to be designed.

TARGET CELL: TARGETING GENE THERAPY TO CANCER

Neoplastic cells have molecular characteristics that distinguish them from normal cells. They have an elevated activity of genes in charge of: 1) accelerating growth and/or inhibiting apoptosis (cell death), 2) degrading the extracellular matrix (to spread itself), 3) accelerating angiogenesis and 4) regulating the immune system to evade it, among others [4]. In a similar way, cancerous cells may possess no activity or low activity of genes in charge of the functions contrary to those just mentioned. Their cellular membrane may also have changes in proportion and types of receptors. These alterations are consequences of changes in the patterns of gene expression or "activation". These molecular peculiarities are taken advantage of to create specific gene therapy strategies against cancer. The idea is to eliminate the cancer by modifying cellular and molecular functions that characterize and maintain the life of neoplastic cells.

One of the advantages of gene therapy with respect to traditional chemotherapy or radiotherapy is the capacity to selectively eliminate neoplastic cells while causing the least possible damage to healthy tissue. Ideally it should also be capable of acting at the systemic level to attack both the primary tumor and metastatic deposits [39]. Molecular characteristics of cancer can serve as a flag to mark the neoplastic cell so that it can preferentially be attacked by gene therapy vectors (targeting). There are various strategies for directing the therapeutic gene to fight cancer [39].

Targeted Delivery

Delivery of the vector directly to the tumor site by intratumoral injection is the simplest manner to direct therapy towards the cancer and thereby largely avoids normal tissues [39]. This option is not useful in systemic treatments or when the tumor is not visible, as in metastasis.

The transfer of genes is entirely dependent on the interaction between the vector and target cell surface [8]. There are differences in the efficiency of each vector for entering into cells. Another simple strategy includes the exploitation of natural viral tropisms, such as those exhibited by adenoviruses to target lung epithelium cancer or by herpes simplex virus to target the nervous system. However, the interaction that naturally occurs between the vector and target cell surface can be modified in order to increase the entrance of the vectors into the cells and/or redirect their tropism (figure 2). Many cancerous cells have an elevated quantity of certain types of receptors in their membranes. A good example is the large quantity of human epidermal growth factor receptor type 2 (HER2) in some types of breast cancer [40]. The proteins of the viral vectors in charge of interaction with cell receptors can be modified so that they specifically unite with a receptor that is mainly found in cancerous cells. Similarly, naked DNA, and even some viral vectors, can form complexes with proteins (like antibodies) or biomolecules, that when acting as specific ligands, facilitate their entrance into a particular type of neoplastic cell through a compatible receptor (figure 2). An example of this is the recent design of an adenovirus that has been modified in its exterior structure so that it is capable of selective delivery of a gene to HER2 positive cancer cells [40].

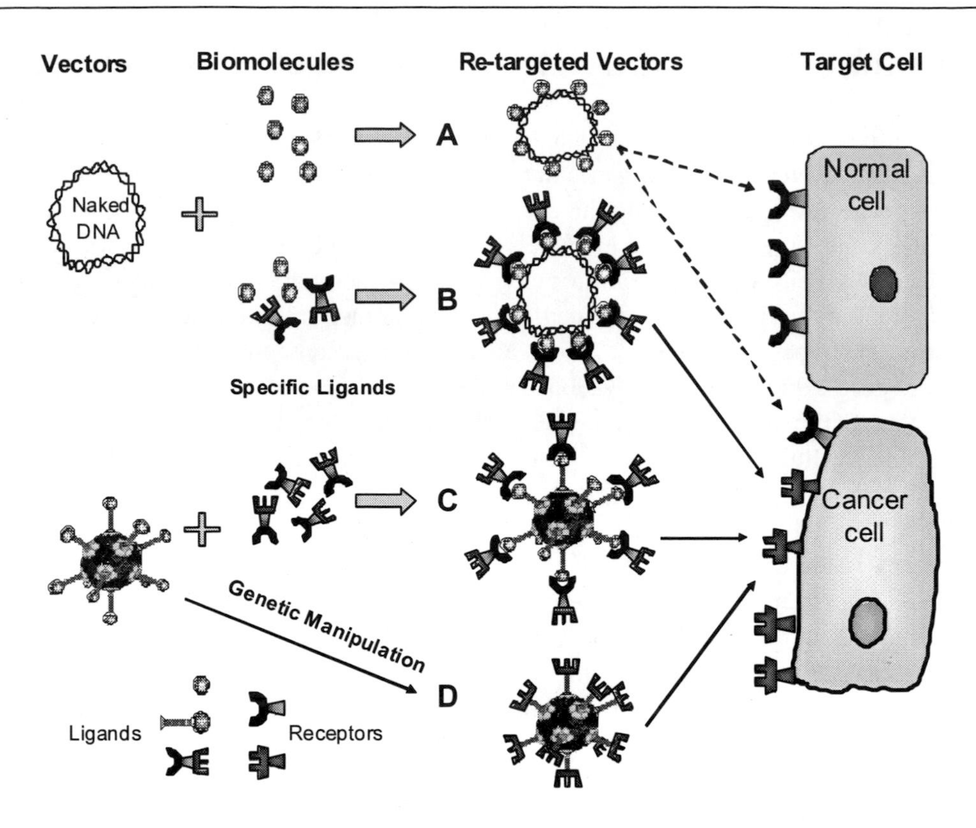

Figure 2. Strategies to target both viral and nonviral delivery agents to tumor cells. These include redirecting vectors A) using biomolecules to direct naked DNA to target cells; B and C) using tissue or cancer-specific ligands or monoclonal antibodies incorporated onto the surface of DNA complexes or viral vectors to change native tropism (redirecting virus to a cancer-specific receptor); D) genetically modifying the virus to ablate native receptor interactions and incorporating a novel ligand into one of the coat proteins of the virus.

Targeted Expression

In a general manner it can be said that a gene is a functional DNA unit that carries codified information and that will make later protein or RNA sequence production possible. The gene contains both "coding" sequences (cDNA) that determine what it does, and "non-coding" sequences that determine when it is active (expressed). In human cells, a gene produces an RNA chain in the nucleus (transcription) that later is translated into a protein in the ribosomes. The expression process involves all the necessary steps for proteins or functional RNA sequences to be produced from the information contained in a gene. A gene is said to have a high level of expression or is over-expressed when large quantities of RNA or protein proceeding from that gene are detected. The promoter is a non-coding region of DNA that regulates when and where a gene is active as well as the quantity of RNA to be produced. In other words, it regulates gene expression [39]. Although other processes may be involved in controlling gene pattern expression, generally it is promoter activity that is principally responsible for its regulation.

In a cancerous cell there are alterations in the expression levels of many genes. There is an over-expression of genes that accelerates the rhythm of cellular growth and an underexpression of genes that blocks growth or favors cell death. In cancer, many promoters responsible for gene over-expression can be used to control therapeutic gene expression within a gene therapy vector. These promoters would be very active in the cancer and would hardly function outside the cancer or the type of tissue giving rise to the neoplasm. A classical example is prostate-specific antigen. It is mainly produced in prostate cells and it increases greatly when these cells are neoplastic – when their promoter is prostate-specific (tissue-specific). It is also very active in prostate cancer (cancer-specific). On the other hand, there can be a vector transporting a gene that produces a toxic protein and promotes cell death. If the toxic gene expression of the vector is controlled by the prostate-specific antigen promoter, the toxic gene will be over-expressed when the vector enters the prostate cancer cells and will for all purposes is inactive if it enters a healthy cell or the cell of another tissue [39]. It will then be possible for this vector to selectively cause the death of tumor cells without affecting healthy tissue.

These cancer-specific promoters or promoters that are very active in cancer may be used to control the expression of any gene or interference RNA that provokes tumor cell death. Moreover, these promoters may be used to control the expression of genes that have a key role in viral vector replication so they can be converted into oncolytic viruses. These vectors replicate themselves selectively in malignant cells, provoking their death (see Oncolytic Agents section). Other expression control mechanisms have also been used in gene therapy against cancer, although to a much smaller degree.

Therapeutic Genes

Even though a gene has the same function in healthy tissue as in cancerous tissue, its activity can affect each type of tissue differently. The therapeutic gene function itself can, to a certain extent, direct its effect towards neoplastic cells. A gene whose product is toxic for cells in proliferation will more intensely affect malignant cells simply because their growth is more accelerated than that of healthy cells. A product that inhibits angiogenesis will have a greater effect in tissues where there is greater formation of new vessels, such as in tumors. However, there are strategies in which the therapeutic gene really directs its effect mainly towards malignant cells. A large number of tumors are secondary to viral oncogenic activity. Neoplasms that are associated with oncogenic viruses express a large quantity of viral proteins that are hardly ever found in healthy cells. These types of protein, viral or not, are called tumor associated antigens (TAA). In experimental animals, the application of vectors transporting TAA genes, along with immunostimulatory genes, has been able to awaken an important specific immune response against TAA-associated cancer, although evaluation of this type of vector in clinical trials has not indicated exceptional tumor protection in a large percentage of patients. Despite this, there is hope for the advent of effective treatment modalities that will prolong tumor-free survival and enhance the quality of life in patients with malignant disease [41].

ACTION MECHANISMS OF GENE THERAPY TO FIGHT CANCER

Various strategies may be developed to eliminate cancerous cells by combining therapeutic genes, the type of vector and the way in which the therapy is directed towards the cancer. Not unlike car designers, only researcher creativity is the limit for creating the best gene vehicle with the best performance.

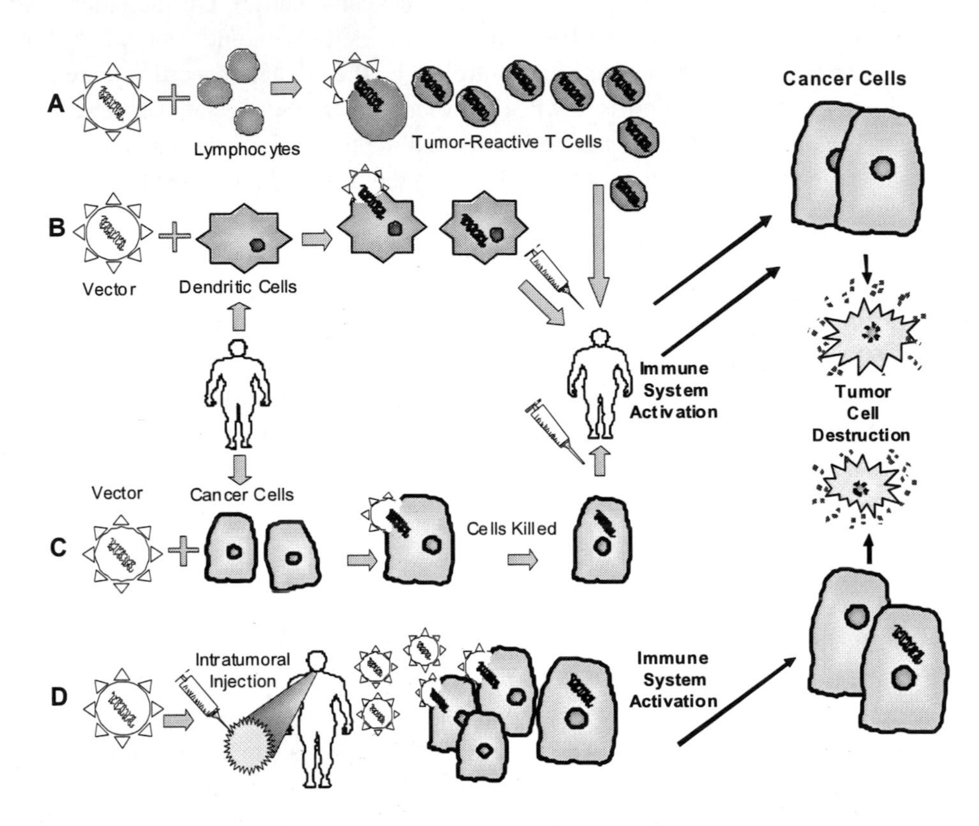

Figure 3. Schematic diagram of immunotherapy. Pathway A represents adoptive therapy using TCR gene therapy. Pathway B represents vaccination with dendritic cells expressing a tumor-associated antigen. Pathway C represents immunotherapy with modified cancer cells. Pathway D represents vaccination with immunostimulatory genes *in vivo.*

Immunotherapy

The establishment of cancer involves not only the escape of tumor cells from normal growth control but also their escape from immunological recognition. The main objective of immunotherapy is to control or eliminate tumors by enhancing the host's immune response to tumor antigens. The term "immunogene therapy" can be defined as genetically manipulating tumor cells or dendritic cells in order to stimulate antitumor immunity; the genes can be transferred *in situ* or *ex vivo* as part of the preparation of an anticancer vaccine (figure 3). Immunogene therapy is emerging as one of the promising treatment modalities for malignant tumors [42].

On the other hand, adoptive transfer of antigen-specific T lymphocytes is an alternative form of immunotherapy for cancer. In this case the strategy relies on cloned T cell receptor (TCR) genes that can be used to produce T lymphocyte populations of desired specificity to recognize cancer antigens and mediate cancer regression *in vivo* [43,44].

Thus, specific strategies of immunotherapy that have been employed to enhance antitumor responses can be grouped into 1) cancer vaccines and 2) adoptive therapy using antigen-specific T lymphocyte transfer (TCR gene therapy).

Cancer Vaccines:

These are used to stimulate both innate immunity and specific immune effectors responses to empower stronger tumor-specific responses. These kinds of vaccines include a) vaccination with tumor cells engineered to express immunostimulatory molecules [45], b) vaccination with recombinant viral vectors encoding tumor antigens [46], c) vaccination with dendritic cells expressing tumor antigens [47,48] and d) naked DNA vaccines [42,49].

The following are various examples of cancer vaccines:

a) Vaccination with Tumor Cells Engineered to Express Immunostimulatory Molecules:

With the use of gene transfer strategies, tumor cells or fibroblasts have been genetically modified *ex vivo* to express high levels of genes encoding for immunostimulatory molecules such as cytokines. This strategy has been considered an attractive tool to induce immune responses against the tumor because of the paracrine adjuvant effects of tumor-released cytokines in the absence of systemic toxic effects [49,50].

Cytokines can impede tumor growth and activate innate and adaptive immune responses, leading to the elimination of cancer cells. Many studies have validated the therapeutic potential of manipulating the cytokine balance in the tumor microenvironment to promote immune-mediated tumor destruction. Cytokine genes that have been used for immunogene therapy of cancer include IL-2, IL-4, IL-7, IL-12, IL-15, IL-18, INFα, INFβ, INFγ, GM-CSF and TNFα alone or combined with genes encoding co-stimulatory molecules, such as B7-1 [51-58]. *In vivo* administration of these immunomodulatory molecules has been extensively investigated in experimental tumor models and is currently being applied in a number of clinical trials [59-61]. Granulocyte macrophage colony stimulating factor (GM-CSF) stimulates the recruitment, maturation and function of dendritic cells, the most potent antigen-presenting cells with the capacity to interact with T cells and initiate their response [62-64]. GM-CSF has been identified in murine models as one of the most potent immunostimulatory molecules that enhance host responses, following gene transfer into tumor cells [65]. Clinical trials of vaccination with irradiated tumor cells engineered to secrete GM-CSF (autologous tumor cells were engineered to secrete GM-CSF by either retroviral or adenoviral mediated gene transfer) were undertaken in patients with solid and hematologic malignancies [66-69]. Although these studies revealed the induction of humoral and cellular reactions that effectuated substantial tumor destruction, most subjects eventually succumbed to progressive disease, implicating the existence of additional immune defects that remain to be addressed. However, the strong evidence for enhanced tumor immunity together with the lack of significant toxicity formed the basis for advancing this vaccination strategy to advanced clinical trials in several diseases [45].

b) Vaccination with Recombinant Viral Vectors Encoding Tumor Antigens:

Active specific immunotherapy is designed to enhance the immunologic response of patients to their own tumors. The recent identification of the genes encoding tumor-associated antigens (TAA) has opened new possibilities for the development of cancer vaccines [70]. Melanoma-associated antigens (MART-1) and gpl00 are recognized by specific tumor infiltrating T lymphocytes (TILs) derived from patients with melanoma and appear to be involved in tumor regression. Therefore they are excellent candidates for the development of antigen-specific vaccines for the treatment of melanoma patients. To develop immunizing vectors for treatment, replication-defective recombinant adenoviruses expressing MART-l and gp100 have been developed. The transduction of tumoral cell lines with such vectors resulted in their recognition by antigen-specific CTLs, as demonstrated by specific target cell lysis and release of cytokines, including IFN-γ, TNF-α, and GM-CSF. Vaccines that use the entire natural antigen or that contain multiple antigenic epitopes (in contrast to peptide vaccines) would be preferable for cancer immunotherapy [71].

A combinatorial approach using a poxvirus-based vaccine encoding prostate-specific antigen (PSA) and radiation therapy has been evaluated in patients with localized or locally advanced prostate cancer. The induction of specific immune response to the vaccine was assessed. Patients treated with radiation and vaccine (but not those treated with radiation alone), had a significant increase in PSA-specific T-cell response, although this trial did not show a benefit in overall survival or disease progression [72].

c) Vaccination with Dendritic Cells Expressing Tumor Antigens:

Dendritic cells (DCs) are potent antigen-presenting cells that exist in virtually every tissue from which they capture antigens and migrate to secondary lymphoid organs where they activate native CD4+ T-helper cells and CD8+ CTLs. Because of their immunoregulatory capacity, the DCs are attractive vehicles for the delivery of therapeutic cancer vaccines. DCs are able to prime T-cells against TAA. The utilization of DC-based cancer vaccines relies on the hypothesis that the lack of efficient tumor antigen presentation to mature DCs that is frequently observed in tumor-bearing individuals can be bypassed by direct loading of DCs with oncoproteins *in vitro*, thus ensuring the transfer of immunostimulatory peptides to the respective antigen-presenting molecules. Several genetic manipulations to enhance loading of DCs with oncoproteins *in vitro* have been shown to be efficient in experimental tumor models. DCs were transfected either with DNA or RNA coding for TAA, or with DNA encoding immunostimulatory cytokines and co-stimulatory molecules. The delivery of genes coding for antigenic epitopes or other molecules with a recombinant retrovirus, adenovirus, poxvirus, or lentivirus into dendritic cells has also been used for transduction and therapy [47,73]. Therefore, genetic engineering of DCs is feasible using both viral and non-viral gene delivery. However, a study that characterized antigen presentation by human DCs genetically modified with plasmid cDNAs, RNAs, adenoviruses, or retroviruses, encoding the melanoma antigen gp100 or the tumor-testis antigen NY-ESO-1, suggests that DCs transduced with viral vectors may be more efficient than DCs transfected with cDNAs or RNAs for the induction of tumor reactive CD8+ and CD4+ T cells *in vitro* and in human vaccination trials [47,73].

d) Naked DNA Vaccines:

An attractive alternative concept of cancer immunotherapy is the direct use of plasmid DNA to elicit humoral and cellular immune responses [74]. Injection of naked DNA has been shown to be effective in the treatment of cancer in several animal tumor models. However, these types of vaccines have been more effective in small animal models than in larger models and humans. The development of new technologies has increased the potential of naked DNA administration, with greatly enhanced immune responses in various species [75]. There are currently several clinical trials underway to investigate the safety of plasmid DNA as a cancer vaccine.

HER2 is over-expressed in 20–30% of human breast cancers and is correlated with more aggressive disease and reduced survival [76]. A comparative study between two human HER2 vaccines, naked DNA and a whole cell vaccine, which encompassed a human ovarian cancer cell line with amplified HER2 was performed in a mouse model. The results suggested that T cell immunity and protection against HER2+ tumors were superior in DNA vaccinated mice [77].

Adoptive Therapy using Antigen-Specific T Lymphocyte Transfer (TCR Gene Therapy):

This is a treatment that uses a cancer patient's own T lymphocytes with anti-tumor activity expanded *in vitro* and re-infused into the patient [78,79]. However, for many patients with cancers it is difficult to obtain tumor-reactive T lymphocytes. A potential solution to this problem is the transduction of genes encoding tumor-reactive T cell receptor (TCR) into patient peripheral blood lymphocytes (PBL) to convert them into tumor-reactive T cells [80,81]. For use in gene therapy, the TCR genes should be incorporated into a retroviral expression system used to transduce PBL *ex vivo*, prior to reinfusion. Experiments in a mouse model showed that T cells transduced with a retrovirus encoding a TCR against a self-expressed ovalbumin antigen can persist and function *in vivo* in transgenic mice [82]. Thus in the last years research has begun on the use of TCR gene therapy as a means to control and eradicate malignancies. Recent findings support the idea that with the use of this technology it is possible to redirect T-cell antigen specificity to produce cytotoxic and helper T cells, which are functionally competent *in vivo* and show promising antitumor effects in humans [43].

Thus, the advances in our ability to genetically modify lymphocytes have opened possibilities for the *in vitro* creation of lymphocytes with appropriate therapeutic properties [81]. High-affinity T cell receptors can be introduced into a patient's normal lymphocytes and the administration of these cells to the lymphodepleted patient has now been shown to be effective in mediating cancer regression [43].

To achieve an antitumor immune response *in vivo*, isolated T cells that recognize tumor antigens with the highest avidity and exhibit high-affinity TCR should be selected, as they most potently induce an *in vivo* antitumor response. In an attempt to identify optimal TCR for gene therapy, MART-1 melanoma antigen-reactive tumor-infiltrating lymphocyte clones were derived from tumors of patients with a wide display of cellular avidities. α and β TCR genes were isolated from these clones, and TCR RNA was introduced into the same non-MART-1-reactive allogeneic donor PBL and TIL. TCR recipient cells gained the ability to recognize both MART-1 peptide and MART-1-expressing tumors *in vitro*, with avidities that closely corresponded to the original TCR clones. The highest-avidity TCR identified, CD8-

independent, holds promise as a candidate for allogeneic TCR gene therapy in metastatic melanoma patients. This TCR was sufficient to transform nonreactive donor CD8+ and CD4+PBL as well as TIL to recognize MART-1-expressing tumors, produce high levels of multiple immunologically relevant cytokine, and lyse tumor cells *in vitro*. Thus, it was proposed that inducing expression of a highly avid TCR in patient PBL has the potential to induce tumor regression in the melanoma patient [83].

The first trial in humans using TCR gene-modified T cells was performed in melanoma patients. High-affinity T cell receptors were introduced into normal lymphocytes from patients and the administration of these cells to the lymphodepleted patient produced cancer regression. This study reported the ability to specifically confer tumor recognition by autologous lymphocytes from peripheral blood by using a retrovirus that encodes the MART-1 TCR alpha and beta chains. High sustained levels of circulating engineered cells were observable 1 year after infusion in two patients, both of whom demonstrated objective regression of metastatic melanoma lesions [43]. The patients experienced cancer regression and are disease free more than 3 years later [84]. This method has potential for use in patients for whom TILs are not available.

Transference Of Toxic Or Tumor Growth Suppression Genes

A wide variety of genes are capable of producing cell death (suicide genes) or of stopping the growth of a cancer (figure 4). A classic example of a suicide gene is the HSV thymidine kinase (HSVtk) gene. HSV infection is treated with non-toxic nucleoside analogues, such as ganciclovir. These drugs eliminate the cells infected by HSV through the following mechanism: HSVtk, together with other enzymes, converts ganciclovir into phosphorylated compounds. These new compounds are incorporated into the newly emerging DNA chains that are created (DNA replication) prior to cell division. However, these phosphorylated compounds act as chain terminators, blocking the DNA replication process and causing cell death [1]. HSVtk activity is indispensable to this process that is specific for cells that require DNA replication, or in other words, dividing cells. In this manner, cells infected by HSV (or that express HSVtk) can be eliminated by ganciclovir.

The HSVtk gene has been placed in gene therapy vectors that have been applied intratumorally in combination with systemic administration of ganciclovir. This treatment has been shown to be effective against prostate and glioblastoma tumors, among others [1]. Its effect is not limited to the cells into which the vector entered since the toxic molecule derived from ganciclovir is exported toward the neighboring cells, killing them, too (bystander effect). This phenomenon is common among different toxic products that are created through gene therapy (figure 4). In addition, when using adenoviral, HSV o vaccinia vectors, an antitumoral immunological stimulus that helps in the systemic control of the disease has been demonstrated [9].

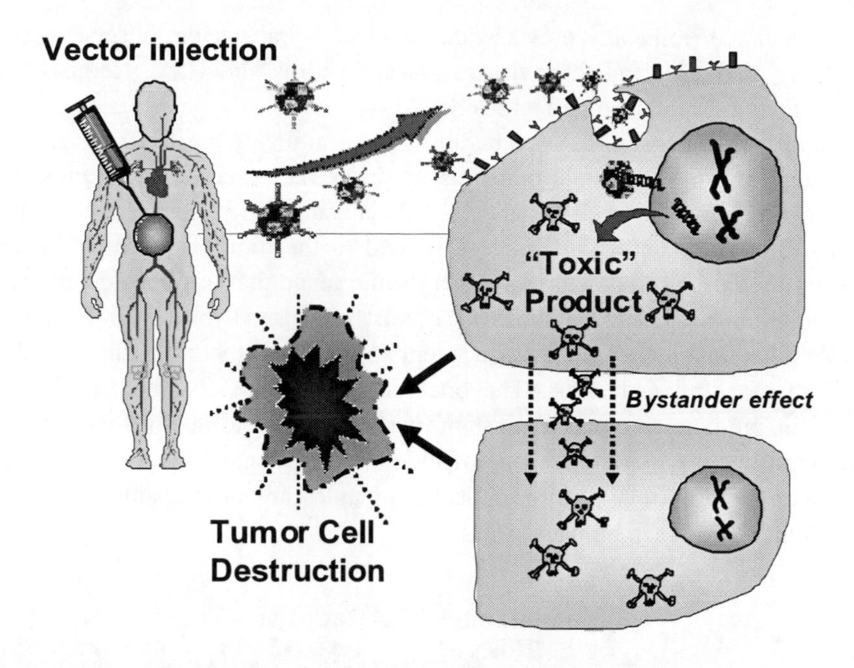

Figure 4. Schematic diagram of gene transfer therapy. Toxic molecule derived from gene transfer is exported toward the neighboring cells, killing them too (bystander effect).

Pro-apoptotic genes, anti-angiogenic genes and genes that increase sensitivity to chemotherapy or radiotherapy have also been introduced, along with interference RNAs that block oncogene activity. Rexin-G, the first injectable gene therapy agent to achieve orphan drug status from the Food and Drug Administration for treatment of pancreatic cancer, is an example [1]. This gene therapy agent contains a gene designed to interfere with the cyclin G1 gene and is delivered via a retroviral vector. The gene integrates into the cancer cell's DNA to disrupt the cyclin G1 gene and causes cell death or growth arrest [1]. In a Phase I trial, 3 out of 3 patients experienced tumor growth arrest with 2 patients experiencing stable disease [1]. Rexin-G is also being evaluated for other cancers.

The introduction of gene p53 is another strategy in which great strides have been made. Two examples are Advexin and Gendicine, which are adenoviral vectors containing p53 for gene transfer [85]. The p53 gene is an important cell cycle regulator that is mutated in 50 to 70% of human tumors. Mutations in this gene are often linked to aggressiveness. It has been shown that restoration of a functional p53 gene in cancer cells results in tumor cell stasis and often in apoptosis [85].

Therapeutic gene expression can be controlled by cancer-specific or tissue specific promoters which are responsible for selective gene expression in cancer cells. This increases vector security, though on occasion it reduces their potency.

Oncolytic Agents

One of the principal short-comings of gene therapy with replication- deficient viral vectors is limited intratumoral dissemination. For the purpose of overcoming this limitation there was a new therapeutic strategy boom called virotherapy or oncolytic viral therapy at the end of the 1990's. Virotherapy uses a wide variety of viral vectors but the most frequently used are those derived from adenoviruses, vaccinia virus and HSV. Neoplastic cell death occurs from the viral replication effect itself [86].

The main characteristic of virotherapy is the utilization of viral vectors that can selectively replicate themselves in tumor tissue under very specific and exclusive molecular conditions of the neoplastic cell (figure 5). This characteristic allows for the elimination of tumor cells through an infectious process limited to the tumor and with few side effects, always when the dose used is within the therapeutic range that has been determined for each vector. In addition, replication amplifies the entrance dose of oncolytic viruses facilitating better dissemination on the part of the agent towards neighboring tumor cells, with the possibility of reaching metastasis. The oncolytic effect can also be strengthened by the creation of an immune response against the vector and the cancerous cells infected by it. Oncolytic viral therapy is presently one of the most promising therapeutic tools in the fight against cancer and different pharmaceutical companies are now testing different oncolytic vectors in clinical studies in humans [86].

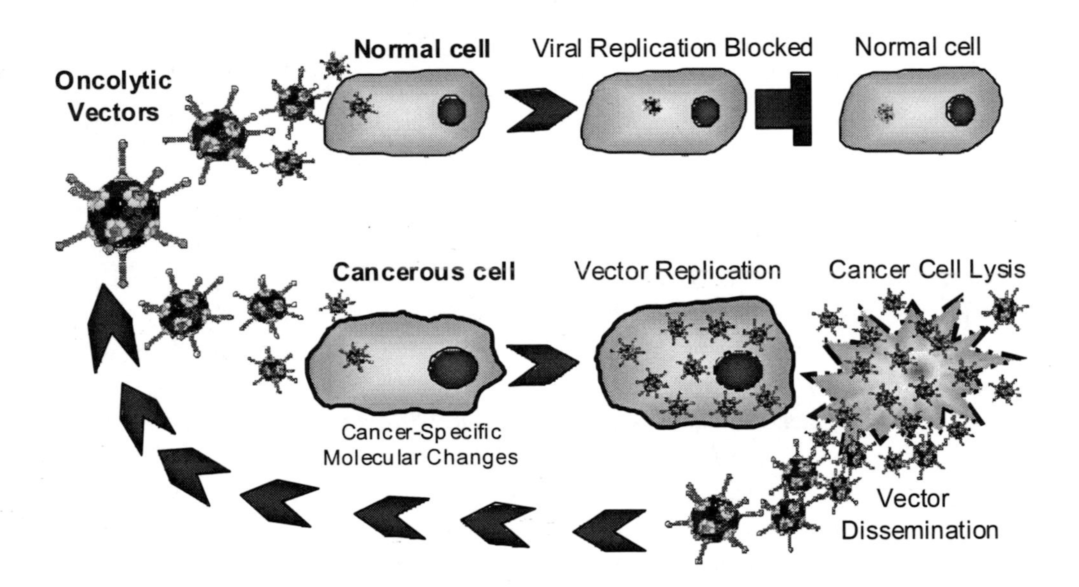

Figure 5. Schematic diagram of oncolytic vectors.

Viral replication is a process that can be manipulated. When a virus enters a cell only some "key" replication genes are initially activated in its genome. Then proteins created by these key genes activate the rest of the viral genes to begin the viral replication process. If these key genes are not activated there is no replication [86]. A viral vector is replication-deficient if these key genes are eliminated from its genome. Likewise if the expression of these key genes is controlled, vector replication can be controlled. The most frequently used strategy for creating controlled replication in neoplastic cells is obtained by having the key gene expression regulated or controlled by a cancer-specific or tissue-specific promoter. In this way the key gene will only be expressed in cells where the promoter is active and if it is only active exclusively in cancer cells there will only be replication in cancerous cells.

In the case of adenoviruses, the key replication gene is called E1A, although the E1B also participates but to a lesser degree [86]. Prostate-specific antigen promoter was used to control E1A expression in one of the first oncolytic vectors. It showed E1A gene activation and viral replication only in prostate cells [87]. Another example is the use of the human papillomavirus (HPV) E6/E7 promoter. HPV is associated with the arising of different neoplasias, especially cervical-uterine and head and neck cancers. These neoplasias are a consequence of HPV E6/E7 oncogene over-expression. E6/E7 is over-expressed in neoplastic cells and is almost undetectable in surrounding healthy tissue [88]. In a similar manner, HPV E6/E7 viral promoter is very active in cancer and practically inactive in healthy cells or cells not infected by HPV. HPV E6/E7 promoter was placed in an adenoviral vector so that it would control E1A gene expression. The resulting vector had E1A expression and viral replication in neoplastic cells with HPV while it had limited activity in HPV-negative cells [88]. There are many vectors that use cancer-specific promoters to control replication.

Another strategy for creating oncolytic vectors is based on eliminating fragments of "key" viral replication genes. These genes have different regions or domains that have definite functions. In healthy cells the cell cycle and rhythm of division are very restricted and/or controlled. Some regions of the key genes of viruses are in charge of confusing or deregulating the cell cycle to facilitate viral replication. If these regions are eliminated, viral replication becomes difficult and very slow in healthy cells since they are not capable of confusing the cell cycle. However, the cell cycle of cancer cells is generally already altered (it is confused by alterations in the gene expression) and certain regions of the "key" genes are not so necessary for viral replication in cancerous cells. In this way, a vector with certain specific mutations (deletions) in the "key" genes can selectively to replicate in cancerous cells [89,90]. Examples of these types of vectors are the ONYX-015 or H101 (Oncorine) viral therapies [1,91].

ONYX-015 and H101 (Oncorine) are adenoviruses that have been engineered to lack the viral E1B protein. Without this protein, the virus is unable to replicate in cells with a normal p53 pathway. Cancer cells often have deficiencies in the p53 pathway due to mutations and thus allow ONYX-015 or H101 to replicate and lyse the cells [1,91]. Both ONYX-015 and H101 have been tested in clinical trials on squamous cell carcinoma of the head and neck that resulted in tumor regression correlating to the p53 status of the tumor. Tumors with an inactive pathway demonstrated a better response. It should be mentioned that oncolytic viruses may also carry therapeutic genes that strengthen their effect.

Clinical Use

It is important to remember the different stages that a drug or therapeutic strategy must pass through to stop being experimental and to be offered for sale. The first stages include experiments in cell cultures and laboratory animals. If the results are satisfactory, the therapy is tried out in humans for the first time in clinical phases. Phase I is usually carried out on a few very well-supervised patients in a dose-escalation study and careful analysis of toxic effects. Phase II is carried out on a larger number of patients and in addition to analyzing adverse effects, benefits of the therapy in different types of disease are also registered in detail to determine its best indication. Phase III carries out multicentric studies on a very large number of patients to evaluate the usefulness and safety of the treatment with exactness and is the last step before the therapy can be commercialized. In Phase IV the drug is now on the market, although its benefits and side effects continue to be monitored. Up to March 2010 only 1,579 gene therapy clinical trials had been initiated. Sixty per cent were in Phase I, 35% in Phase II or I/II, 1% in Phase II/III, 3% in Phase III, and 0.1% in Phase IV (two vectors in China –Gendicine and Oncorine-). Sixty-five per cent were clinical trials for cancer diseases. A general panorama is described on the web page "Gene Therapy Clinical Trials Worldwide" provided by the Journal of Gene Medicine [2,92].

After gene therapy clinical trials began in 1989 [93], the first vector on the market was Gendicine, from Shenzhen SiBiono GeneTech, which was approved in China in 2003 [94]. Used for head and neck cancer, Gendicine is a recombinant human type 5 adenovirus in which the E1 region (where the "key" replication genes are located) is replaced by a human wild-type p53 controlled by a very active promoter (replication-deficient vector) [94].

Gendicine is a wide-spectrum antitumor agent. Significant synergistic effects have been demonstrated for the combination of Gendicine with conventional therapies in clinical applications. An example could be the use of Gendicine in combination with radiotherapy for the treatment of advanced head and neck squamous cell carcinoma. The response rate in the Gendicine-radiotherapy group was 93%, with 64% showing complete regression and 29% partial regression. The response rate in the radiotherapy group was 79%, with 19% of the patients showing complete regression. The complete regression rate in the Gendicine-radiotherapy group was 3 times higher than that in the radiotherapy group [94]. The clinical efficacy of Gendicine may be independent of the endogenous *p53* gene status of tumor cells. Furthermore, Gendicine reduced the side effects caused by conventional chemo- and radiation therapy. A significant observation was that some patients showed improved appetite and general health *status* approximately 2 days after receiving Gendicine treatment. This is a positive clinical development for cancer patients who suffer from severe side effects caused by radio- and chemotherapy [94]. In a general sense, the concept of gene therapy as a new modality for cancer treatment at the gene level has become a reality with the use of Gendicine.

Since the second half of 2009, Ark's drug Cerepro® for the treatment of malignant glioma is rapidly nearing the phase of commercial use in Europe [95]. Cerepro® uses a replication-deficient adenoviral vector to introduce the HSVtk. Following standard surgery to remove the solid tumor mass, Cerepro® is injected through the wall of the cavity left by the surgical removal of the solid tumor into the surrounding healthy brain tissue. In the following days, the healthy cells in the wall of the cavity express TK. Five days after surgery, the drug ganciclovir ("GCV") is given to the patient as part of the overall Cerepro® treatment regimen. Cerepro® administered after surgical removal of the solid tumor mass demonstrated an 81% increase in mean survival (from 39 weeks to 71 weeks) compared with standard care [96].

Introgen's adenoviral p53 gene ADVEXIN (see Toxic Gene Transference section) is a vector that will probably be seen in clinical practice initially for the treatment of head and neck cancer and Li-Fraumeni Syndrome [95,97].

Of the oncolytic vectors, H101 (Oncorine) (see Oncolytic Agents section) was the first on the market in China in 2005 [91]. Shanghai Sunway Biotech Co. Ltd., the company that manufactured H101 reported a 79% response rate for H101 plus chemotherapy (5-fluorouracil and cisplatin), compared with 40% for chemotherapy alone in patients with late stage refractory nasopharyngeal cancer [91,98]. H102 and H103 are other oncolytic agents developed by the same company that are rapidly nearing the phase of commercial use in China [91,98]. In America, vector ONYX-015, developed by Onyx Pharmaceuticals, initiated Phase III clinical trials several years ago for neoplasias such as melanoma and lung cancer [99]. It will probably be available commercially very soon. Although the above-mentioned vectors initially have been used for only certain neoplasias, they are presently being tested for different types of cancer and so their usefulness may grow.

Gene therapy treatment use is increasing significantly. In the second quarter of 2008, a China-based pharmaceutical company sold 2,439 vials of Gendicine, a sequential increase from sales of 1,087 vials sold in the first quarter of 2008 [100]. The cost of gene therapy treatment may vary from one country to another as does the cost of medical service in general. A two-month course of Gendicine in China is reported to cost £20,000 [101]. These treatments may cost more in other countries and with the passing of time their price may go down.

Each year new gene therapy vectors will appear on the market and ideally they will be safer and more efficient. As with any drug, a vector can be taken off the market if serious side effects are seen to develop. All vectors are initially used in combination with previously established standard treatments. Commercial vectors are still something of a novelty and theirs will be a changing market, especially during the first years. At first they will be expensive. They will be used in very specific cancers and patients and even if in the beginning they do not heal the patient they will improve his or her quality of life.

SAFETY

Although, in general, low- and intermediate-dose gene therapy has a good safety record, high doses of replication-deficient or oncolytic vectors are potentially toxic. The death of a patient during a Phase I clinical trial involving a high-dose recombinant adenoviral gene therapy is a tragic reminder that viral vectors are indeed viruses that require careful consideration of safety issues [7]. The death was apparently caused by a vector-induced shock syndrome that included cytokine cascade, disseminated intravascular coagulation, acute respiratory distress, and multi-organ failure. No fatalities have been reported in other cancer gene therapy trials using adenoviral vectors. Oncolytic viruses are a greater safety concern due to the dose increase caused by viral replication in the patient. However, to date, oncolytic adenoviruses have been well-tolerated despite a certain degree of toxicity manifested sometimes by fever and other inflammatory responses [7,98].

Gendicine is the first adenoviral vector against cancer on the market and so has provided more clinical experience outside of research projects than others. The most commonly observed side effects were grade I/II self-limited fever in approximately 32% of Gendicine treated patients. In a few rare cases patient fever reached as high as 40°C [94]. Development of fever was observed as quickly as approximately 3 hr after injection, lasted about 4 hr, and then disappeared spontaneously. On occasion, it lasted more than 10 hr. Gendicine in combination with radiotherapy did not exacerbate any side effects. A few patients receiving intravenous infusion of $1 \text{ X}10^{12}$ viral particles of Gendicine per dose experienced temporary blood pressure decrease (approximately 1.33-kPa drop) when a relatively fast infusion rate was used [94]. So far, no severe side effects have been found in thousands of patients treated with Gendicine administered by different means (including intratumoral injection, intrapleural and intraperitoneal infusion, intravenous injection, hepatic and lung artery infusion, endotracheal and intravesical instillation) [94].

Certain retroviral vectors have caused leukemia in patients (see Retrovirus section). Therefore, long-term vector safety tests are a necessity and an area of intense research within gene therapy. The new vectors created are generally safer than their predecessors. However, since the specific manifestation of toxic effects and the degree of toxicity varies with each vector, individual patients under treatment must remain under close surveillance and their doctor should follow the safety measures recommended by the manufacturer or researcher. The safety of each treatment depends on the type of vector, its genetic modifications, mechanism of action and dose.

Ethics

Like conventional therapy, gene therapy is under the regulation of the Nuremberg Code (1947) and the Declaration of Helsinki (1964) which established the principal research ethics concerning the vulnerability and interest of the patient as well as the benefit of independent review. However, gene therapy also raises specific ethical issues and public concerns [3]. There are national ethics committees and advisory boards such as the USA Recombinant DNA Advisory Committee (RAC), the UK Gene Therapy Advisory committee (GTAC) and the Australian Gene Therapies Research Advisory Panel (GTRAP), to mention a few, that are in charge of providing guidelines for the proper use of gene therapy [3]. Germ cell gene therapy has been prohibited. New therapeutic modalities such as uterus gene therapy as well as the impact of adverse effects are still being discussed – the latter especially since the death of a patient and the appearance of cases of leukemia in gene therapy clinical trials [3]. The dissemination of gene therapy vectors into the environment through patient bodily fluids is also a preoccupation that has caused controversy. Avoiding the dissemination of genetically modified viruses into the environment is a logical rule to follow. The majority of viruses can be eliminated with disinfectant solutions containing hypochlorite. In spite of existing difficulties and obstacles, gene therapy has the potential to become a cornerstone of modern medicine.

Conclusion

Gene therapy against cancer is a reality with a promising future. The hope for a miracle cure for cancer can be felt in the ideas that sustain gene therapy but not yet in its reality. It is a therapeutic area that has practically just begun and this makes the first commercial vectors expensive. Vectors are useful in very specific cancers and patients and although they do not yet provide a cure, they do improve patient quality of life and will continue to do so more and more. This type of therapy seems to be an adequate path to follow to successfully fight malignant tumors. However, there is still a long way to go before the ideal vector is found.

ACKNOWLEDGMENTS

We thank Dr. Fanis Missirlis for his helpful comments on the manuscript. Irma Martínez dedicates this chapter to her beloved family. Iván Delgado dedicates this chapter to Gaby; children Iván Darío and Olivia Delmar; parents Raul and Licho; brothers and sister Omar, Josuel, Osiris; mentors Augusto Rojas, Rocío Ortiz and Hugo A. Barrera; and to all his friends that are fortunately too many to name here -110-.

REFERENCES

[1] Cross D, Burmester JK. Gene therapy for cancer treatment: past, present and future. *Clin Med Res*. 2006;4:218-227.

[2] Edelstein ML, Abedi MR and Wixon Jo. Gene therapy clinical trials worldwide to 2007-an update. *J Gene Med*. 2007; 9:833-842.

[3] Jin X, Yang YD, Li YM. Gene therapy: regulations, ethics and its practicalities in liver disease. *World J Gastroenterol*. 2008;14:2303-2307.

[4] Mbeunkui F, Johann DJ Jr. Cancer and the tumor microenvironment: a review of an essential relationship. *Cancer Chemother Pharmacol*. 2009;63:571-582.

[5] Rojas-Martínez A, Martínez-Dávila IA, Hernández-García A, Aguilar-Córdova E, Barrera-Saldaña HA. Genetic therapy of cancer. *Rev Invest Clin*. 2002;54(1):57-67.

[6] Nemunaitis J, Sterman D, Jablons D, Smith JW 2nd, Fox B, Maples P, Hamilton S, Borellini F, Lin A, Morali S, Hege K. Granulocyte-macrophage colony-stimulating factor gene-modified autologous tumor vaccines in non-small-cell lung cancer. *J Natl Cancer Inst*. 2004;96:326-331.

[7] Shen Y, Post L, Viral vector and their applications. In: Knipe DM, Howley PM, Diane E. Griffin. *Fields virology. Edition 5*. USA. Lippincott Williams & Wilkins 2007. p 540-558.

[8] Nemerow GR. Biology of Adenovirus cell entry. In: Curiel DT and Douglas JT. *Adenoviral vectors for gene therapy*. USA. Academic Press. 2002.p 19-32.

[9] Delgado-Enciso I, Galván-Salazar HR, Coronel-Tene CG, Sánchez-Santillán CF, Enriquez-Maldonado IG, Rojas-Martínez A, Ortiz-López R, Baltazar-Rodriguez LM, Elizalde A, Silva-Platas CI. Preclinical evaluation of the therapeutic effect of adenoviral vectors in human papillomavirus-dependent neoplasias. *Rev Invest Clin*. 2008;60:101-106.

[10] Di Paolo NC, Tuve S, Ni S, Hellström KE, Hellström I, Lieber A. Effect of adenovirus-mediated heat shock protein expression and oncolysis in combination with low-dose cyclophosphamide treatment on antitumor immune responses. *Cancer Res*. 2006;66:960-969.

[11] Vlachaki MT, Hernandez-Garcia A, Ittmann M, Chhikara M, Aguilar LK, Zhu X, Teh BS, Butler EB, Woo S, Thompson TC, Barrera-Saldana H, Aguilar-Cordova E. Impact of preimmunization on adenoviral vector expression and toxicity in a subcutaneous mouse cancer model. *Mol Ther*. 2002;6:342-348.

[12] O'Neal WK, Zhou H, Morral N, Langston C, Parks RJ, Graham FL, Kochanek S, Beaudet AL. Toxicity associated with repeated administration of first-generation

adenovirus vectors does not occur with a helper-dependent vector. *Mol Med.* 2000;6:179-195.

[13] Bangari DS, Mittal SK. Current strategies and future directions for eluding adenoviral vector immunity. *Curr Gene Ther*. 2006;6:215-226.

[14] Segura MM, Alba R, Bosch A, Chillón M. Advances in helper-dependent adenoviral vector research. *Curr Gene Ther*. 2008;8:222-235.

[15] Moroziewicz D, Kaufman HL. Gene therapy with poxvirus vectors. *Curr Opin Mol Ther*. 2005;7:317-325.

[16] Zhang Q, Yu YA, Wang E, Chen N, Danner RL, Munson PJ, Marincola FM, Szalay AA. Eradication of Solid Human Breast Tumors in Nude Mice with an intravenously Injected Light-Emitting Oncolytic Vaccinia Virus. *Cancer Res*. 2007; 67:10038-10046.

[17] Thorne SH, Hwang TH, Kirn DH. Vaccinia virus and oncolytic virotherapy of cancer. *Curr Opin Mol Ther*. 2005;7:359-365.

[18] Essajee S, Kaufman HL. Poxvirus vaccines for cancer and HIV therapy. *Expert Opin Biol Ther*. 2004;4:575-588.

[19] Shen Y, Nemunaitis J. Fighting cancer with vaccinia virus: teaching new tricks to an old dog. *Mol Ther*. 2005;11:180-195.

[20] Gómez CE, Nájera JL, Krupa M, Esteban M. The poxvirus vectors MVA and NYVAC as gene delivery systems for vaccination against infectious diseases and cancer. *Curr Gene Ther*. 2008;8:97-120.

[21] Tartaglia J, Perkus ME, Taylor J, Norton EK, Audonnet JC, Cox WI, Davis SW, van der Hoeven J, Meignier B, Riviere M, et al. NYVAC: a highly attenuated strain of vaccinia virus.*Virology*. 1992;188:217-232.

[22] Gentschev I, Stritzker J, Hofmann E, Weibel S, Yu YA, Chen N, Zhang Q, Bullerdiek J, Nolte I, Szalay AA. Use of an oncolytic vaccinia virus for the treatment of canine breast cancer in nude mice: preclinical development of a therapeutic agent. *Cancer Gene Ther*. 2009;16:320-328.

[23] Kirn DH, Thorne SH. Targeted and armed oncolytic poxviruses: a novel multi-mechanistic therapeutic class for cancer. *Nat Rev Cancer*. 2009;9:64-71.

[24] Park BH, Hwang T, Liu TC, Sze DY, Kim JS, Kwon HC, Oh SY, Han SY, Yoon JH, Hong SH, Moon A, Speth K, Park C, Ahn YJ, Daneshmand M, Rhee BG, Pinedo HM, Bell JC, Kirn DH. Use of a targeted oncolytic poxvirus, JX-594, in patients with refractory primary or metastatic liver cancer: a phase I trial. *Lancet Oncol*. 2008;9:533-542.

[25] Burton EA, Fink DJ, Glorioso JC. Gene delivery using herpes simplex virus vectors. *DNA Cell Biol*. 2002;21:915-936.

[26] Berges BK, Wolfe JH, Fraser NW. Transduction of brain by herpes simplex virus vectors. *Mol Ther*. 2007;15:20-29.

[27] Shah K, Breakefield XO. HSV amplicon vectors for cancer therapy. *Curr Gene Ther*. 2006;6:361-370.

[28] Marconi P, Argnani R, Berto E, Epstein AL, Manservigi R. HSV as a vector in vaccine development and gene therapy. *Hum Vaccin*. 2008;4:91-105.

[29] Cuchet D, Potel C, Thomas J, Epstein AL. HSV-1 amplicon vectors: a promising and versatile tool for gene delivery. *Expert Opin Biol Ther*. 2007;7:975-995.

[30] Nair V. Retrovirus-induced oncogenesis and safety of retroviral vectors. *Curr Opin Mol Ther*. 2008;10:431-438.

[31] Breckpot K, Emeagi PU, Thielemans K. Lentiviral vectors for anti-tumor immunotherapy. *Curr Gene Ther*. 2008;8:438-448.

[32] Wang Q, Liu QY, Liu ZS, Qian Q, Sun Q, Pan DY. Lentivirus mediated shRNA interference targeting MAT2B induces growth-inhibition and apoptosis in hepatocelluar carcinoma. *World J Gastroenterol*. 2008;14:4633-4642.

[33] Wang F, Chen L, Mao ZB, Shao JG, Tan C, Huang WD. Lentivirus-mediated short hairpin RNA targeting the APRIL gene suppresses the growth of pancreatic cancer cells in vitro and in vivo. *Oncol Rep*. 2008;20:135-139.

[34] Park K, Kim WJ, Cho YH, Lee YI, Lee H, Jeong S, Cho ES, Chang SI, Moon SK, Kang BS, Kim YJ, Cho SH. Cancer gene therapy using adeno-associated virus vectors. *Front Biosci*. 2008 Jan 1;13:2653-2659.

[35] Ribas A. Genetically modified dendritic cells for cancer immunotherapy. *Curr Gene Ther*. 2005;5:619-628.

[36] Yu Y, Pilgrim P, Zhou W, Gagliano N, Frezza EE, Jenkins M, Weidanz JA, Lustgarten J, Cannon M, Bumm K, Cobos E, Kast WM, Chiriva-Internati M. rAAV/Her-2/neu loading of dendritic cells for a potent cellular-mediated MHC class I restricted immune response against ovarian cancer.*Viral Immunol*. 2008;21:435-442.

[37] Thorne SH. Oncolytic vaccinia virus: from bedside to benchtop and back. *Curr Opin Mol Ther*. 2008;10:387-392.

[38] Seow Y, Wood MJ. Biological Gene Delivery Vehicles: Beyond Viral Vectors. *Mol Ther*. 2009; 17:767-777.

[39] Dachs GU, Dougherty GJ, Stratford IJ, Chaplin DJ. Targeting gene therapy to cancer: a review. *Oncol Res*. 1997;9:313-325.

[40] Belousova N, Mikheeva G, Gelovani J, Krasnykh V. Modification of adenovirus capsid with a designed protein ligand yields a gene vector targeted to a major molecular marker of cancer. *J Virol*. 2008;82:630-637.

[41] Chaudhuri D, Suriano R, Mittelman A, Tiwari RK. Targeting the immune system in cancer. *Curr Pharm Biotechnol*. 2009;10:166-184.

[42] Parney IF and Chang LJ, Cancer immunogene therapy: a review. *J. Biomed Sci*. 2003;10:37-43

[43] Morgan RA, Dudley ME, Wunderlich JR, Hughes MS, Yang JC, Sherry RM, Royal RE, Topalian SL, Kammula US, Restifo NP, Zheng Z, Nahvi A, de Vries CR, Rogers-Freezer LJ, Mavroukakis SA, Rosenberg SA. Cancer regression in patients after transfer of genetically engineered lymphocytes. *Science* 2006;314:126-129.

[44] Stauss HJ, Thomas S, Cesco-Gaspere M, Hart DP, Xue SA, Holler A, King J, Wright G, Perro M, Pospori C, Morris E.WT1-specific T cell receptor gene therapy: improving TCR function in transduced T cells. *Blood Cells Mol Dis*. 2008;40:113-116.

[45] Jinushi M, Hodi FS, Dranoff G. Enhancing the clinical activity of granulocyte-macrophage colony-stimulating factor-secreting tumor cell vaccines. *Immunol Rev*. 2008;222:287-298.

[46] Lechleider RJ, Arlen PM, Tsang KY, Steinberg SM, Yokokawa J, Cereda V, Camphausen K, Schlom J, Dahut WL, Gulley JL. Safety and immunologic response of a viral vaccine to prostate-specific antigen in combination with radiation therapy when metronomic-dose interleukin 2 is used as an adjuvant. *Clin Cancer Res*. 2008;14:5284-5291.

[47] Lotem M, Zhao Y, Riley J, Hwu P, Morgan RA, Rosenberg SA, Parkhurst MR. Presentation of tumor antigens by dendritic cells genetically modified with viral and nonviral vectors. *J Immunother*. 2006;29:616-627.

[48] Schuurhuis DH, Lesterhuis WJ, Kramer M, Looman MG, van Hout-Kuijer M, Schreibelt G, Boullart AC, Aarntzen EH, Benitez-Ribas D, Figdor CG, Punt CJ, de Vries IJ, Adema GJ. Polyinosinic polycytidylic acid prevents efficient antigen expression after mRNA electroporation of clinical grade dendritic cells. *Cancer Immunol Immunother*. 2009; 58:1109-1115.

[49] Parmiani G, Colombo MP, Melani C, Arienti F. Cytokine gene transduction in the immunotherapy of cancer. *Adv Pharmacol*. 1997;40:259-307.

[50] Musiani P, Modesti A, Giovarelli M, Cavallo F, Colombo MP, Lollini PL, Forni G. Cytokines, tumour-cell death and immunogenicity: a question of choice. *Immunol Today*. 1997;18:32-36.

[51] Niranjan A, Moriuchi S, Lunsford LD, Kondziolka D,Flickinger JC, Fellows W, Rajendiran S, Tamura M, Cohen JB, Glorioso JC. Effective treatment of experimental glioblastoma by HSV vector-mediated TNF alpha and HSV-tk gene transfer in combination with radiosurgery and ganciclovir administration. *Mol Ther* 2000;2:114–120.

[52] Mackensen A, Lindemann A, Mertelsmann R: Immunostimulatory cytokines in somatic cells and gene therapy of cancer. Cytokine Growth Factor Rev 1997;8:119–128.

[53] Qian HN, Liu GZ, Cao SJ, Feng J,Ye X: Experimental study of ovarian carcinoma vaccine modified by human B7-1 and IFN-gamma genes. *Int J Gynecol Cancer* 2002;12:80–85.

[54] Suzuki K, Nakazato H, Matsui H, Hasumi M, Shibata Y, Ito K, Fukabori Y, Kurokawa K, Yamanaka H. NK cell-mediated anti-tumor immune response to human prostate cancer cell, PC-3: immunogene therapy using a highly secretable form of interleukin-15 gene transfer. *J Leukoc Biol*. 2001;69:531-537.

[55] Croce M, Meazza R, Orengo AM, Radić L, De Giovanni B, Gambini C, Carlini B, Pistoia V, Mortara L, Accolla RS, Corrias MV, Ferrini S. Sequential immunogene therapy with interleukin-12- and interleukin-15-engineered neuroblastoma cells cures metastatic disease in syngeneic mice. *Clin Cancer Res*. 2005;11:735-742.

[56] Yoshimura K, Hazama S, Iizuka N, Yoshino S, Yamamoto K, Muraguchi M, Ohmoto Y, Noma T, Oka M. Successful immunogene therapy using colon cancer cells (colon 26) transfected with plasmid vector containing mature interleukin-18 cDNA and the Igkappa leader sequence. *Cancer Gene Ther*. 2001;8:9-16.

[57] Kosaka K, Yashiro M, Sakate Y, Hirakawa K. A synergistic antitumor effect of interleukin-2 addition with CD80 immunogene therapy for peritoneal metastasis of gastric carcinoma. *Dig Dis Sci*. 2007;52:1946-1953.

[58] Parney IF, Chang LJ, Farr-Jones MA, Hao C, Smylie M, Petruk KC. Technical hurdles in a pilot clinical trial of combined B7-2 and GM-CSF immunogene therapy for glioblastomas and melanomas. *J Neurooncol*. 2006 May;78(1):71-80.

[59] Baskar S. Gene-modified tumor cells as cellular vaccine. *Cancer Immunol Immunother*. 1996;43:165-173.

[60] Morini M, Albini A, Lorusso G, Moelling K, Lu B, Cilli M, Ferrini S, Noonan DM. Prevention of angiogenesis by naked DNA IL-12 gene transfer: angioprevention by immunogene therapy. *Gene Ther*. 2004;11:284-291.

[61] Tüting T, Storkus WJ, Lotze MT. Gene-based strategies for the immunotherapy of cancer. *J Mol Med. 1997*;75:478-491.

[62] Huang AY, Golumbek P, Ahmadzadeh M, Jaffee E, Pardoll D, Levitsky H. Role of bone marrow-derived cells in presenting MHC class I-restricted tumor antigens. *Science*. 1994;264:961-965.

[63] Mach N, Gillessen S, Wilson SB, Sheehan C, Mihm M, Dranoff G. Differences in dendritic cells stimulated in vivo by tumors engineered to secrete granulocyte-macrophage colony-stimulating factor or Flt3-ligand. Cancer Res. 2000;60:3239-3246.

[64] Bubeník J. Genetically engineered dendritic cell-based cancer vaccines. *Int J Oncol.* 2001;18:475-478.

[65] Dranoff G. GM-CSF-based cancer vaccines. *Immunol Rev*. 2002;188:147-154.

[66] Soiffer R, Hodi FS, Haluska F, Jung K, Gillessen S, Singer S, Tanabe K, Duda R, Mentzer S, Jaklitsch M, Bueno R, Clift S, Hardy S, Neuberg D, Mulligan R, Webb I, Mihm M, Dranoff G. Vaccination with irradiated, autologous melanoma cells engineered to secrete granulocyte-macrophage colony-stimulating factor by adenoviral-mediated gene transfer augments antitumor immunity in patients with metastatic melanoma. *J Clin Oncol*. 2003;21:3343-3350.

[67] Tani K, Azuma M, Nakazaki Y, Oyaizu N, Hase H, Ohata J, Takahashi K, OiwaMonna M, Hanazawa K, Wakumoto Y, Kawai K, Noguchi M, Soda Y, Kunisaki R, Watari K, Takahashi S, Machida U, Satoh N, Tojo A, Maekawa T, Eriguchi M, Tomikawa S, Tahara H, Inoue Y, Yoshikawa H, Yamada Y, Iwamoto A, Hamada H, Yamashita N, Okumura K, Kakizoe T, Akaza H, Fujime M, Clift S, Ando D, Mulligan R, Asano S. Phase I study of autologous tumor vaccines transduced with the GM-CSF gene in four patients with stage IV renal cell cancer in Japan: clinical and immunological findings. *Mol Ther*. 2004;10:799-816.

[68] Salgia R, Lynch T, Skarin A, Lucca J, Lynch C, Jung K, Hodi FS, Jaklitsch M, Mentzer S, Swanson S, Lukanich J, Bueno R, Wain J, Mathisen D, Wright C, Fidias P, Donahue D, Clift S, Hardy S, Neuberg D, Mulligan R, Webb I, Sugarbaker D, Mihm M, Dranoff G. Vaccination with irradiated autologous tumor cells engineered to secrete granulocyte-macrophage colony-stimulating factor augments antitumor immunity in some patients with metastatic non-small-cell lung carcinoma. *J Clin Oncol.* 2003;21:624-630.

[69] Nemunaitis J, Jahan T, Ross H, Sterman D, Richards D, Fox B, Jablons D, Aimi J, Lin A, Hege K. Phase 1/2 trial of autologous tumor mixed with an allogeneic GVAX vaccine in advanced-stage non-small-cell lung cancer. *Cancer Gene Ther*. 2006;13:555-562.

[70] Kawakami Y, Eliyahu S, Delgado CH, Robbins PF, Sakaguchi K, Appella E, Yannelli JR, Adema GJ, Miki T, Rosenberg SA. Identification of a human melanoma antigen recognized by tumor-infiltrating lymphocytes associated with in vivo tumor rejection. *Proc Natl Acad Sci U S A*. 1994;91:6458-62.

[71] Zhai Y, Yang JC, Kawakami Y, Spiess P, Wadsworth SC, Cardoza LM, Couture LA, Smith AE, Rosenberg SA. Antigen-specific tumor vaccines. Development and characterization of recombinant adenoviruses encoding MART1 or gp100 for cancer therapy. *J Immunol*. 1996;156:700-710.

[72] Gulley JL, Arlen PM, Bastian A, Morin S, Marte J, Beetham P, Tsang KY, Yokokawa J, Hodge JW, Ménard C, Camphausen K, Coleman CN, Sullivan F, Steinberg SM,

Schlom J, Dahut W. Combining a recombinant cancer vaccine with standard definitive radiotherapy in patients with localized prostate cancer. *Clin Cancer Res*. 2005;11:3353-3362.

[73] Gonzalez-Carmona MA, Lukacs-Kornek V, Timmerman A, Shabani S, Kornek M, Vogt A, Yildiz Y, Sievers E, Schmidt-Wolf IG, Caselmann WH, Sauerbruch T, Schmitz V. CD40ligand-expressing dendritic cells induce regression of hepatocellular carcinoma by activating innate and acquired immunity in vivo. *Hepatology*. 2008;48:157-168.

[74] Bodles-Brakhop AM, Draghia-Akli R. DNA vaccination and gene therapy: optimization and delivery for cancer therapy. Expert Rev Vaccines. 2008;7:1085-101.

[75] Heller LC, Heller R. In vivo electroporation for gene therapy. *Hum Gene Ther*. 2006;17:890-897.

[76] Kiessling R, Wei WZ, Herrmann F, Lindencrona JA, Choudhury A, Kono K, Seliger B. Cellular immunity to the Her-2/neu protooncogene. *Adv Cancer Res*. 2002;85:101-144.

[77] Whittington PJ, Radkevich-Brown O, Jacob JB, Jones RF, Weise AM, Wei WZ. Her-2 DNA versus cell vaccine: immunogenicity and anti-tumor activity. *Cancer Immunol Immunother*. 2009;58:759-767.

[78] Rosenberg SA, Restifo NP, Yang JC, Morgan RA, Dudley ME. Adoptive cell transfer: a clinical path to effective cancer immunotherapy. *Nat Rev Cancer*. 2008;8:299-308.

[79] Rosenberg SA. Overcoming obstacles to the effective immunotherapy of human cancer. *Proc Natl Acad Sci U S A*. 2008;105:12643-12644.

[80] Hughes, M. S., Y. Y. Yu, M. E. Dudley, Z. Zheng, P. F. Robbins, Y. Li, J. Wunderlich, R. G. Hawley, M. Moayeri, S. A. Rosenberg, and R. A. Morgan. Transfer of a TCR gene derived from a patient with a marked antitumor response conveys highly active T cell effector functions. *Hum Gene Ther*. 2005;16:457-472.

[81] Morgan, R. A., M. E. Dudley, Y. Y. Yu, Z. Zheng, P. F. Robbins, M. R. Theoret, J. R. Wunderlich, M. S. Hughes, N. P. Restifo, and S. A. Rosenberg. High efficiency TCR gene transfer into primary human lymphocytes affords avid recognition of melanoma tumor antigen glycoprotein 100 and does not alter the recognition of autologous melanoma antigens. *J Immunol*. 2003;171:3287–3295.

[82] de Witte, M. A., M. Coccoris, M. C. Wolkers, M. D. van den Boom, E. M. Mesman, J. Y. Song, M. van der Valk, J. B. Haanen, and T. N. Schumacher. Targeting self antigens through allogeneic TCR gene transfer. *Blood*. 2006;180:870–877.

[83] Johnson LA, Heemskerk B, Powell DJ Jr, Cohen CJ, Morgan RA, Dudley ME, Robbins PF, Rosenberg SA.Gene transfer of tumor-reactive TCR confers both high avidity and tumor reactivity to nonreactive peripheral blood mononuclear cells and tumor-infiltrating lymphocytes. *J Immunol*. 2006;177:6548-6559.

[84] Brower V. Cancer gene therapy steadily advances. *J Natl Cancer Inst*. 2008;100:1276-1278.

[85] Senzer N, Nemunaitis J. A review of contusugene ladenovec (Advexin) p53 therapy. *Curr Opin Mol Ther*. 2009;11:54-61.

[86] Cervantes-García D, Ortiz-López R, Mayek-Pérez N, Rojas-Martínez A. Oncolytic virotherapy. *Ann Hepatol*. 2008;7:34-45.

[87] Rodriguez R, Schuur ER, Lim HY, Henderson GA, Simons JW, Henderson DR. Prostate attenuated replication competent adenovirus (ARCA) CN706: a selective

cytotoxic for prostate-specific antigen-positive prostate cancer cells. *Cancer Res.* 1997;57:2559-2563.

[88] Delgado-Enciso I, Cervantes-García D, Martínez-Dávila IA, Ortiz-López R, Alemany-Bonastre R, Silva-Platas CI, Lugo-Trampe A, Barrera-Saldaña HA, Galván-Salazar HR, Coronel-Tene CG, Sánchez-Santillán CF, Rojas-Martínez A. A potent replicative delta-24 adenoviral vector driven by the promoter of human papillomavirus 16 that is highly selective for associated neoplasms. *J Gene Med.* 2007;9:852-861.

[89] Fueyo J, Gomez-Manzano C, Alemany R, Lee PS, McDonnell TJ, Mitlianga P, Shi YX, Levin VA, Yung WK, Kyritsis AP. A mutant oncolytic adenovirus targeting the Rb pathway produces anti-glioma effect in vivo. *Oncogene*. 2000;19:2-12.

[90] Heise C, Hermiston T, Johnson L, Brooks G, Sampson-Johannes A, Williams A, Hawkins L, Kirn D. An adenovirus E1A mutant that demonstrates potent and selective systemic anti-tumoral efficacy. *Nat Med.* 2000;6:1134-1139.

[91] Garber K. China approves world's first oncolytic virus therapy for cancer treatment. *J Natl Cancer Inst*. 2006;98:298-300.

[92] John Wiley and Sons Ltd. *The Journal of Gene Medicine*. 2010. available from: http://www.wiley.co.uk/genmed/clinical/

[93] Schenk-Braat EA, van Mierlo MM, Wagemaker G, Bangma CH, Kaptein LC. An inventory of shedding data from clinical gene therapy trials. *J Gene Med.* 2007;9:910-921.

[94] Peng Z. Current status of gendicine in China: recombinant human Ad-p53 agent for treatment of cancers. *Hum Gene Ther*. 2005;16:1016-1027.

[95] Researchers record stem cells, transplant organs breakthrough. The Guardian Newspaper. 05 march 2009. Available from: http://www.ngrguardiannews.com/science/article01/indexn2_html?pdate=050309&ptitle=Researchers%20record%20stem%20cells,%20transplant%20organs%20breakthrough

[96] Ark Therapeutics Group plc. 2009. Available from: http://www.arktherapeutics.com/main/ products.php?content=products_cerepro

[97] Introgen therapeutics Inc. 2009. Available from: http://www.introgen.com/our_products/advexin.asp

[98] Sunway Biotech Co.,Ltd. Development and manufacture of bioengineered, adenovirus-based targeted oncolytic immune therapies for the treatment of human cancers. Chinese biopharmaceutical company. 2006. Available from: http://www.sunwaybio.com.cn/e041oat.htm

[99] Cohen EE, Rudin CM. ONYX-015. Onyx Pharmaceuticals. *Curr Opin Investig Drugs.* 2001;2:1770-1775.

[100] PR Newswire. News and information. Benda Pharmaceutical Reports Second Quarter 2008 Financial Results. 2009. from: http://www.prnewswire.com/cgi-bin/ stories.pl?ACCT=104&STORY=/www/story/08-14-2008/0004867947&EDATE=

[101] Hilsum L. Gene therapy tourists. Newstatesman. 05 february 2007. Available from: http://www.newstatesman.com/asia/2007/02/gene-treatment-china-cancer

INDEX

A

B

C

D

E

F

G

H

I

N

Q

R

S

T

U

V